Nurses and Families

A Guide to
Family Assessment
and Intervention

FIFTH EDITION

THE GLEN TAYLOR
NURSING INSTITUTE FOR FAMILY AND SOCIETY

MINNESOTA STATE UNIVERSITY, MANKATO

This book was purchased
through the generous donation
of The Glen Taylor Nursing
Institute for Family and Society
Endowment

SCHOOL OF NURSING
MINNESOTA STATE UNIVERSITY, MANKATO

Nurses and Families

A Guide to Family Assessment and Intervention

FIFTH EDITION

Lorraine M. Wright, RN, PhD
International Lecturer
Professor Emeritus of Nursing
University of Calgary
Calgary, Alberta, Canada

Maureen Leahey, RN, PhD
Manager, Mental Health Outpatient Program
Alberta Health Services, Calgary
Adjunct Associate Professor
Faculties of Nursing and Medicine (Psychiatry)
University of Calgary
Calgary, Alberta, Canada

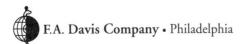
F.A. Davis Company • Philadelphia

F. A. Davis Company
1915 Arch Street
Philadelphia, PA 19103
www.fadavis.com

Printed in the United States of America

Last digit indicates print number: 10 9 8 7 6 5 4 3 2

Publisher, Nursing: Joanne Patzek DaCunha, RN, MSN
Director of Content Development: Darlene D. Pedersen
Senior Project Editor: Padraic J. Maroney
Art and Illustrations Manager: Carolyn O'Brien

As new scientific information becomes available through basic and clinical research, recommended treatments and drug therapies undergo changes. The author(s) and publisher have done everything possible to make this book accurate, up to date, and in accord with accepted standards at the time of publication. The author(s), editors, and publisher are not responsible for errors or omissions or for consequences from application of the book, and make no warranty, expressed or implied, in regard to the contents of the book. Any practice described in this book should be applied by the reader in accordance with professional standards of care used in regard to the unique circumstances that may apply in each situation. The reader is advised always to check product information (package inserts) for changes and new information regarding dose and contraindications before administering any drug. Caution is especially urged when using new or infrequently ordered drugs.

Library of Congress Cataloging-in-Publication Data

Wright, Lorraine M., 1944-
  Nurses and familes : a guide to family assessment and intervention / Lorraine M. Wright, Maureen Leahey. — 5th ed.
    p. ; cm.
  Includes bibliographical references and index.
  ISBN-13: 978-0-8036-2130-5
  ISBN-10: 0-8036-2130-2
  1. Family nursing. 2. Nursing assessment. I. Leahey, Maureen, 1944- II. Title.
  [DNLM: 1. Nursing Assessment. 2. Family Health—Nurses' Instruction. 3. Interviews as Topic—methods—Nurses' Instruction. WY 100 W951n 2009]
  RT120.F34W75 2009
  616.07'5—dc22

                                                                    2008045042

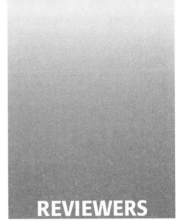

REVIEWERS

Martha M. Colvin,
PhD, MSN, BSN, RN
Professor and Chair of Undergraduate
Department of Nursing
George College and State University
Milledgeville, Georgia

Christine Davis, BScN, Med, MN
Professor
Laurentian University/St. Lawrence
College Collaborative
Brockville, Ontario, Canada

Mary Ann Drake, RN, PhD
Associate Professor
Webster University
Saint Louis, Missouri

Susan DeNisco,
MS, APRN-BC, DNP
Associate Clinical Professor
Sacred Heart University
Fairfield, Connecticut

Nancy Feeley, RN, PhD
Assistant Professor
McGill University
Senior Research
Jewish General Hospital
Kirkland, Quebec, Canada

Nina Hrycak,
RN, BSc N, MEd, PhD
Associate Professor
University of Calgary
Calgary, Alberta, Canada

Peggy Leapley,
PhD, RN, APRN, BC
Professor and Chair
California State University, Bakersfield
Bakersfield, California

Manon Lemonde, RN, PhD
Associate Professor, Faculty of Health
Sciences
University of Ontario Institute of
Technology
Oshawa, ON, Canada

Wilma Schroeder, RN, BN, MMFT
Nursing Instructor
Red River College
Winnipeg, Manitoba, Canada

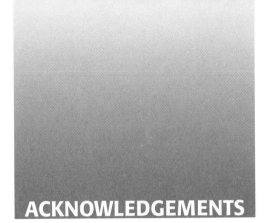

ACKNOWLEDGEMENTS

We are grateful to our many colleagues, local, national, and international, for their continued support, interest, and positive comments about our book over these 25 years as we continue to evolve our ideas of how to best involve and assist families experiencing illness, loss, and/or disability. It continues to amaze and gratify us that, since 1984 when the first edition was published, so many practicing nurses, students, and faculty have joined us in promoting family nursing worldwide.

We are especially grateful to:

- Joanne DaCunha, Publisher, Nursing Department, F.A. Davis, for her unfailing support, promptness, helpfulness, competence, and good nature as we worked on this fifth edition.
- Bob Martone, Publisher, Nursing Department, F.A. Davis, for his vision and support of our work starting with the first edition in 1984.
- Padraic Maroney, Senior Project Editor, Nursing, for his care in readying the manuscript for production.

Finally, we are grateful to each other ... for enduring friendship/colleagueship over some 33 years, for Caffe Beano Saturday morning conversations, fabulous restaurant experiences, and wonderful trips to Provence, Thailand, Iceland, Lake O'Hara...

Lorraine M. Wright and Maureen Leahey

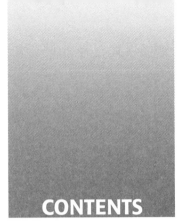

CONTENTS

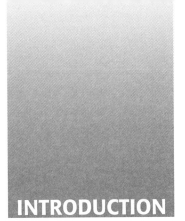

INTRODUCTION

REFLECTIONS ON THE FIRST TO FIFTH EDITIONS

We welcome you to the fifth edition of *Nurses and Families*. Whether you are a nursing student, practicing nurse, or nurse educator, this book is for you. Research evidence and clinical narratives of families experiencing illness make it mandatory and a moral imperative for nurses to include families with care and competence in whatever nursing context we find ourselves. The development and evolution of family nursing has moved beyond the debate of whether families should be included in health care to a more important focus and emphasis on *how to* involve families. Therefore, the main emphasis and thrust of our book is once again to offer ideas of *how to* include families in nursing practice with the specific knowledge and skills to accomplish that. Yes, this is a "how to" book.

The first edition of *Nurses and Families* was published in 1984, the second in 1994, the third in 2000, the fourth 2005, and now the fifth in 2009. Some of the changes and developments in family nursing plus the influence of larger societal differences in the past 25 years are obvious and apparent to us and our text whereas others are more subtle and perhaps tenuous.

One example of the palpable globalization of family nursing is our text having been translated into French, Japanese, Korean, Portuguese, German, and Swedish. As well, we have developed a website *www.familynursingresources.com* for educational resources. We have written and produced five educational DVDs (Wright & Leahey, 2000, 2001, 2002, 2003, 2006). These programs are also available in streaming video (.mov files and Quicktime and Windows Media Player). The programs are:

- *How to Do a 15-Minute (or Less) Family Interview* (2000)
- *Calgary Family Assessment Model: How to Apply in Clinical Practice* (2001)
- *Family Nursing Interviewing Skills: How to Engage, Assess, Intervene, and Terminate with Families* (2002)
- *How to Intervene with Families with Health Concerns* (2003)
- *How to Use Questions in Family Interviewing* (2006)

We are delighted that these DVDs are being utilized by faculties and schools of nursing worldwide; educational programs complement this text, *Nurses and Families,* by demonstrating family interviewing skills in action.

Further tangible evidence of the expansion of family nursing assessment models worldwide is that the Calgary Family Assessment Model (CFAM) continues to be widely adopted in undergraduate and graduate nursing curricula and by practicing nurses. The CFAM is utilized in curricula throughout North America, Australia, Brazil, Chile, England, Iceland, Japan, Korea, Taiwan, Thailand, Finland, Portugal, Scotland, Spain, Hong Kong, Norway and Sweden. With this expansion, we have had to revisit and revise our thinking about the CFAM in order to acknowledge, recognize, and embrace the evolving importance of certain dimensions of family life that influence health and illness, such as class, gender, ethnicity, race, family development, and beliefs.

A significant amplification in our text was the development of a framework and model for interventions, namely the CFIM, which was introduced in the second edition. This was done in recognition of the need to give just as much emphasis to intervention as there had been on assessment of families and to provide a framework within which to capture family interventions. This change was clearly influenced by the advances in family nursing research, education, and practice from a primary emphasis on assessment to an expanding and equal emphasis on intervention.

Perhaps a more subtle but equally significant development is our ever-changing and evolving relationship with the families with whom we work. This change is reflected in our choice of language to describe the nurse–family relationship that we deem most desirable. Our preferred stance/posture with families has evolved into a more collaborative, consultative, relational, and nonhierarchical relationship over the past 25 years. When we adopt this stance, we notice greater equality, respectfulness, and status given to the family's expertise. Therefore, the combined expertise of both the nurse and the family form a new and effective synergy in the context of therapeutic conversations that otherwise did not and could not exist.

Another subtle development evolving throughout our five editions has been the movement toward a postmodernist worldview. We embrace the notion that there are multiple realities in and of "the world," that each family member and nurse see a world that he or she brings forth through interacting with themselves and with others through language. We encourage an openness in ourselves, our students, and the families with whom we work to the many "worlds," differences, and diversity between and among family members and among health-care providers.

We have also been influenced by dramatic restructuring in health care that has occurred over the past 15 years in Canada and the United States. With massive restructuring in health-care institutions and community clinics, budgetary constraints, and managed care, many nurses feel they cannot afford the opportunity to get involved in or attend to the needs of families in health-care settings. Nurses, particularly those in acute-care hospital settings, have expressed their frustration about the substantially reduced time to attend to families' needs and concerns because of increased caseloads, heightened acuity of patients, and short-term stays. To respect and respond to this change, we developed ideas about how to conduct a 15-minute (or less) family interview and introduced them in the third edition.

We have been very gratified by how these ideas have been enthusiastically accepted in both our text and when presenting these ideas at nursing workshops or conferences. More importantly, based on anecdotal reports, the implementation of these ideas has shown great promise. We have been encouraged by nurses' reports of reduced suffering by family members and enhanced health promotion with families in their care. Equally gratifying are reports of increased job satisfaction by practicing nurses when collaborating with families, even if only for 15 minutes or less.

We consider it a great privilege to collaborate and consult with families for health promotion and/or to diminish or soften emotional, physical, or spiritual suffering from illness. We are also grateful for opportunities to teach professional nurses and undergraduate and graduate nursing students about involving, caring for, and learning from families in health care. Through our own clinical practice and teaching of health professionals for over 35 years and personal family experiences with illness, we recognize the extreme importance of nurses' possessing sound family assessment and intervention knowledge, skills, and compassion in order to assist families. We also acknowledge the profound influence that families have upon our own lives and relationships.

A SNAPSHOT OF 25 YEARS OF PROGRESS AND PARADIGM EVENTS IN FAMILY NURSING

Over these 25 years since the publication of the first edition of *Nurses and Families*, there have been paradigm events in family nursing very worthy of celebration. There has been progress, and yet there are other areas where we still need to put "our shoulder to the wheel." We believe one of the most far-reaching paradigm events in family nursing has been the publication of the *Journal of Family Nursing* in 1995. Since its inception, it has been under the very able and competent editorship of Dr. Janice M. Bell. The establishment provided a central place, for the first time, for the uniting of family nurses and the dissemination of family nursing knowledge. Another paradigm event was the offering of the first International Family Nursing Conference in 1988, in Calgary, Canada. Without any formal organization or association, eight International Family Nursing Conferences (IFNC) have been held in North America, South America (Chile) and (in 2007 for the first time) Asia (specifically, Bangkok, Thailand). Conferences being held in Chile and Thailand have enabled a further appreciation of family nursing's global expansion beyond the boundaries of North America. In 2009, the Ninth IFNC will be held for the first time in Europe at Reykjavik, Iceland, and 2011, in Kyoto, Japan.

With each international family nursing conference, there is confirmation of clear, steady progress in the development and expansion of family nursing. It is evident and visible in the presentations, workshops, and keynotes of an observable advancement of knowledge in theory, research, assessment, and interventions in family work. The community of family nurses has expanded to truly be a global force and phenomenon with enduring colleagueships and friendships. Questions are now being raised about the possibility of formally organizing the international conferences and the pros/cons in doing so (Curry, 2007).

The face of families has dramatically changed over the past 25 years as our demographics indicate an ever-increasing aging population; Baby Boomers are approaching retirement with significantly reduced numbers of Generation Xers to care for them. Marriages are being delayed or are nonexistent, as are pregnancies. Diversity in North American populations is clearly evident, demanding ever-increasing respect for a wide array of cultural, religious, and sexual orientation differences in our health-care system. Increased globalization invites the possibility for better health-care practices worldwide but also allows for the universal transmission of diseases, making it much more difficult for health-care providers to isolate, control, and segregate the origins of disease.

Amidst all the changes in demographics, technology, health-care delivery, and diversity, there are also profound changes occurring in our worldviews, from modernism to postmodernism, from secularism to spiritualism. Family nursing has not been immune to these changes, nor have we.

Numerous other paradigm events have influenced families and the development of family nursing. Massive health-care restructuring and downsizing in North America, the growth of managed care in the United States, and the movement to reduce the length of hospitalizations have expanded and enlarged community-based nursing practice in the United States, Canada, and other countries. This movement has directly and indirectly placed more responsibility on the backs of families for the care of their ill family members. Perhaps as a result of these dramatic changes, there is an expanded consumer movement and more collaboration with families about their health-care needs. Adding to this consumer movement is the increased technology, particularly the use of computers, personal digital assistants, instant messaging, and cellular phones. Access to the internet and e-mail enables family members to be more proactive and knowledgeable about their health problems through their ability to obtain current knowledge about their health problems, options for treatments, and traditional and alternative health-care resources.

THE FIFTH EDITION: WHAT IT IS, WHAT IS NEW AND UNIQUE

This revised fifth edition of *Nurses and Families* continues to be a "how-to" basic text for undergraduate, graduate, and practicing nurses. It is the only textbook, of which we are aware, that provides specific *how-to* guidelines for family assessment and intervention. This practical how-to guide for clinical work offers the opportunity for nursing students, practitioners, and educators to deliver better health care to families. Students and practitioners of community and public health nursing, maternal child nursing, pediatric nursing, mental health nursing, geriatric nursing, palliative care nursing, and those specializing in family systems nursing will find it most useful. Nurse educators who currently teach a family-centered approach and/or those who will be introducing the concept of the "family as the client" will find it a valuable resource. Educators involved in continuing education courses or nurse practitioner programs, especially family nurse practitioner programs, will be able to use this book to update and substantially enhance nurses' clinical knowledge and skills in family-centered care.

Our text provides specific guidelines for nurses to consider when preparing for, conducting, and documenting family meetings from the first interview through to discharge or termination. Actual clinical case examples are given throughout the book. These case examples reflect ethnic, cultural, racial, and sexual orientation diversity in conjunction with various family developmental life cycle stages and transitions. Special attention is given to the variety of family forms and structures prevalent in today's society. Issues in a variety of practice settings, including hospital, primary care, community, outpatient, and home are addressed.

The clinical practice ideas are based on solid theory, research, and each of our own 35 years of clinical work with families. The ideas are current best practices. Due to our extensive clinical experience both in our own practice and in the teaching and supervision of nursing and interdisciplinary students, we have been able to adapt the theoretical and clinical ideas so that they can be useful. How to Do a 15-Minute (or Shorter) Family Interview (Chapter 8) remains one of the most popular, well-received, and useful chapters in the book as reported by numerous practicing nurses and nursing students. It assists nurses working in time-pressured environments to offer valuable assistance to families.

The major purposes of this book are to (1) provide nurses with a sound theoretical foundation for family assessment and intervention; (2) provide nurses with clear, concise, and comprehensive, evidence-based family assessment and intervention models for current best practice; (3) provide guidelines for family interviewing skills; (4) offer detailed ideas and suggestions with clinical examples of how to prepare, conduct, use questions, document, and terminate family interviews; (5) provide nurses with an appreciation of the powerful influence of nurse–family collaboration to diminish, soften, or alleviate illness suffering.

In this fifth edition the following features are new and/or unique:

- A new chapter has been added: How to Use Questions in Family Interviewing. We are hopeful that this chapter will give nurses a clear idea of how to best use questions to focus and maximize their time with families.

- The well-known and internationally adopted Calgary Family Assessment Model (CFAM) has been thoroughly updated and expanded with many new references to the most current research, theory, and U.S statistics about families. This will contribute to enhance evidence-based practice. Increased attention is given to diversity issues, including ethnicity, race, culture, sexual orientation, gender, and class. CFAM is an easy-to-apply, practical, and relevant model for busy nurses working with a wide variety of complex issues and family structures and encountering various developmental stages.

- More complex genograms have been added. Recommendations for how to draw genograms for blended families with multiple parents and siblings, lesbian and gay families with children, and other family structures will enable nurses to increase their interviewing skills and take proactive steps to help families.

- The Calgary Family Intervention Model (CFIM) has been updated and revised to continue to make it more user-friendly. It remains, to our knowledge, the only family intervention model for nurses by nurses. It offers clear and specific family nursing interventions to assist with improving and/or sustaining family functioning and coping with illness.

- Increased complex family situations and key intervention skills will foster nurses' competence in dealing with multifaceted clinical issues, such as genetic testing, obesity, intergenerational adoption, and the impact of terrorism.

- Effects of the internet such as health networks, social networking, pornography, cybertherapy and cyberbullying on families have been integrated into information-rich content.

- Specific suggestions for fostering collaborative nurse–family relationships have been added throughout this fifth edition. Sample questions for the nurse to ask herself or himself and the family are also offered.

- New real-life specific clinical vignettes and boxes including questions used in practice are fast and easy reference tools for busy nurses.

TOUR OF THE CHAPTERS

The first five chapters provide the conceptual base for collaborating and consulting with families. To be able to interview families, identify strengths and concerns, and intervene to soften suffering, it is first necessary to have a sound conceptual framework. The specific how-to section of the book is included in Chapters 6 through 12 with numerous clinical examples in a variety of practice settings.

Chapter 1 establishes a rationale for family assessment and intervention. It describes the conceptual shift required in considering the family system, rather than the individual, as the unit of health care. It outlines the indications and contraindications for family assessment and intervention.

Chapter 2 addresses the major concepts of systems, cybernetics, communication, biology of knowing, and change theory that underpin the two models offered in this text, namely the CFAM and CFIM. It also presents a brief description of some of the major worldviews that influence our models, such as postmodernism and gender sensitivity. Clinical examples of the application of these concepts are offered.

Chapter 3 presents the updated and revised CFAM, a comprehensive, three-pronged structural, developmental, and functional family assessment framework. This widely adopted model has been thoroughly updated and expanded to reflect the current range of family forms in North American society and it has increased emphasis on diversity issues such as ethnicity, race, culture, sexual orientation, gender, and class. Ideas of specific questions that the nurse may ask the family are provided. Two structural assessment tools, namely the genogram and ecomap, are delineated, and instructions and helpful hints are given for using them when interviewing families. Excerpts from actual family interviews are presented to illustrate how to use the model in clinical practice.

Chapter 4 describes the updated and revised CFIM. The revisions enable nurses to move beyond assessment and to more easily have available a repertoire of family interventions that will effect or sustain changes in family functioning in cognition, affect, and/or behavior. Actual clinical examples of family work are presented, and a variety of interventions are offered for consideration. Nurses traditionally have primarily focused on family assessment because there have been no family nursing intervention models within nursing to draw on.

Chapter 5 describes the family interviewing skills and competencies necessary in family-centered care. Specifically, perceptual, conceptual, and executive skills necessary for family assessment and intervention are presented. The skills are written in the form of training objectives, and clinical examples are given to help broaden the nurse's understanding of how to use these skills. Nurse educators, in particular, may find this chapter useful in focusing their evaluation of students' family interviewing skills. Ethical considerations in family interviewing are addressed.

Chapter 6 presents clinical guidelines useful when preparing for family interviews. Ideas are given for developing hypotheses, choosing an appropriate interview setting, and making the first telephone contact with the family.

Chapter 7 delineates the various stages of the first interview and the remaining stages of the entire interviewing process: engagement, assessment, intervention, and termination. Actual clinical case examples in a variety of health-care settings illustrate the practice of conducting interviews.

Chapter 8 offers clear, specific suggestions on how to conduct 15-minute (or less) family interviews in a manner that enhances the possibilities for healing or health promotion. These ideas respond to the realities facing many nurses in this era of managed care and health restructuring. It also encourages nurses to adopt the belief that any time spent with families is better than no time.

Chapter 9 is a new chapter in this fifth edition; it emphasizes that questions are one of the most helpful interventions nurses offer to families. Questions to engage, assess, elicit problem-solving skills, intervene, and request feedback are recommended for relational practice in various clinical settings.

Chapter 10 offers ideas on how to avoid the three most common errors made in family nursing. Each error is defined and discussed. A clinical example is given, followed by very specific ideas of how the error could have been avoided. This chapter has proved useful to nurses in improving their care to families as well as enhancing their satisfaction in collaborating with families.

Chapter 11 presents ideas on how to document in a manageable fashion the vast amounts of data generated during family assessment and intervention meetings. Suggestions are given for developing a list of strengths and problems, assessment summary, progress record, and discharge synopsis. Sample documentation is provided so students can compare their writing with a printed example.

Chapter 12 highlights how to terminate with families in a therapeutic manner, whether after only one very short meeting or after several meetings with a family. Ideas are given for family-initiated and nurse-initiated termination as well as for discharges determined by the health-care system.

The major difference between this book and other books on family nursing is that this book's primary emphasis is on how to meet, interview, and collaborate with families to soften suffering and/or promote health. We wish to emphasize, however, that this book does not offer a "cookbook" approach to family meetings and interviews. The real development of skills results from actual clinical practice and supervisory feedback.

We envision this book as a springboard for nursing students, nursing educators, and practicing nurses. With a solid conceptual base and practical how-to ideas for family assessment and intervention, we hope that more nurses will gain confidence and a commitment to engage in the nursing of families. In so doing, they will be reclaiming some aspects of nursing that have been directly or inadvertently given to other health professionals. In the process, nurses will continue to regain an important and expected dimension of nursing practice and be instrumental in the health promotion and healing of families with whom they collaborate.

References

Curry, D.M. (2007). Does international family nursing need a professional organization? *Journal of Family Nursing, 13*(11), 395–402.

Wright, L.M., & Leahey, M. (Producers). (2000). *How to do a 15-minute (or less) family interview.* [Videotape/DVD]. Calgary, Canada: www.familynursingresources.com.

Wright, L.M., & Leahey, M. (Producers). (2001). *Calgary Family Assessment Model: How to apply in clinical practice.* [Videotape/DVD]. Calgary, Canada: www.familynursingresources.com.

Wright, L. M., & Leahey, M. (Producers). (2002). *Family nursing interviewing skills: How to engage, assess, intervene, and terminate with families.* [Videotape/DVD]. Calgary, Canada: www.familynursingresources.com.

Wright, L. M., & Leahey, M. (Producers). (2003). *How to intervene with families with health concerns.* [Videotape/DVD]. Calgary, Canada: www.familynursingresources.com.

Wright, L.M., & Leahey, M. (Producer). (2006). *How to use questions in family interviewing.* [DVD/Videotape]. Calgary, Canada: www.familynursingresources.com.

NEW FEATURES IN FIFTH EDITION

- New chapter: *How to Use Questions in Family Interviewing*
- Calgary Family Assessment Model thoroughly updated with latest research and family statistics
- Increased complex, multiproblem family situations and key intervention skills for evidence-based practice
- Addition of genograms for complex, blended families with multiple parents and siblings, lesbian and gay families with children, and other family structures
- Effects of internet knowledge and expansion on families integrated into information-rich content
- Additional real-life, specific, clinical vignettes and boxes including questions used in practice for fast, easy reference
- New, updated research integrated into the revised Calgary Family Intervention Model

Chapter 1

Family Assessment and Intervention: An Overview

Nurses have a commitment and an ethical and moral obligation to involve families in their own health care. Nursing theory, practice, and research have provided evidence that the family has a significant impact on the health and well-being of individual family members and can also have a considerable influence on the illness of its members. This evidence should compel and obligate nurses to consider family-centered care an integral part of nursing practice. However, family-centered care is achieved responsibly and respectfully only by the enlistment of sound family assessment and intervention as well as relational practices.

A rich tradition of nursing literature about the involvement of families in nursing care has been evolving, most specifically, over the past 35 years. Some of the classic and more recent texts on family nursing have enabled a new language to emerge through naming, describing, and communicating about the involvement of families in health care. Terms such as "family interviewing" (Wright & Leahey, 2005); "family health promotion nursing" (Bomar, 2004); "family health care nursing" (Hanson, Kaakinen, & Gedaly-Duff, 2005; Hanson, 2001; Hanson & Boyd, 1996); "family nursing" (Bell, Watson, & Wright, 1990; Friedman, Bowden, & Jones, 2003; Gilliss, 1991; Gilliss, et al, 1989; Wegner & Alexander, 1993; Wright & Leahey, 1990; Broome, et al, 1998); "family nursing practice," "family systems nursing" (Wright & Leahey, 1990; Wright, Watson, & Bell, 1990); "nursing of families" (Feetham, et al, 1993); and "family nursing as relational inquiry" (Doane & Varcoe, 2005) have all helped to bring forth the emergence of a vital aspect of nursing practice heretofore overlooked, neglected, or minimized. Perhaps the most significant, but not necessarily well-known, publication about family nursing is the monograph published by the International Council of Nurses titled *The Family Nurse: Frameworks for Practice* developed by Madrean Schober and Fadwa Affara (2001). It is a convincing validation for an emerging new role and specialty to have the influential International Council of Nurses identify the "family nurse" and "family nursing" as one of the important new trends in nursing.

As nurses theorize about, conduct research on, and involve families more in health care, they modify their usual patterns of clinical practice. The implication for this change in practice is that nurses must become competent in assessing and intervening with families through collaborative nurse–family relationships. Nurses who embrace the belief that illness is a family affair can most efficiently learn the knowledge and clinical skills required to conduct family interviews (Wright & Bell, in press). This belief leads nurses to thinking interactionally, or reciprocally, about families. The dominant focus of family nursing assessment and intervention must be the reciprocity between health and illness and the family.

It is most helpful and enlightening for nurses to assess the impact of illness on the family and the influence of family interaction on the cause, course, and cure of illness. Additionally, the reciprocal relationship between nurses and families is also a significant component of both softening suffering and enhancing healing.

EVOLUTION OF THE NURSING OF FAMILIES

Throughout history, family involvement has always been part of nursing, but it has not always been labeled as such. Because nursing originated in patients' homes, family involvement and family-centered care were natural. With the transition of nursing practice from homes to hospitals during the Great Depression and World War II, families became excluded not only from involvement in caring for ill members, but also from major family events such as birth and death. After having undergone all these developmental changes, the practice of nursing has now come full circle, with an emphasis on and an obligation to invite families once again to participate in its own health care. However, this invitation is being made with much more knowledge, research evidence, sophistication, respect, and collaboration than at any other time in nursing history.

The history, evolution, and theory development of the nursing of families in North America have been discussed in depth in the literature (Anderson, 2000; Feetham, et al, 1993; Ford-Gilboe, 2002; Friedman, Bowden, & Jones, 2003; Gilliss, 1991; Gilliss, et al, 1989; Hartrick, 2000; Hanson, Kaakinen, & Gedaly-Duff, 2005; Hartrick Doane, 2003). These authors have made significant contributions to the advancement of family nursing knowledge by contextualizing nursing care with families. A landmark work by Broome, et al (1998) synthesizes the research literature on nursing of children and their families, particularly in the areas of health promotion, acute illness, chronic illness, and the health-care system. This text methodically reviews the assessment and intervention models used in other research reports.

It is also very heartening that the evolution, development and practice of family nursing is being documented in countries outside of North America, such as Scotland, Hong Kong (Simpson, et al, 2006), and Nigeria (Irinoye, Ogunfowokan, Olaogun, 2006).

Perhaps the boldest and most ambitious global effort to enhance the care to families by implementing and improving the education and practice of nurses is the World Health Organization Family Health Nurse Multinational Study (World Health Organization, 2006). Eighteen European countries were involved in this multinational study whose aim was to implement and evaluate the concept of Family Health Nurse (FHN) within their various health and educational systems. The inclusion of countries such as Slovenia, Kyrgyzstan, Tajikistan, Republic of Moldova, and Lithuania in this study is an indication of the continued global expansion of family nursing. An FHN was defined as a skilled, generalist family/community nurse combining the elements of illness prevention and management as well as multifaceted duties determined by family/community needs.

In 2006, there was an evaluation and final meeting in Berlin, Germany, 6 years after the start of the study. At this meeting, the conclusion was that "the project was very much an action research and action learning process. Participants showed great enthusiasm and commitment to the research aims. Implementing a new nursing service is a change management process and in-country change cycles at the time of the multinational study were diverse. Some had developed a fully functional FHN programme and had advanced into a second phase. Some countries had not yet implemented the FHN programme whilst others were in the process of their implementation" (pg. 10). One example of a country that had an impressive report and a vision for the future was Slovenia. In 2003 the FHN role was further developed, and in 2004 the College for Nurses implemented a new curriculum for family health nursing specialists. The education program lasts 1 year (40 weeks) and consists of 53% clinical practice, 39% seminars, and 8% lectures. In 2005 eight students received their diploma in family health nursing. In 2006 six students were expected to finish their education. The aim is to educate 200 FHNs by the year 2010.

The evolution of family nursing is most evident in the textbooks utilized in the field. It is exciting and encouraging to report that five major textbooks on family health nursing in North America referenced throughout this text are now in their second to fifth editions. We are also aware that the history and evolution of family health nursing exists in journal articles and books in the language of their country in places such as Brazil, Finland, Germany, Iceland, Portugal, Sweden, Thailand, and Japan. Providing nurses with a clear framework for family assessment and the necessary interventions to treat families can facilitate the transition from thinking in a more traditional, individualistic manner toward thinking interactionally or thinking family.

FAMILY ASSESSMENT

Numerous disciplines have attempted to define and conceptualize the concept of *family*. Each discipline has its own point of view or frame of reference for viewing the family, and all have an ever-increasing appreciation of diversity issues. Economists, for example, have been concerned with how the family works together to meet material needs. Sociologists, on the other hand, are concerned with the family as a specific group in society. Mischke-Berkey, Warner, and Hanson (1989); Hanson and Boyd (1996); and Tarko & Reed (2002) have identified and described several family assessment models and instruments developed by both nurses and non-nurses. Although it is helpful for nurses to be aware of the many models offered by various disciplines and the distinct variables emphasized in each model, we believe no one assessment model, however, explains all family phenomena.

In any clinical practice setting, nurses benefit from adopting a clear conceptual framework or map of the family. This framework encourages the synthesis of data so that family strengths and problems can be identified and a useful management plan devised. When no conceptual framework exists, it is extremely difficult for the nurse to group disparate data or to examine the relationships among the multiple variables that impact the family. Use of a family assessment framework helps to organize this massive amount of seemingly disparate information. It also provides a focus for intervention.

CALGARY FAMILY ASSESSMENT MODEL: AN INTEGRATED FRAMEWORK

The Calgary Family Assessment Model (CFAM) was one of the four models identified in *The Family Nurse: Frameworks for Practice* monograph by the International Council of Nurses (Schober & Affara, 2001). The CFAM is a multidimensional framework consisting of three major categories: structural, developmental, and functional (see Chapter 3). The model is based on a theory foundation involving systems, cybernetics, communication, and change. It was adapted from Tomm and Sanders' (1983) family assessment model and has been substantially embellished since the first edition of this textbook in 1984. The model is also embedded within larger worldviews of postmodernism, feminism, and biology of cognition. Diversity issues are also emphasized and appreciated within our particular model. See Chapter 3 for a detailed description of CFAM.

INDICATIONS AND CONTRAINDICATIONS FOR A FAMILY ASSESSMENT

It is important to identify guidelines for determining which families will automatically be considered for family assessment. Because families now tend to have increased health-care awareness and knowledge, nurses are encountering families who present themselves as a family unit for assistance with family health and illness issues. Frequently, however, the illness is presented as isolated within a particular family member. Therefore, with each illness situation, a judgment must be made about whether that particular problem should be approached within a family context.

Here are some examples of indications for a family assessment:

- A family is experiencing emotional, physical, or spiritual suffering or disruption caused by a family crisis (e.g., acute or end-of-life illness, injury, death).

- A family is experiencing emotional, physical, or spiritual suffering or disruption caused by a developmental milestone (e.g., birth, marriage, youngest child leaving home).

- A family defines an illness or problem as a family issue and a motivation for family assessment is present.

- A child or adolescent is identified by the family as having difficulties (e.g., cyberbullying, fear of cancer treatment).

- The family is experiencing issues that jeopardize family relationships (e.g., terminal illness, addictions).

- A family member is going to be admitted to the hospital for psychiatric or mental health treatment.

- A child is going to be admitted to the hospital.

Conducting and completing a family assessment does not absolve nurses from assessing serious risks, such as suicide and homicide, or serious illnesses in individual family members. Family assessment is neither a panacea nor a substitute for an individual assessment. In advanced nursing practice, particularly family systems nursing, assessment of individuals and assessment of the family system occur simultaneously (Wright & Leahey, 1990).

Some situations contraindicate family assessment, including when:

- family assessment compromises the individuation of a family member (For example, if a young adult has recently left home for the first time, a family interview may not be desirable.)

- the context of a family situation permits little or no leverage (For example, the family might have a fixed belief that the nurse is working as an agent of some other institution, such as the court.)

During the engagement process, nurses must explicitly present the rationale for a family assessment. (Suggestions for how to do this are given in Chapters 6 and 7.) A nurse's decision to conduct a family assessment should be guided by sound clinical principles and judgment. The nurse can take advantage of opportunities to consult with peers and supervisors if questions exist about the suitability of such an assessment.

After the nurse has completed the family assessment, he or she must decide whether to intervene with the family. In the next section of this chapter, general ideas about intervention are discussed. Specific ideas for nurses to consider when making clinical decisions about interventions with particular families are presented in Chapters 4, 8, and 9. The three most common errors in working with families are discussed in Chapter 10.

NURSING INTERVENTIONS: A GENERIC DISCUSSION

Numerous terms are used to distinguish and ultimately label the treatment portion of nursing practice, including intervention, treatment, therapeutics, action, activity, moves, and micromoves (Bulechek & McCloskey, 1992b, 2000; Wright & Bell, in press). In our clinical practice and research with families, we prefer the designation *intervention*. The most rigorous effort to standardize the language for nursing interventions is the work of Bulechek and McCloskey (1992a, 1992b, 2000) and their colleagues at the University of Iowa. More recently, these authors have worked to build taxonomies such as the Nursing Interventions Classification, which is based on nurses' reports of their practice (Bulechek, Butcher, & McCloskey Dochterman, 2007).We applaud their ambitious and needed efforts to develop and validate nursing intervention labels.

Our practice differs in that after assessing a family, we prefer to generate a list of strengths and problems rather than diagnoses. We conceptualize the list as one observer's perspective, not the "truth" about a family. We view the problem list as presenting problems that nurses can treat. It has been our experience that nursing diagnoses have unfortunately become too rigid and do not include enough consideration of ethnic and cultural issues. We prefer to identify the strengths of a family and list them along-side the problems (see Chapter 11). The advantage of this type of listing is that it gives a balanced view of a family. It also asks nurses not to be blinded by a family's problems but to realize that every family has strengths, even in the face of potential or actual health problems.

Definition of a Nursing Intervention

Bulechek and McCloskey (2000) define nursing interventions as "any treatment, based upon clinical judgment that a nurse performs to enhance patient/client outcomes. Nursing interventions include both direct and indirect care; those aimed at individuals, families, and the community; including nurse-initiated, physician-initiated treatments and other provider-initiated treatment" (p. xix). Wright and Bell (in press) offer an alternate definition: "any action or response of the clinician, which includes the clinician's overt therapeutic actions and internal cognitive-affective responses, that occurs in the context of a clinician-client relationship offered to effect individual, family, or community functioning for which the clinician is accountable." Wright & Bell (in press) expand on their definition of intervention by suggesting that an intervention "usually implies a one-time act with clear boundaries, frequently offering something or doing something to someone else." Interventions are normally purposeful and conscious and usually involve observable behaviors of the nurse.

Context of a Nursing Intervention

Nursing interventions should focus on the nurse's behavior and the family response. This differs from nursing diagnoses and nursing outcomes, which focus on client behavior (Bulechek & McCloskey, 1992a, 2000). We believe that nurse behaviors and client behaviors are contextualized in the nurse–client relationship. Therefore, an interactional phenomenon occurs whereby the responses of a nurse (interventions) are invited by the responses of clients (outcome) which, in turn, are invited by the responses of a nurse. To focus on only client behaviors or nurse behaviors does not take into account the relationship between nurses and clients. All of our nursing interventions are interactional; that is, not doing to or for the patient, but *with* the patient. Nursing interventions are actualized only in a relationship.

Intent of Nursing Interventions

The intent of any nursing intervention is to effect change. Therefore, effective nursing interventions are those to which clients and families respond because of the "fit," or meshing, between the intervention offered by the nurse and the biopsychosocial-spiritual structure of family members. In relational practice with families, we do not have a predetermined, standardized intervention to use across a number of families. Rather, the nurse, in collaboration with a specific family, would determine what interventions are most useful for a family experiencing a particular illness.

NURSING INTERVENTIONS FOR FAMILIES: A SPECIFIC DISCUSSION

Nurses can intervene with families in numerous ways. This section discusses some specific aspects of family interventions. It also presents indications for and contraindications to family interventions.

Conceptualization of Interventions with Families

Notions about reality gleaned from postmodernism and social constructionism are helpful when conceptualizing ideas about interventions. It is unwise to attempt to ascertain what is "really" going on with a particular family or what the "real" problem or suffering is. Rather, nurses should recognize that what is "real" to them as nurses is always a consequence of the nurse's construction of the world. Maturana (1988) presents an intriguing notion of reality by submitting that individuals (living systems) bring forth reality—they do not construct it and it does not exist independent of them. This concept has implications for nurses' clinical work with families; specifically, what nurses perceive about particular situations with families is influenced by how nurses behave (i.e., their interventions), and how they behave depends on what they perceive.

Therefore, one way to change the "reality" that family members have constructed is to assist them with developing new ways of interacting in the family. The interventions that we use in this endeavor focus on changing cognitive, affective, or behavioral domains of family functioning. As family members' perceptions about each other and the illness in their family change, so do their behaviors.

The effectiveness of family interventions in the treatment of physical illness has been examined in two integrative reviews conducted by Campbell and Patterson (1995) and Campbell (2003). These reviews included only studies that used a control group. Support was found for the effectiveness of interventions directed to the family rather than just the individual diagnosed with the illness.

Weihs and colleagues (2002) reported the efforts of a multidisciplinary group who reviewed and collated existing literature about family interventions in chronic illness. Three general goals for family-focused interventions were identified: helping families cope with the challenges of chronic illness management, mobilizing family support, and reducing intrafamilial hostility and suffering. Evidence has been found for a significant reduction in the use of health-care services following individual, marital, and family therapy (Law, Crane, & Berge, 2003). This study substantiates the need for more family intervention research in nursing. Unfortunately, data from the National Institute for Nursing Research suggest that only 25% of all funded nursing research is focused on family and even fewer studies are focused on family intervention.

Family nurse clinicians are grounded in the everyday complexities and uniqueness of each family they serve. While clinicians may benefit from the research literature that offers a description of family responses in health and illness, they are intimately involved in *doing* intervention and consequently find themselves wanting to know about the specific practice offered to families.

It is encouraging that there are now a few studies that have begun to uncover family interventions with families experiencing illness, particularly about the usefulness of family interventions that target family interactions and examine the influence of each family member's illness experiences on other family members (Duhamel & Talbot, 2004; Duhamel & Dupuis, 2004; Noiseux & Duhamel, 2003; O'Farrell, Murray, & Hotz, 2000).

Documentation of clinical experience indicates that interventions normally directed at challenging the meanings or beliefs that families give to behavioral events or their experience of illness tend to have the most sustaining changes (Bohn, Wright, & Moules, 2003; Duhamel & Talbot, 2004; Houger Limacher & Wright, 2003, 2006; Moules, 2002; Moules, Thirsk, & Bell, 2006; Moules, et al, 2007; Wright & Bell, in press).

Efforts to develop and identify intervention strategies for family health promotion are also being made, although little documentation of their effectiveness is evident (Loveland-Cherry & Bomar, 2004). Reports of family interventions to promote diet and exercise behavior indicate some limited success (Nicklas, et al, 2001). Family health promotion is an area of family nursing in which there are tremendous opportunities for the development and testing of family interventions.

Nurses must also keep in mind the element of time with regard to interventions. Interventions do not begin just with the intervention stage of family work. Rather, they are an integral part of family interviewing, spanning engagement to termination. Normally, interventions used during family interviewing are based on the nurse's and family's influence on the experience of suffering, a problem, or an illness. If engagement and assessment have been adequate, the interventions are generally more effective. For example, if a nurse working with a Latino family perpetually addresses family members other than the father first, the family may disengage. The opportunity to further intervene will be eliminated. In this example, the nurse needs not only to possess family interviewing skills but also to possess sensitivity to ethnic issues before embarking on specific goal-oriented interventions.

Indications and Contraindications for Family Interventions

After a family assessment, a nurse must decide whether to intervene with a family. The nurse should consider the family's level of functioning, his or her own skill level, and the resources available. We recommend intervention in the following circumstances:

- **A family member presents with an illness that has an obvious detrimental impact on other family members.** For instance, a grandfather's Alzheimer's disease may cause his grandchildren to be afraid of him, or a young child's cyberbullying behavior may be related to his mother's deterioration from multiple sclerosis.

- **A family member contributes to another family member's symptoms or problems.** For example, lack of visitation from adult children exacerbates physical or psychological symptoms in an elderly parent.

- **One family member's improvement leads to symptoms or deterioration in another family member.** For example, decreased asthma symptoms in one child correlate with increased abdominal pain in a sibling.

- **A child or an adolescent develops an emotional, a behavioral, or a physical problem in the context of a family member's illness.** For example, an adolescent with diabetes suddenly requests that his mother administer his daily insulin injections even though he has been injecting himself for the past 6 months.

- **Illness is first diagnosed in a family member.** If family members have no previous knowledge or experience with a particular illness, they require information and may also require reassurance and support.

- **A family member's condition deteriorates markedly.** Whenever deterioration occurs, family patterns may need restructuring and intervention is indicated.
- **A chronically ill family member moves from a hospital or rehabilitation center back into the community.**
- **An important individual or family developmental milestone is missed or delayed.** For example, an adolescent is unable to move out of the home at the anticipated time.
- **A chronically ill patient dies.** Although the patient's death may be a relief, the family might feel a tremendous void when the caregiving role is lost.

After the nurse and family have decided that intervention is indicated, they must then collaboratively decide on the duration and intensity of the family sessions. If sessions occur too frequently, the family may have insufficient time to recalibrate and process the change. The optimal number of days, weeks, or months between sessions is difficult to state categorically. We recommend that nurses ask family members when they would like to have another meeting. Families are much better judges than nurses of how frequently they need to be seen to resolve a particular problem. Furthermore, nurses should be aware that the duration and intensity of sessions depend on the context in which the family is seen. For example, if a hospital nurse is working with a family, he or she may have the opportunity for only one or two meetings before discharge, whereas a community health nurse may be able to schedule a series of meetings. The context in which the nurse encounters families commonly dictates the frequency and number of family meetings. Whether a nurse has 1 or 10 meetings with a family for assessment or intervention, there are important considerations for terminating with families. Additional information on termination is discussed in Chapter 12.

Family intervention is not always required, and contraindications for family intervention exist, including:

- All family members state that they do not wish to pursue family meetings or treatment even though it is recommended.
- Family members state that they agree with the recommendation for family meetings or treatment but would prefer to work with another professional.

These contraindications are generally evident to the nurse immediately after the family assessment. Sometimes during the course of intervention, however, families indicate a desire to stop treatment. This situation will be discussed more fully in Chapter 12.

Nurses working with patients and families in a variety of health-care settings need to have a good understanding of when family involvement is indicated and when it is contraindicated. Not only for their own benefit but also for each family's benefit, nurses should distinguish between family assessment and family intervention. Families are often willing to come for an assessment when they can see the nurse face to face and make their own assessment of the nurse's competence. When a nurse does a careful, credible assessment, he or she has an easier time initiating family interventions.

DEVELOPMENT AND IDENTIFICATION OF NURSING INTERVENTIONS WITH FAMILIES

We believe that the slow pace of the development of nursing interventions with families has been due in part to the lack of appreciation of the connection between illness and family dynamics (i.e, the interactional aspect of families and illness). We also believe that the lack of specific interventions with families has been caused by the lack of nurse educators who are skilled family clinicians. Because interventions related to the family are independent nursing actions for which nurses are accountable, nurse-educators and researchers must begin to name, specify, explore, understand, and test interventions related to the family. Very few nursing interventions with families have been tested. This fact is not surprising given that the nursing profession is at a very early stage in simply identifying and describing family interventions.

In a thoughtful and thought-provoking editorial about evidence-based nursing, interventions, and family nursing, Hallberg (2003) offers specific recommendations for nursing interventions with individuals and families. Specifically, the author recommends that nurses develop and examine "interventions that acknowledge family members as experts and that acknowledge their role as primary caregivers; interventions directed at older people, especially those between 80 and 100 years and those dependent on others as opposed to independent older people; and interventions that elaborate on ways in which professionals can cooperate with families caring for older people in their homes and that apply a perspective of family caregiving as more complex than only a burden or a strain" (p. 21). Hallberg strongly emphasizes the belief that interventions with older people and their families are the most urgent need of the three. Nurses in direct clinical contact with families perceive family interventions differently from nurses who predominantly conduct research or engage in theory development. The education and training of undergraduate students in clinical work with families primarily focus on the family as context (Wright & Leahey, 1990). Nursing students who specialize in family systems nursing do so at the graduate or advanced-practice level (Wright & Leahey, 1990; Wright, & Bell, in press). Thus, it is extremely important that efforts to label interventions be consistent within a particular practice framework (e.g., within the family as context, within family systems nursing, within family therapy). However, some interventions labeled as being in one domain of clinical practice with families might also be identifiable in another domain of clinical practice.

FAMILY RESPONSES TO INTERVENTIONS

The previous discussion of interventions in family nursing practice primarily focused on the behaviors of the nurse. However, interventions are actualized only in a relationship. Therefore, it is equally important to ascertain the responses of family members to interventions that are offered. Since the last edition of this text, more intervention studies have been conducted. These studies increase nurses' understanding of what is helpful to families and what is not. Bell & Wright (2007) challenge the predominant belief within "good science" that before intervention research can be designed and conducted, there first must be a thorough understanding of the phenomena, (i.e., an in-depth knowledge of what the variables are that mediate families' response to health and illness). They offer an alternate view that in daily nursing practice, nurses encounter families suffering in a variety of clinical settings that require immediate care and intervention. Therefore, family nursing practice as it occurs in the daily life of nurses needs to be described, explored, and evaluated to gain an understanding of what is working in the moment. What are nurses actually doing and saying that is helpful to families in their experience of illness?

The study by Robinson and Wright (1995) identified what nurses do that makes a positive difference to families. They found that families who experienced difficulty managing a member's chronic condition and sought assistance in an outpatient nursing clinic could readily identify interventions that alleviated or softened their suffering. The nursing interventions that made a difference for these families fell within two stages of the therapeutic change process:

- Bringing the family together to engage in new and different conversations (this fell within the stage of "creating the circumstances for change")
- Establishing a therapeutic relationship between the nurse and family, particularly in the areas of providing comfort and demonstrating trust. (Within the stage of "creating the circumstances for change").

Within the stage of "moving beyond and overcoming problems," families identified four interventions that promoted healing:

- Inviting meaningful conversation
- Noticing and distinguishing family and individual strengths and resources
- Paying careful attention to and exploring concerns
- Putting illness problems in their place.

Recent studies indicate that nurses are eager to learn more about the usefulness of family interventions that target family interactions and examine the influence of each family member's illness experiences on other family members (O'Farrell, Murray, & Hotz, 2000).

A few qualitative studies have been useful in examining particular family interventions, such as commendations (Houger Limacher & Wright, 2003, 2006), spiritual practices (McLeod, 2003), therapeutic letters (Moules, 2002, 2003), interventions for parents with children experiencing bone marrow transplants (Noiseux & Duhamel, 2003), interventions in perinatal family care (Goudreau & Duhamel, 2003) interventions for families experiencing chronic illness (Robinson, 1998; Robinson & Wright, 1995), interventions for families experiencing heart disease (Tapp, 2001), and interventions that are significant for therapeutic change (Wright & Bell, in press; Duhamel & Talbot, 2004).

Duhamel and Talbot (2004) conducted an ambitious, labor-intensive study to evaluate the usefulness of a family systems nursing approach utilizing the CFAM and Calgary Family Intervention Model (CFIM) with families experiencing cardiovascular and cerebrovascular diseases. Because interventions are actualized only within the context of a relationship between the nurse and the family, it is important to study the process itself rather than simply the results. The Duhamel and Talbot (2004) study was extremely beneficial because it was based on a participatory research design that allowed for continuous feedback and improvement of the interventions throughout the study.

In such a study, the participants are all people concerned with the problem: nurses, patients, their spouses, and caregivers. Family members described the "humanistic attitude of the nurse, constructing a genogram, interventive questioning, offering educational information, normalization, and exploring the illness experience in the presence of other family members" (Duhamel & Talbot, 2004, p. 21) as the most useful interventions. Although all of these interventions are part of CFAM and CFIM, Duhamel and Talbot's (2004) study results provide interesting insights to substantiate their usefulness.

The study also had a positive impact on the nurses involved as co-investigators—a revealing finding. For example, the nurses indicated that they gained a better understanding of the impact of the illness on the family members' relationships; acquired an appreciation of the importance of active listening and a humanistic and personalized approach; centered on family members' specific concerns to reduce their anxiety; and integrated new family systems nursing interventions into their practice.

Nurses are also being creative in their efforts to implement family nursing interventions. For example, a study by Davis (1998) examined the effectiveness of telephone-based skill building for reducing caregiver stress and improving coping among family members providing care to individuals with dementia. Her findings suggest that "telephone-based skill building may increase dementia caregivers' sense of social support, reduce their depressive symptoms, and improve their life satisfaction in the midst of caregiving" (p. 265).

The identification of these interventions offers incredibly useful ideas for improving the care of families experiencing illness. However, many more studies are needed to ascertain families' responses to the interventions offered.

CALGARY FAMILY INTERVENTION MODEL: AN ORGANIZING FRAMEWORK

The CFIM is an organizing framework for conceptualizing the relationship between families and nurses that helps change to occur and healing to begin. Specifically, the model highlights the family–nurse relationship by focusing on the intersection between family member functioning and interventions offered by nurses (see Chapter 4). It is at this intersection that healing can take place. The CFIM is a resilience and strength-based, collaborative, nonhierarchical model that recognizes the expertise of family members experiencing illness and the expertise of nurses in managing illness and promoting health. The model is rooted in notions from postmodernism and the biology of cognition. It can be applied and used with patients and families from diverse cultures because it emphasizes fit of particular interventions from a particular cultural viewpoint. It remains, to the best of our knowledge, the only family nursing intervention model that is currently documented.

NURSING PRACTICE LEVELS WITH FAMILIES: GENERALIST AND SPECIALIST

Schober and Affara (2001) emphasize that nursing practice with families is directed by whether the concept of the family is defined as *family as context* or *family as client*. One way to alleviate potential confusion of practice levels is to clearly distinguish two levels of expertise in nursing with regard to clinical work with families: generalists and specialists. Typically, generalists are nurses at the baccalaureate level who predominantly use the concept of the family as context (Wright & Leahey, 1990), although upper-level baccalaureate students begin to conceptualize the family as the unit of care. Specialists, on the other hand, are nurses at the graduate (master's or doctoral) level who predominantly use the concept of family as the unit of care. This requires specialization in family systems nursing (Wright & Leahey, 1990). Family systems nursing specialization requires that "the focus is always on interaction and reciprocity. It is not 'either/or' but rather 'both/and'" (Wright & Leahey, 1990, p. 149).

Family systems nursing integrates nursing, systems, cybernetics, and family therapy theories (Wright & Leahey, 1990). It requires familiarity with an extensive body of knowledge: family dynamics, family systems theory, family assessment, family intervention, and family research. It also requires accompanying competence in family interviewing skills. Family systems nursing simultaneously focuses on both the family system and the individual system (Wright & Leahey, 1990). All nurses should be knowledgeable about and competent in involving families in health care across all domains of nursing practice. Consequently, the emphasis in the practice of family nursing at the generalist level is on the family as context.

In contrast, the practice of family systems nursing at the specialist level emphasizes the family as the unit of care. However, these boundaries can become blurred, with upper-level baccalaureate students recognizing the importance of a focus on interaction and reciprocity. These students often develop nursing competence and are able to deal with individual and family systems simultaneously.

CONCLUSIONS

We consider it a great privilege to work with families experiencing illness and/or suffering, loss, and disability. We are also grateful for opportunities to teach professional nurses and nursing students how to involve families in health care. Through this process, we recognize the extreme importance of nurses having sound family assessment and intervention knowledge and compassion. The remainder of this textbook is our effort to help nursing students, practicing nurses, and nurse-educators learn new ways to heal families.

References

Anderson, K.H. (2000). The family health system approach to family systems nursing. *Journal of Family Nursing, 6*, 103–119.

Bell, J.M., Watson, W.L., & Wright, L.M. (Eds.) (1990). *The cutting edge of family nursing.* Calgary, Alberta: Family Nursing Unit Publications.

Bell, J.M., & Wright, L.M. (2007). La recherche sur la pratique des soins infirmiers a la famille. In F. Duhamel (Ed.) La sante et la famille: Une approache systemique en soins infirmieres (2nd ed.) Montreal, Quebec, Canada: Gaetan Morin editeru, Cheneliere Education.

Berkey, K.M., & Hanson, S.M.H. (1991). *Pocket guide to family assessment and intervention.* St. Louis: Mosby.

Bohn, U., Wright, L.M., & Moules, N.J. (2003). A family systems nursing interview following a myocardial infarction: The power of commendations. *Journal of Family Nursing, 9*(2), 151–165.

Bomar, P.J. (Ed.). (2004) *Promoting health in families: applying family research and theory to nursing practice* (3rd ed.) Philadelphia: W.B. Saunders.

Broome, M.E., et al (Eds.) (1998). *Children and families in health and illness.* Thousand Oaks, CA: Sage Publications.

Bulechek, G.M., Butcher, H., & McCloskey Dochterman, J. (2007). *Nursing interventions classification (NIC)* (5th ed.) New York: Elsevier.

Bulechek, G.M., & McCloskey, J.C. (Eds.) (1992a). Defining and validating nursing interventions. *Nursing Clinics of North America, 27*(2), 289–299.

Bulechek, G.M., & McCloskey, J.C. (Eds.) (1992b). *Nursing interventions: Essential nursing treatments.* Philadelphia: W.B. Saunders Company.

Bulechek, G.M., & McCloskey, J.C. (2000). *Nursing interventions classification (NIC).* St. Louis: Mosby.

Campbell, T.L. (2003). The effectiveness of family interventions for physical disorders. *Journal of Marital and Family Therapy, 29*(2), 545–583.

Campbell, T.L., & Patterson, J.M. (1995). The effectiveness of family interventions in the treatment of physical illness. *Journal of Marital and Family Therapy, 21*(4), 545–583.

Cousins, N. (1979). *Anatomy of an illness as perceived by the patient: Reflections on healing and regeneration.* New York: Bantam Books.

Davis, L.L. (1998). Telephone based interventions with family caregivers: A feasibility study. *Journal of Family Nursing, 4,* 255–270.

Doane, G.H., & Varcoe, C. (2005). *Family nursing as relational inquiry.* Philadelphia: Lippincott Williams & Wilkins.

Dorothee, J.H., et al. (2004). Family nursing in Scotland. *Journal of Family Nursing, 10*(8), 323–337.

Duhamel, F. & Dupuis, F. (2004). Guaranteed returns: Investing in conversations with families of cancer patients. *Clinical Journal of Oncology Nursing,* 8(1), 68-71.

Duhamel, F., Dupuis, F., & Wright, L.M. (in press). Families and nurses answers to the "One question question": Helpful directions for clinical practice, education, and research in family nursing. *Journal of Family Nursing.*

Duhamel, F., & Talbot, L.R. (2004). A constructivist evaluation of family systems nursing interventions with families experiencing cardiovascular and cerebrovascular illness. *Journal of Family Nursing, 10*(1), 12–32.

Feetham, S.L., et al. (1993). *The nursing of families: Theory, research, education, and practice.* Newbury Park, CA: Sage Publications.

Ford-Gilboe, M. (2002). Developing knowledge about family health promotion by testing the developmental model of health and nursing. *Journal of Family Nursing, 8*(2), 140–156.

Friedman, M.M., Bowden, V.R., & Jones, E.G. (2003). Family nursing: Research, theory and practice (5th ed.). Upper Saddle River, NJ: Prentice Hall.

Gilliss, C.L. (1991). Family nursing research, theory and practice. *Image: Journal of Nursing Scholarship, 23*(1), 19–22.

Gilliss, C.L., et al. (Eds.) (1989). *Toward a science of family nursing.* Menlo Park, CA: Addison-Wesley.

Goudreau, J., Duhamel, F. (2003). Interventions in perinatal family care: A participatory study. *Families, Systems, & Health, 21*(2), 165–180.

Hallberg, I.R. (2003). Evidence-based nursing, interventions, and family nursing: Methodological obstacles and possibilities. *Journal of Family Nursing, 9*(3), 3–22.

Hanson, S.M.H. (2001). *Family health care nursing: Theory, practice, and research* (2nd ed.). Philadelphia: F. A. Davis.

Hanson, S.M.H., & Boyd, S.T. (1996). *Family health care nursing: Theory, practice, and research.* Philadelphia: F. A. Davis.

Hanson, S.M.H., Kaakinen, J.R., & Gedaly-Duff, V. (2005). *Family health care nursing: Theory, practice, and research* (3rd ed.). Philadelphia: F. A. Davis.

Hartrick, G. (2000). Developing health promoting practice with families: One pedagogical experience. *Journal of Advanced Nursing, 31*(1), 27–34.

Hartrick Doane, G. (2003) Through pragmatic eyes: Philosophy and the re-sourcing of family nursing. *Nursing Philosophy, 4*(1), 25–33.

Houger Limacher, L., & Wright, L.M. (2003). Commendations: Listening to the silent side of a family intervention. *Journal of Family Nursing, 9*(2), 130–135.

Houger Limacher, L., & Wright, L.M. (2006). Exploring the therapeutic family intervention of commendations: Insights from research. *Journal of Family Nursing, 12,* 307–331.

Irinoye, O., Ogunfowokan, A., & Olaogun, A. (2006). Family nursing education and family nursing practice in Nigeria. *Journal of Family Nursing, 12*(11), 442–447.

Janosik, E., & Miller, J. (1979). Theories of family development. In D. Hymovich & M. Barnard (Eds.), *Family health care—general perspectives* (vol. 1, 2nd ed.) (pp. 3–16). New York: McGraw-Hill.

Law, D.D., Crane, D.R., & Berge, J.M. (2003). The influence of individual, marital, and family therapy on high utilizers of health care. *Journal of Marital and Family Therapy, 29*(3), 353–363.

Loveland-Cherry, C.J., & Bomar, P.J. (2004). Family health promotion and health protection. In P.J. Bomar (Ed.), *Promoting health in families: Applying family research and theory to nursing practice* (3rd ed.). Philadelphia: Saunders.

Maturana, H. (1988). Reality: The search for objectivity or the quest for a compelling argument.*The Irish Journal of Psychology, 6*(1), 25–83.

McCloskey, J.C., & Bulechek, G.M. (1994). Standardizing the language for nursing treatments: An overview of the issues. *Nursing Outlook, 42*(2), 56–63.

McCloskey, J.C. & Bulechek, G.M. (1996). *Nursing intervention classification (NIC),* (2nd ed.). St. Louis: Mosby.

McLeod, D.L. (2003). Opening space for the spiritual: Therapeutic conversations with families living with serious illness. Unpublished doctoral thesis, University of Calgary, Alberta, Canada.

Mischke-Berkey, K., Warner, P., & Hanson, S. (1989). Family health assessment and intervention. In P.J. Bomar (Ed.), *Nurses and family health promotion: Concepts, assessment, and interventions.* Baltimore: Williams & Wilkins.

Moules, N.J. (2002). Nursing on paper: Therapeutic letters in nursing practice. *Nursing Inquiry, 9*(2), 104–113.

Moules, N.J. (2003). Therapy on paper: Therapeutic letters and the tone of relationship. *Journal of Systemic Inquiries, 22*(1), 33–49.

Moules, N.J., et al. (2007). The soul of sorrow work: Grief and therapeutic interventions with families. *Journal of Family Nursing, 13*(2), 117–141.

Moules, N.J., Thirsk, L.M., & Bell, J.M. (2006) A Christmas without memories: Beliefs about grief and mothering—A Clinical Case Analysis. *Journal of Family Nursing, 12*(11), 426–441.

Nicklas, T.A., et al. (2001). Family and child-care provider influences on preschool children's fruit, juice, and vegetable consumption. *Nutritional Reviews, 59*(7), 224–235.

Noiseux, S., & Duhamel, F. (2003). La greffe de moelle osseuse chez l'enfant. Evaluation constructiviste de l'intervention aupres des parents. [Bone marrow transplantation in children. Constructive evaluation of an intervention for parents]. *Perspective Infirmiere, 1*(1), 12–24.

O'Farrell, P., Murray, J., & Hotz, S.B. (2000). Psychological distress among spouses of patients undergoing cardiac rehabilitation. *Heart and Lung, 29*(2), 97–104.

Robinson, C.A. (1998). Women, families, chronic illness, and nursing interventions: From burden to balance. *Journal of Family Nursing, 4*(3), 271–290.

Robinson, C.A., & Wright, L.M. (1995). Family nursing interventions: What families say makes a difference. *Journal of Family Nursing, 1*(3), 327–345.

Schober, M. & Affara, F. (2001). *The family nurse: Frameworks for practice.* Geneva: International Council of Nurses.

Simpson, P., et al. (2006). Family systems nursing: A guide to mental health care in Hong Kong. *Journal of Family Nursing, 12*(8), 276–291.

Tapp, D.M. (2001). Conserving the vitality of suffering: Addressing family constraints to illness conversations. *Nursing Inquiry, 8*(4), 254–263.

Tarko, M.A., & Reed, K. (2002). *Taxonomy of family nursing diagnosis based upon the Neuman systems model of nursing* [Unpublished manuscript]. New Westminster, British Columbia, Canada: Douglas College

Tomm, K., & Sanders, G. (1983). Family assessment in a problem oriented record. In Hansen, J.C. & Keeney, B.F. (Eds.). *Diagnosis and assessment in family therapy.* London: Aspen Systems Corporation, pp. 101–102.

Wegner, G.D., & Alexander, R.J. (Eds.) (1983). *Readings in family nursing.* Philadelphia: J.B. Lippincott Company.

Weihs, K., Fisher, L., & Baird, M. (2002). Families, health, and behavior. *Families, Systems, & Health, 20*(1), 7–46.

World Health Organization (2006). *Fifth workshop on the WHO Family Health Nurse Multinational Study: Evaluation six years after the Munich declaration.* Copenhagen, Denmark: World Health Regional Office for Europe, Author.

Wright, L.M. & Bell, J.M. (in press). *Beliefs and illness: A model for healing.* Calgary, AB: 4th Floor Press.

Wright, L.M., & Leahey, M. (1990). Trends in nursing of families. *Journal of Advanced Nursing, 15*(2), 148–154.

Wright, L.M., & Leahey, M. (2005). *Nurses and families: A guide to family assessment and intervention* (4th ed.). Philadelphia: F.A. Davis.

Wright, L.M., Watson, W.L., & Bell, J.M. (1990). The family nursing unit: A unique integration of research, education, and clinical practice. In J.M. Bell, W.L. Watson, & L.M. Wright (Eds.), *The cutting edge of family nursing* (pp. 95–109). Calgary, Alberta: Family Nursing Unit Publications.

Chapter **2**

Theoretical Foundations of the Calgary Family Assessment and Intervention Models

Models are useful ways to bring clusters of ideas, notions, and concepts into our awareness. However, models cannot stand alone. For example, nursing practice models are built on a foundation of many worldviews, theories, beliefs, premises, and assumptions. These models are more comprehensible and meaningful if the underlying theories, assumptions, and premises are articulated. Therefore, to comprehend and use the Calgary Family Assessment Model (CFAM) (see Chapter 3) and the Calgary Family Intervention Model (CFIM) (see Chapter 4) in nursing practice with individuals, couples, and families, nurses must know the theoretical assumptions underlying these models. The underlying theoretical assumptions of any family assessment and intervention model are important to declare because they become evident when the models are applied in clinical practice.

The six theoretical foundations and worldviews that inform the CFAM and CFIM and the family nursing practice guidelines presented in the rest of this textbook are postmodernism, systems theory, cybernetics, communication theory, change theory, and biology of cognition. Each theory or worldview and some of its distinguishing concepts are presented and related to clinical practice with individuals, couples, and families. We wish to emphasize that no one overall model of family nursing exists. "No one theoretical or conceptual framework adequately describes the complex relationships of family structure, function, and process. No single theoretical perspective gives nurses a sufficiently broad base of knowledge and understanding for use as a guide to family assessment and interventions with families. Thus there is no single theoretical basis that guides nursing care of families. Rather, nurses must draw on multiple theories and frameworks to guide their work with families and take an integrated approach to practice, research, and education in family nursing" (Kaakinen & Hanson, 2004, p. 111). We concur.

POSTMODERNISM

Humans seem to delight in rethinking, reexamining, reconstructing, and deconstructing their history and culture. One popular way to do this is through the lens of postmodernism. Anything before the present "enlightened" worldview is considered modernist and therefore less desirable to those who rigidly hold postmodernist beliefs. Consequently, the influence of the ideas, conditions, and beliefs of postmodernism have been demonstrated in art, literature, architecture, science, culture, religion, philosophy and, more recently, nursing (Burnard, 1999; Glazer, 2001; Kermode & Brown, 1996; Moules, 2000; Tapp & Wright, 1996). The popularity and increasing acceptance of postmodern ideas are evident in the literature.

We, too, have been influenced by and have embraced many of the notions of postmodernism. These ideas have proved useful in our clinical nursing practice with families. However, we do not wish to imply that we have been able to successfully distance ourselves from all modernist ideas, nor would we want to. We concur with Glazer (2001), who criticizes the postmodern movement for abandoning the biological underpinnings of nursing. We cannot deny our history and culture and how they are a function of who we were and are. Therefore, we acknowledge the previous and continuing influences of both modernist and postmodernist paradigms on our lives, our relationships, and our practice of relational family nursing.

CONCEPT 1

Pluralism is a key focus of postmodernism.

Postmodernism offers the end of a single world view and a resistance to single explanations, and a respect for difference. One of the major notions of postmodern thinking is the idea of pluralism, or a belief in multiplicity—in other words, that there are as many ways to understand and experience the world as there are people who experience it (Moules, 2000; Wright & Bell, in press). In family nursing practice, this idea becomes operational by recognizing that there are as many ways to understand and experience illness as there are families experiencing illness. In an ethical and relational family nursing practice, it becomes operational by acknowledging the multiplicity of cultural, ethnic, and religious beliefs and their influence on various complex family structures.

CONCEPT 2

Postmodernism is a debate about knowledge.

Postmodernism is partly a reaction to the modernist claim that knowledge primarily emerges from science and technology (Glazer, 2001). The belief that progressive technology necessarily leads to a better world has become open to reexamination, questioning, and doubt (Tapp & Wright, 1996). Therefore, an intense critique is being made of the meta-narratives and grand belief systems that have formed the foundation of many of our scientific, religious, and political movements and institutions. As these grand narratives are questioned, opportunities arise to deconstruct or uncover certain "taken-for-granted" beliefs and practices, to hear voices of marginal groups, and to value knowledge from a variety of domains heretofore not legitimized (Tapp & Wright, 1996). In encounters with families experiencing illness, much more emphasis is now given to the illness narratives and experiences of family members within their particular cultural context, not just to medical narratives. Honoring the voices of families about their illness narratives has profound implications for nursing practice with families. It invites collaboration and consultation between nurses and families to honor the knowledge and expertise of both nurses and family members. These practices are the cornerstone of relational nursing. Inviting the illness narratives of families also enhances the possibilities for healing as their stories are heard, understood, and witnessed.

Some offshoots of postmodernism include constructivism, social constructionism, and biology of cognition (also called "bring forthism") (Maturana & Varela, 1992; Moules, 2000; Wright & Bell, in press). The latter, biology of cognition, is the offshoot that we have found most useful in our clinical work and, therefore, is discussed in more detail later in this chapter.

The postmodernist movement has been strongly critiqued by feminists, who claim that women's voices continue to be diminished or ignored because of the grand narrative of patriarchy and oppression (Kermode & Brown, 1996). This has not been our experience in working with families. Evidence for the importance of acknowledging women's voices and their illness burden in family systems nursing practice can be found in Robinson's (1998) study. She discovered that women in families experiencing chronic illness are vulnerable to the demands of illness responsibility, illness work, and illness problems. As a more equitable balance of illness demands was sought by the nurse and by family members, the women in this study found better lives for themselves and were able to live beyond illness and the problems they experienced. They also took on new views of their situations and thus behaved differently. This study's recognition of women's voices as distinct and different from a collective "family voice" seems in keeping with the best that the postmodernist movement has to offer.

SYSTEMS THEORY

Health professionals have applied general systems theory, introduced in 1936 by von Bertalanffy, to the understanding of families for a number of years. In addition to the original writings on systems theory by von Bertalanffy (1968, 1972, 1974), numerous articles and chapters in books have been written on systems theory and its concepts. This proliferation of systems information is also evident within nursing literature. We concur with Kaakinen and Hanson (2004) in their belief that "systems theory and its extrapolation to the family has been the most influential of all the family frameworks" (p. 100).

One of the most useful analogies that highlights systems concepts as applied to families is offered by Allmond, Buckman, and Gofman (1979). They suggest that, when thinking of the family as a system, it is useful to compare it to a mobile:

> Visualize a mobile with four or five pieces suspended from the ceiling, gently moving in the air. The whole is in balance, steady yet moving. Some pieces are moving rapidly; others are almost stationary. Some are heavier and appear to carry more weight in the ultimate direction of the mobile's movement; others seem to go along for the ride. A breeze catching only one segment of the mobile immediately influences movement of every piece, some more than others, and the pace picks up with some pieces unbalancing themselves and moving chaotically about for a time. Gradually the whole exerts its influence in the errant part(s) and balance is reestablished but not before a decided change in direction of the whole may have taken place. You will also notice the changeability regarding closeness and distance among pieces, the impact of actual contact one with another, and the importance of vertical hierarchy. Coalitions of movement may be observed between two pieces. Or one piece may persistently appear isolated from the others; yet its position of isolation is essential to the balancing of the entire system (p. 16).

Keeping the analogy of the mobile in mind, some of the most useful concepts of systems theory, which have frequent application in clinical practice with families, are highlighted in the following paragraphs. These systems concepts provide a theoretical foundation for understanding the family as a system. A *system* can be defined as a complex of elements in mutual interaction. When this definition is applied to families, it allows us to view the family as a unit and thus focus on observing the interaction among family members, and between the family and the illness or problem rather than studying family members individually. However, remember that each individual family member is both a subsystem and a system in his or her own right. An individual system is both a part and a whole, as is a family.

CONCEPT 1

A family system is part of a larger suprasystem and is composed of many subsystems.

The concept of hierarchy of systems is very useful when applied to families. It is especially helpful for nurses struggling with how to conceptualize complex family situations. A family is composed of many subsystems, such as parent–child, marital, and sibling subsystems. These subsystems are also composed of subsystems of individuals. Individuals are extremely complex systems composed of various subsystems, some of which are physical (such as the cardiovascular and reproductive systems) or psychological (cognitive, affective, and behavioral systems). At the same time, the family is just one unit nested in larger suprasystems, such as neighborhoods, organizations, or church communities. Drawing a large circle and placing elements, parts, or variables inside the circle can be a helpful way to visualize a system. Inside the circle, lines can be drawn among the component parts to represent relationships between elements. Outside the circle is the larger context, where all other factors impinging on the system can be placed. Thus, a nurse can draw a circle to visualize a family and then place the individual family members within it (Fig. 2–1).

Systems are arbitrarily defined by their boundaries, which aid in specifying what is inside or outside the system. Normally, boundaries associated with living systems are physical in nature, such as the number of people in a family or the skin color of an individual. It is also possible to construct a boundary and, therefore, create a system around ideas, beliefs, expectations, or roles. For example, a person may have a system of multiple roles, such as daughter, partner, colleague, wife, sister, nurse, mother, and grandmother. From time to time, however, it may be useful to draw an imaginary boundary and create, for example, a system of parental beliefs about the use of non-medical drugs by their children.

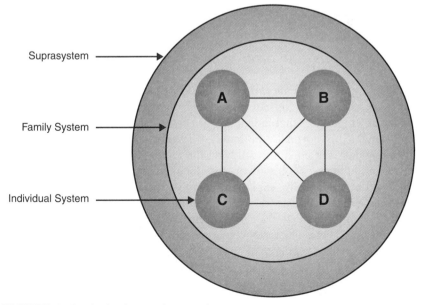

FIGURE 2-1: The family as it relates to other systems.

When working with families, nurses should initially consider:

- Who is in this family system?
- What are some of the important subsystems?
- What are some of the significant suprasystems to which the family belongs?

In addition, within family systems and their subsystems, nurses should assess the permeability of the boundaries. In family systems, the boundaries must be both permeable and limiting. If the family boundary is too permeable, the system loses identity and integrity (for example, members may be too open to input from the outside environment, such as extended family, friends, or health professionals) and therefore does not allow the family to use its own resources in decision making. However, if the boundary is too closed or impermeable, necessary interaction with the larger world is shut off (for example, an immigrant family from Afghanistan that relocates to Pennsylvania may inadvertently remain closed initially because of great differences in language and culture). With increased use of cellular phones, the internet, Personal Digital Assistants, email, Skype, chat rooms, social networking sites such as Facebook, Twitter, and similar technology, the permeability of boundaries has changed dramatically in the last decade.

Hierarchy of systems and the boundaries that create systems are useful concepts to apply when working with and attempting to conceptualize the uniqueness of each particular family. Among certain ethnic groups— for example, Iranian families—honoring hierarchies and boundaries is essential.

CONCEPT 2

The family as a whole is greater than the sum of its parts.

When applied to families, this concept of systems theory emphasizes that the family's "wholeness" is more than simply the addition of each family member. It also emphasizes that individuals are best understood within their larger context, which is normally the family. To study individual family members separately does not equate to studying the family as a unit. By studying the whole family, it is possible to observe interaction among family members, which often more fully explains individual family member functioning. Consider this clinical scenario: a young Filipino mother whose 3-year-old child has temper tantrums that she cannot control asks a community health nurse (CHN) for guidance. The CHN could intervene in a variety of ways:

- See the mother individually and discuss some behavioral methods that could be used to assist in controlling her child's temper tantrums.
- See the child individually and do an individual assessment.

■ See the whole family (mother, father, and child) and perform a child-and-family assessment (see Chapter 3) in order to understand the child, the child's behavior in the family context, and the Filipino family's beliefs about discipline.

Because the CHN understood the importance of Concept 2, she chose to see the whole family. During the first session with the family, the child was well behaved for the first half hour of the interview. Then the child had a temper tantrum, in response to which the mother became annoyed and the father withdrew. The CHN was astute enough to observe the sequence of interaction before the temper tantrum. When the child had the temper tantrum, the parents were in a heated argument about their parenting styles. Once the tantrum started, the parents stopped arguing and focused on the child. This child might have been responding to the tension between the parents and using the temper tantrums to stop the parents' conflict. Thus, the temper tantrums were understood quite differently in the context of the family than they would have been if the child had been assessed in isolation. In this example, the family is the client, but an individual family member is the reason for initiating care (Schober & Affara, 2001). Any time a family seeks assistance because of a concern or problem with an individual family member, the nurse can initiate family nursing with the entire family unit.

Therefore, when possible, nurses should see whole families and observe family interaction to more fully understand family member functioning. This type of observation enables assessment of the relationships among family members as well as individual family member functioning. We cannot understand the parts of a body, a family, a practice, a theory, unless we know how the whole works, for the parts can be understood only in relation to the whole. Conversely, we cannot grasp how the whole works unless we have an understanding of its parts.

CONCEPT 3

A change in one family member affects all family members.

This concept aids the recognition that any significant event or change in one family member affects all family members to varying degrees, as illustrated in the analogy of the mobile. It can be most useful to nurses considering the impact of illness on families. For example, the father of a Malaysian family experienced a myocardial infarction. This event affected all family members and various family relationships. The father and mother were unable to continue their joint participation in sports, and the mother increased her employment from part-time to full-time to supplement the substantially reduced income during the father's convalescence. The eldest daughter, who had been isolated from the family since her marriage, began visiting her father more often. The youngest daughter, by providing emotional support, became closer to her mother. Thus, all family members were affected, and the organization and functioning of the family changed.

This concept can also be used to understand how a nurse can change the family system by implementing family interventions. That is, if one family member changes, other family members cannot respond as they previously did because the individual family member now behaves differently.

CONCEPT 4

The family is able to create a balance between change and stability.

Over the past few years, there has been a shift away from the belief that families tend toward maintaining equilibrium. Instead, the popular belief now is that families are really in constant states of flux and are always changing. The pendulum has now swung to the other end of the continuum. However, von Bertalanffy (1968) warned many years ago to avoid this polarized view of families. He suggested that systems, in this case family systems, can achieve balance among the forces operating within them and on them and that change and stability can coexist in living systems (see "Change Theory" later in this chapter).

However, when change occurs in a family, the disturbance can cause a shift to a new position of balance. The family reorganizes in a way that is different from any previous organization of the family. For example, if a family member is diagnosed with a long-term chronic illness, such as multiple sclerosis, the entire family must reorganize itself in ways that are totally different from the ways it was organized before the diagnosis. The balance between change and stability constantly shifts during periods of remission and exacerbation; however, a balance between change and stability is most common.

The concept of change and stability coexisting is perhaps one of the most difficult concepts of systems theory for nurses to understand. This is partly because, in actual clinical practice, families frequently present themselves as being either in rigid equilibrium or in constant change rather than manifesting an observable balance between the two. However, the more experienced one becomes in family nursing, the greater appreciation one has for the complexity of families. In many cases, when families are "stuck" or experiencing severe difficulties, they are polarized in maintaining rigid equilibrium or are in a phase of too much change. Eventually, the family needs to find ways to obtain a more equal balance between the phenomena of stability and change. In our own practice over the last several years, we have noticed how military families and other families directly affected by terrorism and war have developed creative solutions to cope with the fluctuations of stability and change.

CONCEPT 5

Family members' behaviors are best understood from a view of circular rather than linear causality.

One method of dealing with the massive amounts of data presented in a family interview is to observe for patterns. Tomm (1981) offers a very useful discussion of the differences between linear and circular patterns:

> One major difference between linear and circular patterns lies in the overall structure of the connections between elements of the pattern. Linear patterns are limited to sequences (e.g., A → B → C) whereas circular patterns form a closed loop and are recursive (e.g., A → B → C → A → ... or A → B, B → C, C → A). A less obvious but more significant difference lies in the relative importance usually given to time and meaning when making the connections or links in the pattern. Linearity is heavily rooted in a framework of a continuous progression of time ... Circularity ... is more heavily dependent on a framework of reciprocal relationships based on meaning (p. 85).

Linear causality, defined as a relationship in which one event causes another, can serve a useful and helpful function for individuals and families. For example, when the clock strikes 6 PM, a family routinely eats supper. This is an example of linear causality because event A (the clock striking 6 PM) is seen as the cause of event B (the eating of supper), or A → B; whereas event B does not affect event A.

However, circular causality occurs when event B does affect event A. For example, if a husband takes an interest in his wife's ostomy care (event A) and the wife responds by explaining the daily procedures (event B), then it is likely to result in the husband continuing to take an interest and offer support regarding his wife's ostomy care and his wife continuing to feel supported; thus, the cycle continues (A → B → A). Each individual's behavior has an effect on and influences the other individual's behavior. A method for diagramming these very useful circular interactional patterns is discussed in Chapter 3.

The application of these concepts in clinical practice affects the nurse's style of questioning during a family interview. Linear questions tend to explore descriptive characteristics (such as, "Is the father fearful of another heart attack?"), whereas circular questions tend to explore interactional characteristics. Types of circular questions include difference questions (such as, "Who is most worried about Sunil having another heart attack?"), behavioral effect questions (such as, "What do you do Amal, when your wife's pain becomes unbearable for you?"), hypothetical or future-oriented questions (such as, "What might you do in the future to prevent your elderly father from falling?"), and triadic questions (such as, "When your Dad shows support to your sister Manisha, how does your Mom feel?") (Selvini-Palazzoli, et al. 1978; Loos & Bell, 1990; Tomm, 1984, 1985, 1987a, 1987b, 1988; Wright, & Bell, in press). Bateson (1979) offers the idea that "information consists of differences that make a difference" (p. 99). Tomm (1981) connects the idea of "differences" to relationships:

> Differences between perceptions, objects, events, ideas, etc. are regarded as the basic source of all information and consequent knowledge. On closer examination, one can see that such relationships are always reciprocal or circular. If she is shorter than he, then he is taller than she. If she is dominant, then he is submissive. If one member of the family is defined as being bad, then the others are being defined as being good. Even at a very simple level, a circular orientation allows implicit information to become more explicit and offers alternative points of view. A linear orientation on the other hand is narrow and restrictive and tends to mask important data (p. 93).

Various types of assessment and interventive questions that could be asked during a family interview are highlighted in Chapters 3, 4, 6, 7, 8, and 9.

With regard to family member interaction, the assumption is made that each person contributes to adaptive as well as maladaptive interaction. For example, in geriatric health care facilities, it is common for elderly parents to complain that their adult children do not visit enough and therefore to withdraw; on the other hand, the adult children complain that their elderly parents constantly nag them when they visit. Each family member is "correct" in the perception of the other, but neither recognizes how his or her own behavior influences the behavior of the other family member.

Normally, families and individual family members need help to move from a linear perspective of their situation to a more interactional, reciprocal, and systemic view. This shift is possible only if the nurse avoids linear thinking when attempting to understand family dynamics.

The five concepts listed above are by no means inclusive of all systems concepts, but they reflect those that are deemed most significant and important to the theoretical foundation for working with families.

CYBERNETICS

Cybernetics is the science of communication and control theory. The term cybernetics was originally coined by the mathematician Norbert Weiner. We believe it is important to differentiate between general systems theory and cybernetics, and we do not use the terms synonymously, although some people regard each as a branch of the other. Systems theory is primarily concerned with changing our conceptual focus from parts to wholes, whereas cybernetics is concerned with changing focus from substance to form.

CONCEPT 1

Family systems possess self-regulating ability.

Interpersonal systems, particularly family systems, "may be viewed as feedback loops, since the behavior of each person affects and is affected by the behavior of each other person" (Watzlawick, Beavin, & Jackson, 1967, p. 31). We have found this idea to be one of the most useful in family work because recognizing that each family member's behavior affects other family members and, in turn, that person is affected by other family members' behavior removes any tendency or impulse of a nurse to blame one person in a family for the difficulties that an entire family is facing. For any substantial change to occur in a relationship, the regulatory limits must be adjusted so that a new range of behaviors is possible or an entirely new pattern can emerge (transformation). Tomm (1980) offers a useful method of applying cybernetic regulatory concepts to actual clinical interviewing. His method of diagramming circular patterns of communication is discussed in Chapter 3.

CONCEPT 2

Feedback processes can simultaneously occur at several systems levels with families.

Initially, the application of cybernetic concepts in family work began by observations of simple phenomena (for example, a wife criticizes, the husband withdraws); this is generally referred to as simple cybernetics. However, as cyberneticians began examining more complex orders of phenomena, they recognized different orders of feedback (such as feedback of feedback and change of change). Maturana and Varela (1980) suggest a higher-order cybernetics that links the organization of living process and cognition.

Therefore, the simple feedback phenomenon observed in the interactional pattern of criticizing wife–withdrawing husband may also be understood to be part of a larger feedback loop involving the couple's relationship to their families of origin, which may recalibrate the lower-order loop of the couple's interaction. This concept can be especially helpful to nurses working with complex family situations. Thus, cybernetics of cybernetics moves into a larger context that includes both the observer and the observed.

COMMUNICATION THEORY

The study of communication focuses on how individuals interact with one another. Within families, the function of communication is to assist family members in clarifying family rules regarding behavior, to help them learn about their environment, to explicate how conflict is resolved, to nurture and develop self-esteem for all members, and to model expressions of feeling states constructively within the family as a unit. One of the most significant contributions to the understanding of interpersonal processes is the classic book *Pragmatics of Human Communication* (1967) by Watzlawick, Beavin, and Jackson. The concepts presented here are primarily drawn from this important book on communication and have been updated by the research studies of Dr. Janet Beavin Bavelas in 1992.

CONCEPT 1

All nonverbal communication is meaningful.

This concept helps us to realize that there is no such thing as not communicating because all nonverbal communication by a person carries a message in the presence of another (Watzlawick, Beavin, & Jackson, 1967). In personal communications and in her 1992 publication, Dr. Beavin Bevelas states that she now distinguishes between nonverbal behavior (NVB) and nonverbal communication (NVC). NVC is viewed as a subset of NVB. NVB involves an "inference-making observer," whereas NVC involves a "communicating person" (encoder). In the original text by Watzlawick, Beavin, and Jackson, the concept was presented that all NVB is meaningful.

A significant component of this concept is context. Behavior is relevant and meaningful only when the immediate context is considered. For example, if a mother complains to a CHN that she has been experiencing insomnia for 2 months and finds herself irritable because of the prolonged sleep deprivation, the mother's behavior must be understood in her immediate context. On further exploration, the nurse discovered that this mother has a child on an apnea monitor and that the father sleeps soundly. Also, the family apartment is close to a subway. With this additional context information, the mother's insomnia can be more fully understood and treated by the CHN.

CONCEPT 2

All communication has two major channels for transmission: digital and analog.

Digital communication is commonly referred to as verbal communication. It consists of the actual content of the message, or the brute facts. For example, a man might proudly say, "I lost 15 pounds this past month," or a 10-year-old girl might say, "I can now give myself my own insulin." However, when the analogical communication is also taken into account, the meaning of these statements may change dramatically.

Analogical communication consists not only of the usual types of NVC, such as body posture, facial expression, and tone, but also of music, poetry, and painting. For example, a man who is obese and proudly states that he lost 15 pounds in a month sends a more positive message, both digitally and analogically, than a man who is emaciated and states that he lost 15 pounds.

In discussing the two types of communication, we do not wish to imply that separate channels are dedicated to verbal and nonverbal communication When discrepancies exist between analogical and digital communication, then the analogical message is considered more pertinent to the nurse's observing eye. For example, a teenager who has been placed in a cumbersome cast for a fractured femur might state, "It doesn't bother me," but her eyes are filled with tears. In this situation, the nurse must recognize the importance of the analogical message. To the teenager's boyfriend, the digital communication may be the most relevant. He may not perceive the significance of the analogical communication. More suggestions for operationalizing this concept are included in the CFAM in Chapter 3.

CONCEPT 3

A dyadic relationship has varying degrees of symmetry and complementarity.

The terms *symmetry* and *complementarity* are useful in identifying typical family interaction patterns. Jackson (1973) defined these terms:

> A complementary relationship consists of one individual giving and the other receiving. In a complementary relationship, the two people are of unequal status in the sense that one appears to be in the superior position, meaning that he initiates action and the other appears to follow that action. Thus the two individuals fit together or complement each other. The most obvious and basic complementary relationship would be the mother and infant. A symmetrical relationship is one between two people who behave as if they have equal status. Each person exhibits the rights to initiate action, criticize the other, offer advice and so on. This type of relationship tends to become competitive; if one person mentions that he has succeeded in some endeavor, the other person mentions that he has succeeded in an equally important endeavor. The individuals in such a relationship emphasize their equality or their symmetry with each other. The most obvious symmetrical relationship is a pre-adolescent peer relationship (p. 189).

Both complementary and symmetrical relationships are appropriate and healthy in certain situations. For example, a staff nurse must take a "one-down" position to her nurse-manager most of the time. If the staff nurse cannot do this, conflict could result and the relationship could become predominantly symmetrical. This symmetrical escalation could result in the nurse-manager filing incident reports about the staff nurse or the staff nurse quitting on unpleasant terms. An example of a healthy symmetrical relationship is one between spouses, who may for example debate where to spend their next vacation.

In family relationships, predominance of either complementary or symmetrical behavior usually results in problems. Some cultural groups may prefer one style over another. Couples need to balance symmetry and complementarity in their various experiences. Parent-child relationships, however, typically gradually shift from a predominantly complementary relationship to a more symmetrical, egalitarian relationship as the child moves into the teenage and young adult years.

CONCEPT 4

All communication has two levels: content and relationship.

Communication consists of not only what is being said (content) but also information that defines the nature of the relationship between those interacting. For example, a father might say to his son, "Come over here, son. I want to tell you something," or he might say, "Get over here. I've got something to tell you!" These statements are similar in content, but each implies a very different relationship. The first statement could be viewed as part of a loving relationship, whereas the second statement implies a conflictual relationship. In this instance, it is the tone of the content that gives evidence to a particular kind of relationship. Therefore, "family communication not only reveals a message about 'who is saying what and when,' it also conveys a message about the structure and functions of family relationships in relation to the power base, decision-making processes, affection, trust, and coalitions" (Crawford & Tarko, 2004, p. 162).

CHANGE THEORY

The process of change is a fascinating phenomenon, and researchers have a variety of ideas about how and what constitutes change in family systems. In the discussion of change theory that follows, the most profound and salient points from an extensive review of the literature are synthesized and presented along with our own beliefs about change and the conditions that affect the change process.

Systems of relationships appear to possess a tendency toward progressive change. However, a French proverb states, "the more something changes, the more it remains the same." This paradox beautifully highlights the dilemma frequently faced in working with families. The nurse must learn to accept the challenge of the paradoxical relationship between persistence (stability) and change. Maturana (1978) explains the recursiveness of change and stability in this way: Change is an alteration in the family's structure that occurs as compensation for perturbations and has the purpose of maintaining structure and stability. Change itself is experienced as a perturbation to the system, so change generates further change as well as stability. A change in state is exhibited as behavior; therefore, differences in family interactional patterns must be explored. Changes in behavior may or may not be accompanied by insight. However, "the most profound and sustaining change will be that which occurs within the family's belief system (cognition)" (Wright & Bell, in press).

Watzlawick, Weakland, and Fisch (1974) were the first to suggest that persistence and change must be considered together despite their opposing natures. These researchers offer a widely accepted notion of change and suggest that two different types or levels of change exist. They refer to one type as change occurring within a given system that remains unchanged itself. In other words, the system itself remains unchanged, but its elements or parts undergo some type of change. This type of change is referred to as first-order change. It is a change in quantity, not quality. First-order change involves using the same problem-solving strategies over and over again. Each new problem is approached mechanically. If a solution to the problem is difficult to find, more old strategies are used and are usually more vigorously applied. An example of first-order change is the learning of a new behavioral strategy to deal with a child's excessive use of the computer. A parent who formerly disciplined his child by restricting the child's access to the computer is said to have undergone first-order change when he then limits the child's spending money.

The second type of change, referred to as second-order change, is one that changes the system. Second-order change is thus a "change of change." It appears that the French proverb is applicable only to first-order change. For second-order change to occur, actual changes in the rules governing the system must occur and, therefore, the system is structurally transformed. It is important to note that second-order change is often in the nature of a discontinuity or jump and can be sudden and radical. Other times, second-order change occurs in a logical sequence with the person almost seemingly unaware of the change until it is noted by others.

This type of change represents a quantum jump in the system to a different level of functioning. Second-order change can be said to occur, for example, when a family now spends more time together and is able to raise conflictual issues with one another as a result of resolving their teenager's refusal to eat with the family.

Watzlawick, Weakland, and Fisch (1974) also refer to the most obvious type of change, spontaneous change. In spontaneous change, problem resolution occurs in daily living without the input of professionals or sophisticated theories. For example, an anorexic young woman suddenly and apparently spontaneously begins to eat regularly after 2 years of not doing so, or a man suffering from shingles (herpes zoster) reports that his chronic pain disappeared overnight.

Bateson (1979) offers a most thought-provoking statement with regard to change when he proposes that we are almost always unaware of changes. He suggests that changes in our social interactions and in our environment are dramatically and constantly occurring but that we become accustomed to the "new state of affairs before our senses can tell us that it is new" (p. 98). Bateson (1979) also offers the idea that, with regard to the perception of change, the mind can only receive news of difference. Therefore, as Bateson (1979) states, change can be observed as "difference which occurs across time" (p. 452). These ideas concur with those of Maturana and Varela (1992), who offer the idea that change occurs in humans from moment to moment. This change is either triggered by interactions or perturbations from the environment in which the system (family member) exists or is a result of the system's (family member's) own internal dynamics.

Our own view of change in family work draws from the above authors as well as our own clinical experience in working with families. In summary, we agree with Bateson and with Maturana and Varela that change is constantly evolving in families and that people frequently are unaware of it. This type of continuous or spontaneous change occurs with everyday living and progression through individual and family stages of development. These changes may or may not occur with professional input.

We also believe that major transformation of an entire family system can occur and can be precipitated by major life events, such as serious illness, disability, divorce, unemployment, addictions, terrorism, displacement from home as a result of terrorism, war, hurricanes or tsunamis, or death of a family member; or through interventions offered by nurses. Change within a family can occur within the cognitive, affective, or behavioral domains, but change in any one domain impacts the other domains. Therefore, family nursing interventions can be aimed at any domain or all three domains. Interventions are discussed further in Chapter 4, in which the CFIM is presented. We believe that directly correlating interventions with resulting changes is impossible; therefore, predicting outcomes or the types of change that will occur within families is also impossible.

An important role for nurses (operating from a systems perspective) is to carefully observe the connections between systems. To effect change within the original system (the individual), it is necessary to intervene at a higher systems level or at the metalevel (the family system [see Fig. 2–1]). In other words, if nurses wish to effect change within family systems, they need to be able to maintain a metaposition to each family. They must simultaneously conceptualize both the family system interactions and their own interactions with the family. However, if a problem arises between the nurse and the family, this problem must be resolved at a higher level than the nurse–family system, preferably by a supervisor, who can examine the problem from a further metaposition.

CONCEPT 1

Change is dependent on the perception of the problem.

In a now-famous statement, Alfred Korzybski proclaimed that "the map is not the territory." In other words, the name is different from the thing named and the description is different from what is described. In applying this concept to family interviewing, our "mapping" of a particular situation or our perception of a problem or problems follows from how we, as nurses, choose to see it. How we perceive a particular problem has profound implications for how we will intervene and, therefore, how change will occur and whether it will be effective.

One of the most common traps for nurses working with families is acceptance of one family member's perception or perspective as the "truth" about the family. There is no one "truth" or "reality" about family functioning, or perhaps it is more accurate to say that there are as many "truths" or "realities" as there are members of the family (Maturana & Varela, 1992). The error of taking sides in relational family nursing is discussed in Chapter 10. The important task for the nurse is to accept all family members' perceptions, perspectives, and beliefs and offer the family another view of their health concerns, illness, or problems. Individual family members construct their own realities of a situation based on their history of interactions with people throughout their lives and their genetic history (Maturana & Varela, 1992). Maturana, in an interview with Simon (1985), offers an even more radical idea with regard to different family members' perceptions:

> Systems theory first enabled us to recognize that all the different views presented by the different members of a family had some validity. But, systems theory implied that these were different views of the same system. What I am saying is different. I am not saying that the different descriptions that the members of a family make are different views of the same system. I am saying that there is no one way which the system is; that there is no absolute, objective family. I am saying that for each member there is a different family; and that each of these is absolutely valid (p. 36).

Maturana and Varela (1992) emphasize that human systems "bring forth" reality, in language and living with others. We concur that problems can be perceived in very different, yet valid ways. However, as nurses, we are part of a larger societal system and thus are bound by moral, legal, cultural, and societal norms that require us to act in accordance with these norms regarding illegal or dangerous behaviors (Wright & Bell, in press).

If a nurse does not conceptualize human problems from a systems or cybernetics perspective, the nurse's perceptions of the family and their illness, problems, and concerns will be based on a completely different conception of "reality" based on different theoretical assumptions. We wish to emphasize different theoretical assumptions as opposed to more correct or "right" views of problems.

CONCEPT 2

Change is determined by structure.

Changes that occur in living systems (i.e., human systems), are governed by the present structure of that system. The concept of structural determinism (Maturana & Varela, 1992) offers the notion that each individual's biopsychosocial-spiritual structure is unique and is a product of the individual's genetic history (phylogeny) as well as his or her history of interactions over time (ontogeny).

The implication for nursing practice is that an individual's present structure determines the interpersonal, intrapersonal, and environmental influences that are experienced as perturbations (i.e., trigger structural changes). Therefore, we cannot say beforehand which family nursing interventions will be useful in promoting change for this particular family member at this time and which will not. Individuals, therefore, are selectively perturbed by the interventions that are offered by nurses according to what does or does not "fit" their own unique biopsychosocial-spiritual structures. We cannot predict which family nursing interventions will fit for a particular person and which will disturb that person's structure. This theoretical assumption is why we prefer interventions be tailored to each family rather than standardized interventions for particular kinds of problems.

A deep respect for, awe for, and curiosity about family members develops in nurses who are cognizant of the notion of structural determinism. When structural determinism is applied to clinical work with families, Wright and Levac (1992) suggest that the description of families as noncompliant, resistant, or unmotivated is not only "an epistemological error but a biological impossibility" (p. 913). This concept has made a dramatic difference in the way in which we think about families and the interventions that we offer.

CONCEPT 3

Change is dependent on context.

Efforts to promote change in a family system must always take into account the important variable of context. Interventions must be planned with sufficient knowledge of the contextual constraints and resources. This is particularly important considering the emphasis in the health-care industry on accountability, cost-effectiveness, efficiency, and time-effective intervention. Nurses need to be aware of their position in the health-care delivery system vis-à-vis the family. For example, are other professionals involved with the family and, if so, what are their roles with the family? How do these roles differ from the nurse's role, and how are the nurse and family influenced by and influential on the context in which they find themselves, be it a hospital, a primary care clinic, or an extended-care facility? We find it particularly useful to underscore the positive contributions each health-care stakeholder can make to the family's care rather than attributing or assuming self-serving motives to stakeholders who have different vested interests in family care (such as limiting costs).

Larger systems (e.g., schools, mental health agencies, hospitals, public service delivery systems) frequently impose certain "rules" on families that ultimately serve to maintain the larger system's stability and impede change (Imber Coppersmith, 1983; Imber-Black, 1991). One example is the rule of *linear blame*. That is, institutions tend to blame families for difficulties (e.g., lack of motivation) and tend to make referrals for family treatment in order to "cure" the family. This process is similar to the one that families use to refer another family member to be "cured."

Because members of some larger systems, particularly nursing staff, become intensely involved in a patient's or family member's life, they commonly tend to go beyond the immediate concerns. The end result is that patients in hospitals and their families find themselves inundated with services that commonly usurp the family's own resources. This then places the family in a "one-down" position in terms of articulating what they perceive their present needs to be. When a nurse is asked to complete a family assessment, the nurse may become one more irritant in the life of the family and can be hamstrung before even beginning because of the number of professionals involved. This is another reason why nurses should carefully assess the larger context in which the family and the staff find themselves. In some cases, the more serious problem is at the interface of the family with other professionals rather than within the family itself. Thus, interventions aimed at the family–professional system would need to occur before those addressing problems at the family system level.

Another situation that can arise is unclear expertise and leadership. Families may find themselves in a larger system, such as an outpatient drug assessment and treatment clinic. They may receive different ideas on how to deal with a particular problem (e.g., cocaine addiction) depending on whether they are seen at the clinic, at home, or in a class. This usually occurs because no one clinic or educational program offered within a hospital setting has more decision-making power than another regarding a particular family's treatment plan.

Conflicts can also occur between larger systems or between families and larger systems. Unacknowledged or unresolved conflicts commonly result in triads, which inhibit healthy behavior. For example, if parents wish to send their adolescent son to a drug rehabilitation center but the nurse and rehabilitation director have been in conflict over rehabilitation policies, the family is placed in a situation in which pressure from the larger system (nurse–rehabilitation director system) leads them to align or take sides with either the nurse or the rehabilitation director.

How the family is being influenced by and is exerting influence on their involvement with these suprasystems is important information. Change within a family can be thwarted, sabotaged, or impossible if the issue of context is not addressed.

CONCEPT 4

Change is dependent on co-evolving goals for treatment.

Change requires that goals between nurses and families co-evolve within a realistic time frame. In many cases, the main reason for failure in working with families is either the nurse's or family's setting of unrealistic or inappropriate goals. Frank and open discussions with family members regarding treatment goals can help avoid misunderstandings and disappointments on both sides.

Because one of the primary goals of family intervention is to alter the family's views or beliefs of the problem or illness (Wright & Bell, in press), nurses should help family members to search for alternative behavioral, cognitive, and affective responses to problems. Therefore, one of the goals of the nurse is to help the family discover or reclaim its own solutions to problems.

The task of setting specific goals for treatment is accomplished in collaboration with the family. Part of the assessment process is to identify the current suffering or problems with which the family is most concerned and the changes they would like to see. This provides a baseline for the goals of family interviews and becomes the therapeutic contract.

Contracts with families can be either verbal or written. In our own clinical practice and in the practice of our nursing students, we typically make verbal contracts with families that state which specific problems will be tackled during what specified period of time or number of sessions. At the end of that period, progress is evaluated and either contact with the family is terminated or a new contract is made if further therapeutic work is required.

In most instances, clear goals (in the form of a contract) can be set with families with verbal commitments by family members to work on the problems outlined. On conclusion of the contract, evaluation should consist of assessing changes in the family system in addition to changes in the identified patient.

In summary, family assessment and intervention are often more effective and successful if they are based on clear therapeutic goals. However, families rarely come to family interviews with the understanding that family change is required. Therefore, in addition to goal setting, the nurse must help the family to obtain a different view of their problems. First, the nurse needs to engage the family; this can most easily be accomplished by first focusing on understanding and exploring their current suffering, the presenting problems and concerns, and the changes the family desires in relation to it. More detailed information about goal setting, contracts, and termination is given in Chapters 7 and 12.

CONCEPT 5

Understanding alone does not lead to change.

Changes in family work rarely occur by increasing a family's understanding of problems but rather through effecting changes in their beliefs and behavior. Too often, health professionals engaged in family work assume that understanding a problem brings about a solution by the family. From a systems perspective, however, solutions to problems come about as beliefs about health and illness, problems and patterns change, regardless of whether this is accompanied by insight (Wright & Bell, in press).

There has been a tendency in nursing to believe that one must understand "why" in order to solve a problem. Thus, nurses with good intentions spend many hours attempting to obtain masses of data (usually historical) in order to understand the "why" of a problem. In many cases, patients and families encourage the nurse in this quest and participate in it. For example, a patient might ask: "Why did I have my heart attack?" "Why won't my son give up crack?" or "Why did my wife have to die so young?" We strongly discourage searching for the answers because we do not feel that this is a precondition for change; rather, it steers one away from effective efforts at change. We strongly suggest that the prerequisite or precondition for change is not understanding the "why" of a situation but rather understanding the "what." Therefore, we recommend that nurses ask, "What is the effect of the father's heart attack on him and his family?" and "What are the implications of the father's heart attack on his employment?" These questions serve a much more useful purpose in paving the way for possible interventions than do those focusing on the "why" of the situation.

"Why" questions seem to be entrenched in psychoanalytic roots that bring forth psychopathologies. These perspectives are not congruent with a systems or cybernetic foundation of understanding family dynamics that focuses on human problems such as the experience of illness, loss, or disability as interpersonal crises or dilemmas. Even if the "why" of a problem is occasionally understood, it rarely contributes to a solution. Therefore, it is more useful to explore what is being done in the here and now that perpetuates the problem and what can be done in the here and now to effect a change. The search for causes should be avoided because it inadvertently can invite family members to view problems from a linear rather than a systemic perspective. In other words, we prefer to believe that problems reside between persons rather than within persons.

CONCEPT 6

Change does not necessarily occur equally in all family members.

Recall the analogy of the mobile previously presented in this chapter. Imagine the mobile after a wind has passed it. Some pieces turn or react more rapidly or energetically than do others. This is similar to change in family systems in that one family member may begin to respond or change more rapidly than others and, by this very process, set up an opportunity for change throughout the rest of the family. This occurs because other family members cannot respond in the same way to the family member who is changing and, therefore, a ripple effect of change occurs through the system. We have observed this phenomenon in practice with military families when a spouse returns home from war or a peace-keeping mission. The desire for family members to "return to normal" (in other words, to their pre-posting functioning) often conflicts with the returning armed forces member's experience of change. This event typically precipitates a time of intense adjustment for all family members.

Robinson's (1998) research also highlighted the concept that when families experience chronic illness, all family members are affected but not necessarily equally. In her study, women suffered more emotionally than other family members whether the illness was their own, their spouse's, or their child's.

Change depends on the recursive (cybernetic) nature of a family system. Therefore, a small intervention can lead to a variety of reactions, with some family members changing more dramatically or quickly than others.

CONCEPT 7

Facilitating change is the nurse's responsibility.

We believe that it is the nurse's responsibility to facilitate change in collaboration with each family. Facilitating change does not imply that a nurse can predict the outcome, and a nurse should not be invested in a particular outcome. However, there is a distinct difference between facilitating change and being an expert in resolving family problems or assuming what must change. We believe that families possess expertise about their experiences of their health, illness, and disabilities, whereas nurses have expertise in ideas about health promotion and management of serious illness and disability. It is also crucial for nurses to avoid making value judgments about how families should function. Otherwise, the changes or outcomes in a family system may not be satisfying to the nurse if they are incongruent with how the nurse perceives a family should function. It is more important that the family be satisfied with their new level of functioning than that the nurse be satisfied.

From time to time, nurses must evaluate the level or degree of responsibility they feel for treatment. The level of responsibility is out of proportion if a nurse feels more concerned, more worried, or more responsible for family problems than the families feel themselves. In the opposite response, there is a detachment or a lack of concern, compassion, or responsibility on the part of the nurse for facilitating change within families. Both of these extreme responses indicate the need to obtain clinical supervision.

How much change nurses should expect to be able to facilitate in family work depends on their own competence, their capacity for compassion, the context of family treatment, and the response of the family. Nurses need to be cognizant that they are not change agents; they cannot and do not change anyone (Wright & Levac, 1992). Changes in family members are determined by the members' own biopsychosocial-spiritual structures, not by those of others (Maturana & Varela, 1992). Therefore, it is the nurse's responsibility to facilitate a context for change.

CONCEPT 8

Change occurs by means of a "fit" or meshing between the therapeutic offerings (interventions) of the nurse and the biopsychosocial-spiritual structures of family members.

The concept of "fit" arises from the notion of structural determinism (Maturana & Varela, 1992). That is, the family member's structure, not the nurse's therapeutic offering, determines whether the intervention is experienced as a perturbation that triggers or stimulates change. This concept is aligned with the guiding principle that the nurse is not a change agent (Wright & Levac, 1992) but rather one who, among other things, creates a context for change (Wright & Bell, in press). In our clinical experience, family members who respond to particular therapeutic offerings do so because of a fit, or meshing, between their current biopsychosocial-spiritual structures and the family nursing intervention offered. (For more information on this, see Chapter 4 and the discussion of the CFIM.) This includes nurse sensitivity to the family's race, ethnicity, sexual orientation, and social class.

The concept of "fit" allows nurses to be non-blaming of patients and themselves when "non-fit" and, therefore, "non-adherence" and "non-follow-through" occur (Wright & Bell, in press; Wright & Levac, 1992). Nurses operating from a therapeutic stance appreciative of fit can be highly curious about ways to increase the suitability of interventions for particular family members at a specific time. When the concept of fit is overlooked, neglected, or not appreciated, nurses operate with more lecturing, prescribing behaviors and often labeling family members as noncompliant, not ready for change, or defiant of the professional system.

CONCEPT 9

Change can have myriad causes.

Change is influenced by so many different variables that, in most cases, knowing specifically what precipitated, stimulated, or triggered the change is difficult. Change is not always a result of well thought-out intervention. Commonly, it can be the result of the method of inquiry into family problems. Asking interventive questions (see Chapter 4 for an in-depth discussion about questions within the CFIM and Chapter 9 for how to use questions in family interviewing) may in and of itself promote change. It is more important for nurses to attribute change to families than to concern themselves with what they did to create change (see Chapter 12 for more information on concluding meetings with families). To search for or take undue credit for change is inappropriate at this stage of our knowledge of the change process in families.

BIOLOGY OF COGNITION

The biology of cognition has been described and articulated by two neurobiologists, Maturana and Varela (1992), in their landmark publication *The Tree of Knowledge: The Biological Roots of Human Understanding.* They offer the idea that humans bring forth different views to their understanding of events and experiences in their lives. This idea is not new, but Maturana and Varela's perspective on how we humans make and claim observations is much more radical: it is based on biology and physiology, not philosophy (Wright & Bell, in press; Wright & Levac, 1992). If a nurse adopts a particular view of reality, it follows then that a nurse now encompasses a particular view of people and their functioning, relationships, and illnesses.

CONCEPT 1

Two possible avenues for explaining our world are objectivity and objectivity-in-parentheses (Maturana & Varela, 1992; Wright & Levac, 1992; Wright, Watson, & Bell, 1990).

The view of objectivity assumes that one ultimate domain of reference exists for explaining the world. Within this domain, entities are assumed to exist independent of the observer. Such entities are as numerous and broad as imagination might allow and may be explicitly or implicitly identified as mind, knowledge, truth, and so on. Within this avenue of explanation, we come to believe we have access to a true and correct view of the world and its events, an objective reality. From this "objectivist" view, "a system and its components have a constancy and a stability that is independent of the observer that brings them forth" (Mendez, Coddou, & Maturana, 1988, p. 154). Nursing diagnoses, emotional conflict, pride, and politics are all products of an "objective" view of reality.

When objectivity is "placed in parentheses," people recognize that objects do exist but that they are not independent of the living system that brings them forth. The only "truths" that exist are those brought forth by observers, such as nurses and family members. Each person's view is not a distortion of some presumably correct interpretation. Instead of one objective universe waiting to be discovered or correctly described, Maturana has proposed a "multiverse," where many observer "verses" coexist, each valid in its own right. To increase options and possibilities for families to cope with illness using a variety of strategies or to improve their well-being, nurses need to help family members drift toward objectivity-in-parentheses. When nurses are able to maintain an objective stance, they are increasingly able to invite family members to resist the "sin of certainty," that is, to resist the notion that there is only one true or correct way to manage health or illness, loss, or disability.

CONCEPT 2

We bring forth our realities through interacting with the world, ourselves, and others through language.

Reality does not reside "out there" to be absorbed; rather, people exist in many domains of the realities that they bring forth to explain their experiences (Maturana & Varela, 1992). The ability to bring forth personal meaning and to respond to and interact with the world and with each other, but always with reference to a set of internal coherences, can be seen as the essential quality of living. Maturana and Varela (1980) assert that this statement applies to all organisms, with or without a nervous system. They further suggest that it is best to think of cognition as a continual interaction between what we expect to see (our unconscious premises or beliefs) and what we bring forth. In a telephone interview, Maturana (1988) embellished this notion of reality as follows:

> We exist in many domains of realities that we bring forth ... What I'm saying in the long-run is that there is no possibility of saying absolutely anything about anything independent from us. So whatever we do is always our total responsibility in the sense that it depends completely on us, and all domains of reality that we bring forth are equally legitimate although they are not equally desirable

> or pleasant to live in. But they are always brought forth by us, in our coexistence with other human beings. So if we bring forth a community in which there is misery, well, this is it. If we bring forth a community in which there is well-being, this is it. But it is us always in coexistence with others that … are bringing forth reality. Reality is indeed an explanation of the world that we live [in] with others.

In sum, the world everyone sees is not the world but a world that they bring forth with others (Maturana & Varela, 1992). When nurses adopt this particular ethical stance, they find themselves more curious about the world each family member brings forth and how this "world" influences the person's ability or inability to cope with or manage their illness.

CONCLUSIONS

Nursing is striving to articulate and describe more clearly the theories that inform clinical practice models. In an important and useful review of family studies and interventions, Hallberg (2003) found "a lack of congruence between the theoretical framework, the intervention, and the outcome measure" (p. 9). This chapter is our effort to be more transparent about the theories that provide the foundations of the CFAM and CFIM. We hope that our practice models have more relevance, more meaning, and of course more usefulness in clinical practice with families because of this transparency. Nurses need to continue to conduct research-based practice and practice-based research that enhance our understanding of which theories are most significant to inform practice, especially the offering of interventions.

References

Allmond, B.W., Buckman, W., & Gofman, H.F. (1979). *The family is the patient: An approach to behavioral pediatrics for the clinician.* St. Louis: Mosby.

Bateson, G. (1979). *Mind and nature.* New York: E.P. Dutton.

Bavelas, J.B. (1992). Research into the pragmatics of human communication. *Journal of Strategic and Systemic Therapies, 11*(2), 15–29.

Becvar, D.S., & Becvar, R.J. (1992). *Family therapy: A systemic integration.* Boston: Allyn and Bacon, Inc.

Burnard, P. (1999). Carl Rogers and postmodernism: Challenges in nursing and health sciences. *Nursing and Health Sciences, 1*(4), 241–256.

Crawford, J.A., & Tarko, M.A. (2004). Family communication. In P.J. Bomar (Ed.), *Promoting health in families: applying family research and theory to nursing practice* (3rd ed.). Philadelphia: Saunders.

Furth, H.G. (1987). *Knowledge as desire: An essay on Freud and Piaget.* New York: Columbia University Press.

Glazer, S. (2001). Therapeutic touch and postmodernism in nursing. *Nursing Philosophy, 2*(3), 196–230.

Hallberg, I.R. (2003). Evidence-based nursing, interventions, and family nursing: Methodological obstacles and possibilities. *Journal of Family Nursing, 9*(3), 3–22.

Imber-Black, E. (1991). The family-larger-system perspective. *Family Systems Medicine, 9*(4), 371–396.

Imber Coppersmith, E. (1983). The place of family therapy in the homeostasis of larger systems. In M. Aronson & R. Wolberg (Eds.), *Group and family therapy: An overview* (pp. 216–27). New York: Brunner/Mazel.

Jackson, D.D. (1973). Family interaction, family homeostasis and some implications for conjoint family psychotherapy. In D.D. Jackson (Ed.), *Therapy, communication and change* (4th ed.) (pp. 185–203). Palo Alto, CA: Science & Behavior Books.

Kaakinen, J.R. & Hanson, S.M.H. (2004). Theoretical foundations for family health nursing practice. In P.J. Bomar (Ed.), *Promoting health in families: Applying family research and theory to nursing practice* (3rd ed.). Philadelphia: Saunders.

Kermode, S., & Brown, C. (1996). The postmodernist hoax and its effects on nursing. *International Journal of Nursing Studies, 33*(4), 375–384.

Loos, F., & Bell, J.M. (1990). Circular questions: A family interviewing strategy. *Dimensions in Critical Care Nursing, 9*(1), 46–53.

Maturana, H. (1978). Biology of language: The epistemology of reality. In G.A. Miller & E. Lenneberg (Eds.), *Psychology and biology of language and thought* (pp. 27–63). New York: Academic Press.

Maturana, H.R. (1988). *Telephone conversation: Calgary/Chile coupling* [Telephone transcript]. Calgary, Canada: University of Calgary.

Maturana, H.R., & Varela, F.J. (1980). *Autopoiesis and cognition: The realization of the living*. Dordrecht, Holland: D. Reidl Pub. Co.

Maturana, H.R., & Varela, F. (1992). *The tree of knowledge: The biological roots of human understanding*. Boston: Shambhala Publications, Inc.

Mendez, C.L., Coddou, F., & Maturana, H.R. (1998). The bringing forth of pathology. *Irish Journal of Psychology, 9*(1), 144–172.

Moules, N.J. (2000). Postmodernism and the sacred: Reclaiming connection in our greater-than-human worlds. *Journal of Marital and Family Therapy, 26*(2), 229–240.

Robinson, C.A. (1998). Women, families, chronic illness, and nursing interventions: From burden to balance. *Journal of Family Nursing, 4*(3), 271–290.

Schober, M., & Affara, F. (2001). *The family nurse: Frameworks for practice*. Geneva: International Council of Nurses.

Selvini-Palazzoli, M., et al. (1978). A ritualized prescription in family therapy: Odd days and even days. *Journal of Marriage and Family Counseling, 4*(3), 3–9.

Simon, R. (1985). Structure is destiny: An interview with Huberto Maturana. *Family Therapy*, May–June, 32–43.

Tapp, D.M., & Wright, L.M. (1996). Live supervision and family systems nursing: Postmodern influences and dilemmas. *Journal of Psychiatric and Mental Health Nursing, 3*(4), 225–233.

Tomm, K. (1980). Towards a cybernetic-systems approach to family therapy at the University of Calgary. In D.S. Freeman (Ed.), *Perspectives on family therapy* (pp. 3–18). Toronto: Butterworths.

Tomm, K. (1981). Circularity: A preferred orientation for family assessment. In A.S. Gurman (Ed.), *Questions and answers in the practice of family therapy* (Vol. 1) (pp. 874–887). New York: Brunner/Mazel.

Tomm, K. (1984). One perspective on the Milan systemic approach: Part II. Description of session format, interviewing style and interventions. *Journal of Marital and Family Therapy, 10*(3), 253–271.

Tomm, K. (1985). Circular interviewing: A multifaceted clinical tool. In D. Campbell & R. Draper (Eds.), *Applications of systemic family therapy: The Milan approach* (pp. 33–45). London: Grune & Stratton.

Tomm, K. (1987a). Interventive interviewing: Part I. Strategizing as a fourth guideline for the therapist. *Family Process, 26*(1), 3–13.

Tomm, K. (1987b). Interventive interviewing: Part II. Reflexive questioning as a means to enable self-healing. *Family Process, 26*(6), 167–183.

Tomm, K. (1988). Interventive interviewing: Part III. Intending to ask lineal, circular, strategic, or reflexive questions? *Family Process, 27*(1), 1–15.

Varela, F.J. (1979). *Principles of biological autonomy.* New York: Elsevier North Holland.

von Bertalanffy, L. (1968). *General systems theory: Foundations, development, applications.* New York: George Braziller.

von Bertalanffy, L. (1972). The history and status of general systems theory. In G.J. Klir (Ed.), *Trends in general systems theory.* New York: Wiley-Interscience.

von Bertalanffy, L. (1974). General systems theory and psychiatry. In S. Arieti (Ed.), *American handbook of psychiatry* (pp. 1095–1117). New York: Basic Books.

von Glaserfeld, E. (1984). An introduction to radical constructivism. In P. Watzlawick (Ed.), *The invented reality: Contributions to constructivism* (pp. 17–40). New York: Norton.

Watzlawick, P. (Ed.). (1984). *The invented reality: Contributions to constructivism.* New York: Norton.

Watzlawick, P., Beavin, J.H., & Jackson, D.D. (1967). *Pragmatics of human communication: a study of interactional patterns, pathologies, and paradoxes.* New York: Norton.

Watzlawick, P., Weakland, J.H., & Fisch, R. (1974). *Change: Principles of problem formulation and problem resolution.* New York: Norton.

Wright, L.M., & Bell, J.M. (in press). Beliefs and illness: A model for healing. Calgary, AB: 4th Floor Press.

Wright, L.M., & Levac, A.M. (1992). The non-existence of non-compliant families: The influence of Humberto Maturana. *Journal of Advanced Nursing, 17*(8), 913–917.

Wright, L.M., & Watson, W.L. (1988). Systemic family therapy and family development. In C.J. Falicov (Ed.), *Family transitions: Continuity and change over the life cycle* (pp. 407–430). New York: Guilford Press.

Wright, L.M., Watson, W.L., & Bell, J.M. (1990). The family nursing unit: A unique integration of research, education, and clinical practice. In J.M. Bell, W.L. Watson, & L.M. Wright (Eds.), *The cutting edge of family nursing* (pp. 95–109). Calgary, Alberta: Family Nursing Unit Publications.

Chapter 3

The Calgary Family Assessment Model

The Calgary Family Assessment Model (CFAM) is an integrated, multidimensional framework based on the foundations of systems, cybernetics, communication, and change theory and influenced by postmodernism and biology of cognition. This fifth edition includes a discussion of the distinction between using CFAM to assess a family and using CFAM as an organizing framework, or template, for working with families to help them resolve issues.

CFAM has received wide recognition since the first edition of this book in 1984. It has been adopted by many faculties and schools of nursing in Australia, Great Britain, North America, Brazil, Hong Kong, Japan, Finland, Sweden, Korea, Taiwan, Portugal, Singapore, Spain, Iceland, and Thailand. It has been referenced frequently in the literature, especially the *Journal of Family Nursing*. In addition, the International Council of Nurses has recognized it as one of the four leading family assessment models in the world (Schober & Affara, 2001). Originally adapted from a family assessment framework developed by Tomm and Sanders (1983), CFAM was substantially revised in 1994, 2000, and 2005 and is now more embellished in this fifth edition.

CFAM consists of three major categories:

1. Structural

2. Developmental

3. Functional

Each category contains several subcategories. It is important for *each* nurse to decide which subcategories are relevant and appropriate to explore and assess with *each* family at *each* point in time. That is, not all subcategories need to be assessed at a first meeting with a family, and some subcategories need never be assessed. If the nurse uses too many subcategories, he or she may become overwhelmed by all the data. If the nurse and the family discuss too few subcategories, each may have a distorted view of the family's strengths or problems and the family situation.

It is useful to conceptualize these three assessment categories and their many subcategories as a branching diagram (Fig. 3-1). As the nurse uses the subcategories on the right of the branching diagram, the nurse collects more and more microscopic data. It is important for nurses to be able to move back and forth on the diagram to draw together all of the relevant information into an integrated assessment. This process of synthesizing data helps nurses working with complex family situations.

It is also important for a nurse to recognize that a family assessment is based on the nurse's personal and professional life experiences, beliefs, and relationships with those being interviewed. "It should not be considered as

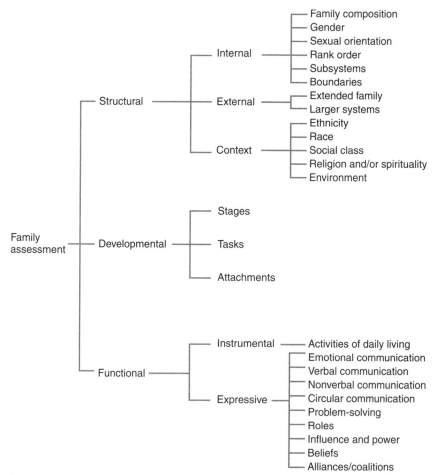

FIGURE 3-1: Branching diagram of CFAM.

'the truth' about the family, but rather one perspective at a particular point in time" (Levac, Wright, & Leahey, 2002, p. 12).

We believe it is useful for nurses to determine whether they are using CFAM as a model to assess a family or as an organizing framework for clinical work with a specific family to help the family address a health issue. When learning CFAM, students and practicing nurses new to family work will likely find the model helpful for directly assessing families. Similarly, researchers seeking to assess families will find the model useful. This use of the model involves asking the family questions about themselves for the express purpose of gaining a snapshot of the family's structure, development, and functioning at a particular point in time.

However, how we have used CFAM is not in a research manner but rather in a clinical manner. Once a nurse becomes experienced with the categories and subcategories of CFAM, he or she can use CFAM as a clinical organizing framework to help families solve problems or issues. For example, a single-parent family in the developmental stage of families with adolescents will have many positive experiences from earlier developmental stages to draw from in coping with their teenager's unexpected illness. The nurse, being reminded of family developmental stages by using CFAM, will draw forth those resiliencies. She will ask questions and collaboratively develop interventions with the family to enhance their functioning during this health-care episode.

Families do not generally present to health-care professionals to be "assessed." Rather, they present themselves or are encountered by nurses while coping with an illness or seeking assistance to improve their quality of life. CFAM helps guide nurses in helping families.

In this chapter, each assessment category is discussed separately. Terms are defined and sample questions relevant to each CFAM category are proposed for the nurse to ask family members. We do not suggest that nurses ask these questions in a disembodied way. Rather, real-life clinical examples are provided in Chapters 4, 7, 8, 9, and 10 so that readers can see how to use the sample questions and apply CFAM. The *"How to" Family Nursing Series* available in DVD (see Appendix 1) provides actual clinical interviews demonstrating the use of CFAM (www.familynursingresources.com). The use of assessment and interventive questions will be discussed in Chapter 4 (The Calgary Family Intervention Model [CFIM]). Again, we wish to emphasize that not all questions about various subcategories of the model need to be asked at the first interview, and questions about each subcategory are not appropriate for every family. Families are obviously composed of individuals, but the focus of a family assessment is less on the individual and more on the interaction *among* all of the individuals within the family.

STRUCTURAL ASSESSMENT

In assessing a family, the nurse needs to examine its structure—that is, who is in the family, what is the connection among family members vis-à-vis those outside the family, and what is the family's context. Three aspects of family structure can most readily be examined: internal structure, external structure, and context. Each of these dimensions of family structural assessment is addressed separately.

Internal Structure

Internal structure includes six subcategories:

1. Family composition
2. Gender
3. Sexual orientation
4. Rank order
5. Subsystems
6. Boundaries

Family Composition

The subcategory family composition has many meanings because of the many definitions given to family. Wright and Bell (in press) define family as a group of individuals who are bound by strong emotional ties, a sense of belonging, and a passion for being involved in one another's lives. There are five critical attributes to the concept of family:

1. The family is a system or unit.
2. Its members may or may not be related and may or may not live together.
3. The unit may or may not contain children.
4. There is commitment and attachment among unit members that include future obligation.
5. The unit caregiving functions consist of protection, nourishment, and socialization of its members.

Using these ideas, the nurse can include the various family forms that are prevalent in society today, such as the biological family of procreation, the nuclear family (family of origin), the sole-parent family, the stepfamily, the communal family, and the lesbian, gay, bisexual, queer, intersexed, transgendered, or twin-spirited (LGBQITT) couple or family. Designating a group of people with a term such as "couple," "nuclear family," or "single-parent family" specifies attributes of membership, but these distinctions of grouping are not more or less "families" by reason of labeling. Rather, attributes of affection, strong emotional ties, a sense of belonging, and durability of membership determine family composition.

Nurses need to find a definition of family that moves beyond the traditional boundaries that limit membership using the criteria of blood, adoption, and marriage. We have found the following definition of family to be most useful in our clinical work: the family is who they say they are. With this definition, nurses can honor individual family members' ideas about which relationships are significant to them and their experience of health and illness. For example, does the family include the surrogate mother and the commissioning couple? The unknown sperm donor? Dolbin-Macnab and Rausch (2006) have discussed the variability among different countries with respect to the anonymity of the donor. Some countries will release identifying information about the donor to the adult offspring, if there is a health consent, while other countries will release identifying information when the child reaches adulthood.

Research has shown that there is a powerful and reciprocal connection between health and the nature of a person's long-term relationships (Post & Neimark, 2007). It is not just the length of a relationship that is important, but the quality of the relationship. One study found that a spouse who suppresses his or her anger when verbally attacked by the other has a higher risk of early death compared to spouses who express their anger (Harburg, Kaciroti, & Gleiberman, 2008).

Although we recognize the dominant North American type of separately housed nuclear families, our definition allows us to address the emotional past, present, and anticipated future relationships within the family system. For example, we support the American Academy of Pediatrics (2002) policy advocating that children who are born or adopted by one member of a same-sex couple deserve the security of two legally defined parents. We know that gays and lesbians often refer to their friendship network as "family," and that for many gays and lesbians this "family" is often as crucial and influential as their family of origin and at times, even more so.

Other family configurations include grandparents as primary caregivers for their grandchildren, an arrangement that has risen over 40 percent since 1990 (Brown-Standridge & Floyd, 2000), sometimes with negative effects on the grandmother's health (Haglund, 2000). In the United States, 4.5 million children live with a grandparent as primary caregiver (Haskell, 2003).

Some authors, such as Penn (2007), have questioned the commonly held belief that all couples want to live together. He discusses "commuter couples," an alternate form of relationship in which each partner retains his or her own separate living quarters while remaining in a committed, monogamous, loving relationship. A rhythm that ensures both solitude and passionate connection is highly valued by these couples. Dual-dwelling duos (DDDs) and other new alternative pair-bonding structures, such as cohabitation and nonmarital coparenting, have also emerged. Our definition of family is based on the family's conception of family rather than on who lives in the household.

Changes in family composition are important to note. These changes could be permanent, such as the loss of a family member or the addition of a new person such as a new baby, an elderly parent, a nanny, or a border. Changes in family composition can also be transient. For example, stepfamilies commonly have different family compositions on weekends or during vacation periods when children from previous relationships cohabit. Families with a child in placement or those experiencing homelessness often live temporarily with other relatives and then move on. In New York City in 2002, more than 13,000 children spent their nights shuttling between shelters and other living accommodations (Egan, 2002).

Losses tend to be more severe depending on how recently they have occurred, the younger some of the family members are when loss occurs, the smaller the family, the greater the numerical imbalance between male and female members of the family resulting from the loss, the greater the number of losses, and the greater the number of prior losses. The circumstances surrounding the loss may be of exquisite concern for the nurse. For example, some parents of severely mentally ill children have reported that they were encouraged to give up custody of their children to foster care as a way of securing intense health-care treatment for them.

Serious illness or death of a family member, especially by violence or war, can lead to profound disruption in the family. The simultaneous deaths of both parents by car or plane crash, murder/suicide, natural disasters such as Hurricane Katrina, war, terrorist acts such as September 11, domestic terrorism such as the Virginia Tech killings, or the absence of one parent in jail and the death of the other parent can result in aunts and uncles raising nieces and nephews, or grandparents raising grandchildren, an often undernoticed family structural arrangement. Other family arrangements can occur when one parent is in a rehab facility owing to military injuries. The extent of the impact of a death on the family depends on the social and ethnic meaning of death, the history of previous losses, the timing of the death in the life cycle, and the nature of the death (Becvar, 2001, 2003). Research by Bowse et al (2003) indicates that the extent of human immunodeficiency virus risk-taking in adulthood is positively related to unexpected deaths experienced early in life and related inadequate mourning. We agree with their recommendation that prevention efforts need to be more family-based and family-focused.

Our own reflections in the aftermath of September 11 and those of the families we work with have only increased our sensitivity to loss, its meaning in our culture, and its very specific meaning for each family in terms of how they cope and deal with uncertainty. Every family touched by tragedy faces the task of making sense of what happened, why it happened, and how to adjust to the changed landscape. Families can find inspiration from many sources to cope with unprecedented tragedy.

The position and function of the person who died in the family system and the openness of the family system must also be considered. We have found it useful to note the family's losses and deaths during the structural assessment process, but do not immediately assume that these losses are of major significance to the family. By taking this stance, we disagree with the position taken by some clinicians who assert that it is important to track patterns of adaptation to loss as a routine part of family assessment even when it is not initially presented as relevant to chief complaints.

In our clinical practice with families, we have found it useful to ask ourselves these questions to determine the composition of families: Who is in *this* family? Who does *this* family consider to be "family"?

Questions to Ask the Family. Could you tell me who is in your family? Does anyone else live with you, for example, grandparents, boarders? So, your family consists of you and Faris, your 35-year-old son who just returned from Afghanistan—anyone else? Has anyone recently moved out? Is there anyone else you think of as family who does not live with you? Anyone not related biologically?

Gender

The subcategory of gender is a basic construct, a fundamental organizing principle. We believe in the constructivist "both/and" position—that is, we view gender as both a universal "reality" operational in hierarchy and power and as a reality constructed by ourselves from our particular frame of reference. We recognize gender as both a fundamental basis for all human beings and as an individual premise. Gender is important for nurses to consider because the difference in how men and women experience the world is at the heart of the therapeutic conversation. We can help families by assuming that differences between women and men can be changed, discarding unhelpful cultural scripts for women and men, and recognizing and attending to hidden power issues.

In couple relationships, the problems described by men and women commonly include unspoken conflicts between their perceptions of gender—that is, how their family and society or culture tell them that men and women should feel, think, or behave—and their own experiences.

We argue on behalf of the integration of male and female attributes in each person. Human development is a process of increasingly complex forms of relatedness and integration rather than a progression from attachment to separation. Gender is, in our view, a set of beliefs about or expectations of male and female behaviors and experiences. These beliefs have been developed by cultural, religious, and familial influences as well as by class and sexual orientation. They are in some ways more important than anatomic differences although persons with ambiguous genitalia are often referred to as having an intersex orientation.

Gender plays an important role in family health care, especially child health care. Differences in parental roles in caring for an ill child may be significant sources of family stress. For example, when a child is ill, the majority of help-seeking is initiated by the mother. Robinson (1998) found role strain among families in which chronic illness became an unwelcome, dominant, powerful burden: "It became clear that the women—the wives and mothers in these families—were responsible for day-to-day, 24-hour, day-in, day-out protection" (p. 277). The women carried both the burden of responsibility and the majority of the workload. Gender can also be an important variable in designing health-care interventions. For example, Hoff et al (2005) found differential treatment effects as a function of parental gender in their study of interventions to decrease uncertainty and distress for parents of children newly diagnosed with type I diabetes.

Levac, Wright, and Leahey (2002) recommend that assessment of the influence of gender is especially important when societal, cultural, or family beliefs about male and female roles are creating family tension. In this situation, couples may desire to establish more equal relationships, with characteristics such as:

■ Partners hold equal status (e.g., equal entitlement to personal goals, needs, and wishes).

■ Accommodation in the relationship is mutual (e.g., schedules are organized equally around each partner's needs).

■ Attention to the other in the relationship is mutual (e.g., equal displays of interest in the other's needs and desires by both partners).

■ Enhancement of the well-being of each partner is mutual (e.g., the relationship supports the psychological health of each equally).

In our clinical supervision with nurses doing relational family practice, we have found it useful to have them consider their own ideas about male, female, intersexed, and transgendered persons. Examples of questions we ask them to consider include: As a woman, how do you believe you should behave toward men? How do you expect them to behave toward you? How do you believe men should behave toward ill family members? What ways have you noticed that men express emotion? What are your thoughts about couples who choose a child's sex? Whose work do you express more interest in: husband's or wife's? Who do you feel more comfortable inviting to an interview: husband or wife? If a father answers the phone, who do you ask to set the appointment with: father, mother, or both?

Questions to Ask the Family. Sabeen, what effect did your parents' ideas have on your own ideas of masculinity and femininity? If your arguments with your male children were about how to stay connected rather than how to separate, would your arguments then be different? If you would show the feelings you keep hidden, Hashim, would your wife think more or less of you? How did it come to be that Mom assumes more responsibility for the dialysis than Dad does?

Sexual Orientation

The subcategory of sexual orientation includes sexual majority and sexual minority populations. *Heterosexism*, the preference of heterosexual orientation over other sexual orientations, is a form of multicultural bias that has the potential to harm both families and health-care providers. Sexual minority populations include LGBQITT persons. This acronym is used to refer to the sexually diverse community of lesbian, gay, bisexual, queer, intersexed, transgender, and two-spirited people. It is an attempt to be an inclusive acronym but is not defininitve. Queer refers to an individual whose gender identity doesn't strictly conform with societal norms traditionally ascribed to either male or female and who defines themselves outside of these definitions. Intersexed describes someone with ambiguous genitalia or chromosomal abnormalities. Two-spirited denotes an individual in the Aboriginal culture with close ties to the spirit world and who may or may not identify as being lesbian, gay, bisexual, or transgender. Overall, it indicates a duality existent in a person.

Discrimination, lack of knowledge, stereotyping, and insensitivity about sexual orientation are being addressed in North American society. Discussions about gay marriage, however, have at times clouded the issue of equal treatment. Despite the fact that approximately 1% of all U.S. households are identified as consisting of same-sex couples (USA Today, 2003), the topic of sexual orientation is one that nurses approach with varying levels of acceptance, comfort, and knowledge. For example, nurses' first encounters with transgendered persons often pose unfamiliar challenges. Lesbians, gay men, queers, and heterosexual women and men live in partially overlapping but partially separate cultures, and their gender role development often follows distinctive trajectories leading to different outcomes. In addition, immigrants may have also been exposed to varying beliefs about gay culture. Samir (2002) states "there's absolutely no gay culture in Iraq. Not a hint of it. The only Arab country establishing a gay culture is Lebanon...Homosexuality in most Arab countries is frowned upon and in some it is a crime punishable by extreme sentences" (p. 98).

In our clinical supervision of relational family nursing, we have found it useful to reflect critically on attitudes about sexual orientation. When comparing lesbian couples with heterosexual couples, we use parallel terms as opposed to "normal" couples. That is, we do not say that lesbian couples as compared to "normal" couples have more coping skills. Rather, we say that lesbian couples believe this and heterosexual couples believe that. We do not assume that what applies to gay relationships can be applied to lesbian relationships or that a patient is heterosexual if the patient says that he or she is dating. We believe that nurses should be able to support a patient along whatever sexual orientation path he or she takes and that the patient's sense of integrity and interpersonal relatedness are the most important goals of all. If a health-care provider is not able to support a patient's explorations or decision to live as a heterosexual, homosexual, bisexual, queer, intersexed, or transgendered person, the nurse should excuse himself or herself from treating such patients.

Questions to Ask the Family. Elsbeth, at what age did you first engage in sexual activity (rather than at what age did you first have intercourse)? When LaCheir first told your mom that she was lesbian, what effect did it have on your mom's caregiving with her? When your brother, LeeArius, announced that he was gay and leaving his marriage, how did your parents respond? What did your parents tell you, Lilah, about your ambiguous genitals?

Rank Order

The subcategory rank order refers to the position of the children in the family with respect to age and gender. Birth order, gender, and distance in age between siblings are important factors to consider when doing an assessment. Toman (1988) has been a major contributor to research about sibling configuration. In his main thesis, the duplication theorem, he asserts that the more new social relationships resemble earlier intrafamilial social relationships, the more enduring and successful they are. For example, the marriage between an older brother (of a younger sister) and a younger sister (of an older brother) has good potential for success because the relationships are complementary. If the marriage is between two firstborns, a symmetrical competitive relationship might exist, with each one vying for the position of leadership.

The following factors also influence sibling constellation: the timing of each sibling's birth in the family history, the child's characteristics, the family's idealized "program" for the child, and the parental attitudes and biases regarding sex differences. For example, we have found that siblings of children with attention deficit hyperactivity disorder (ADHD) felt victimized by their ADHD sibling and that their experiences were often minimized or overlooked in the family.

Although we believe that sibling patterns are important to note, we urge nurses to remember that different child-rearing patterns have also emerged as a result of increased use of birth control, the women's movement, the large number of women in the workforce, and the great variety of family configurations. We hold the view that sibling position is an organizing influence on the personality, but it is not a fixed influence. Each new period of life brings a reevaluation of these influences. An individual transfers or generalizes familial experiences to social settings outside the family, such as kindergarten, schools, and clubs. Given the availability and powerful influence of the internet, the universe of available relationships and experiences is greatly expanded. As an individual is influenced by the environment, his or her relationships with colleagues, friends, and spouses are also generally affected. With time, multiple influences in addition to sibling constellation can affect personality organization.

Prior to meeting with a family, we encourage nurses to hypothesize about the potential influence of rank order on the reason for the family interview. For example, nurses could ask themselves, "If this child is the youngest in the family, could this be influencing the parents' reluctance to allow him to give his own insulin injection?" The nurse could also consider the influence of birth order on motivation, achievement, and vocational choice. For example, is the firstborn child under pressure to achieve academically? If the youngest child is starting school, what influence might this have on the couple's persistent attempts with in vitro fertilization? We urge clinicians not only to consider rank order when children are young but also its relevance when working with siblings in later life. Overlooking the fact that individuals may be influenced by old or ongoing conflicts may lead to missed opportunities for healing.

Questions to Ask the Family. How many children do you have, Amber? Who is the eldest? How old is he or she? Who comes next in line? Have there been any miscarriages or abortions? If your older sister, Gerda, showed more softness and were less controlling of your mom, might you be willing to talk more with your mom? Would you be willing to talk about difficult issues such as her giving up driving because of her macular degeneration?

Subsystems

Subsystems is a term used to discuss or mark the family system's level of differentiation; a family carries out its functions through its subsystems. Dyads, such as husband–wife or mother–child, can be seen as subsystems. Subsystems can be delineated by generation, sex, interest, function, or history.

Each person in the family belongs to several different subsystems. In each, that person has a different level of power and uses different skills. A 65-year-old woman can be a grandmother, mother, wife, and daughter within the same family. An eldest boy is a member of the sibling subsystem, the male subsystem, and the parent-child subsystem. In each of the subsystems, he behaves according to his position. He has to concede the power that he exerts over his younger brother in the sibling subsystem when he interacts with his stepmother in the parent–child subsystem. An only girl living in a single-parent household has different subsystem challenges when she lives on alternate weekends with her father, his new wife, and their two daughters. The ability to adapt to the demands of different subsystem levels is a necessary skill for each family member.

In our clinical practice we have found it useful to consider whether clear generational boundaries are present in the family. If they are, does the family find them helpful or not? For example, we ask ourselves whether one child behaves like a parent or husband surrogate. Is the child a child, or is there a surrogate-spouse subsystem? By generating these hypotheses before and during the family meeting, we are able to connect isolated bits of data to either confirm or negate a hypothesis.

Questions to Ask the Family. Some families have special subgroups; for example, the women do certain things while the men do other things. Do different subgroups exist in your family? If so, what effect does this have on your family's stress level? When Mom and your sister, DeRong, stay up at night and talk about Dad's use of crack, what do the boys do? Which subgroup in the family is most affected by Cleve's crack problem and how?

Who gets together in the family to talk about Shabana's self-mutilating behaviors?

Parent-child: How has your relationship with Caitylin changed since her diagnosis with severe acute respiratory syndrome?

Marital: How much couple time can you and Sherwinn carve out each month without talking about the children?

Sibling: On a scale of 1 to 10, with 10 being the most, how scared were you when AhPoh developed congestive heart failure?

Boundaries

The subcategory boundaries refers to the rule "defining who participates and how" (Minuchin, 1974, p. 53). Family systems and subsystems have boundaries, the function of which is to define or protect the differentiation of the system or subsystem. For example, the boundary of a family system is defined when a father tells his teenage daughter that her boyfriend cannot move into the household. A parent–child subsystem boundary is made explicit when a mother tells her daughter, "You are not your brother's parent. If he is not taking his medication, I will discuss it with him."

Boundaries can be diffuse, rigid, or permeable. As boundaries become diffuse, the differentiation of the family system decreases. For example, family members may become emotionally close and richly cross-joined. These family members can have a heightened sense of belonging to the family and less individual autonomy. A diffuse subsystem boundary is evident when a child is "parentified," or given adult responsibilities and power in decision making.

When rigid boundaries are present, the subsystems tend to become disengaged. A husband who rigidly believes that only wives should visit the elderly and whose wife agrees with him can become disengaged from or peripheral to the senior adult–child subsystem. Clear, permeable boundaries, on the other hand, allow appropriate flexibility. Under these conditions, the rules can be modified. We do not support the pathologizing of coalitions or subsystems just because they exist. In working with families from different cultures, races, and social classes or those from rural settings, we have found that fostering other central ties may be most beneficial for the family.

Boundaries tend to change over time. Boss (2002) suggests that family boundaries become ambiguous during the process of reorganization after acquisition or loss of a member. This is particularly evident with families experiencing separation or divorce. As couples make the transition to parenthood, they may experience the desired child as a family member who is psychologically present but physically absent. This is particularly relevant if there is a surrogate mother or a known sperm donor involved during the pregnancy. Families caring for a member with Alzheimer's disease may experience the opposite phenomenon: the member is physically present but may often be psychologically absent.

Other variations include the ambiguity experienced by some families when a family member is in prison and then returns home. With approximately 650,000 ex-cons leaving state or federal American prisons in 2006 (Penn, 2007), the impact on families is significant. Family boundaries can also be challenged when family members, especially young parents, are soldiers at war, or live in a rehab hospital following a tour of duty. The concept of ambiguous boundaries was quite evident in the days shortly following 9/11 or Hurricane Katrina, when people were missing. Boss (2002) named the situation "ambiguous loss" and further described it as the most difficult loss there is, because families and friends feel helpless and the cultural tendency in the United States is to seek closure. During the early days post-9/11 there was little closure for families who had relatives missing. Many Arab-Americans and other immigrant groups experienced flashbacks of terror and connected to a history of oppression in the Middle East.

Boundary styles can facilitate or constrain family functioning. For example, an immigrant family that moves into a new culture may be very protective of its members until it gradually adapts to the cultural milieu. Its boundaries vis-à-vis outside systems may be quite firm and rigid but may gradually become more flexible. For example, some Muslim families' preference for greater connectedness, more hierarchical family structure, adhering to traditional dress, and an implicit communication style can be a challenge for their teens adjusting to a North American urban lifestyle.

The closeness-caregiving dimension of boundaries is another aspect for nurses to consider. The relative sharing of territory can be assessed along aspects of contact time (time together), personal space (physical nearness, touching), emotional space (sharing of affects), information space (information known about each other), shared private conversations separate from others, and decision space (extent to which decisions are localized within various individuals or subsystems). The closeness-caregiving dimension of a boundary may be very significant for nurses to assess when dealing with older people with chronic illnesses and their adult children.

In our clinical supervision with nurses, we encourage them to consider how each family differentiates itself from other families in the neighborhood and in the city. The nurse considers whether there is a parental subsystem, a marital subsystem, a sibling subsystem, and so forth. Are the boundaries clear, rigid, or diffuse? Does the boundary style facilitate or constrain the family? If there are multiple stepfamilies, which boundary predominates?

Questions to Ask the Family. The nurse can infer the boundaries, for example, by asking a husband if there is anyone with whom he can talk when he feels stressed by his upcoming retirement. The nurse can ask the wife the same question. To whom would you go if you felt happy? If you felt sad? Would there be anyone in your family opposed to your talking with that person? Who would be most in favor of your talking with that person? What impact might it have on your mom's ability to deal with your dad's illness if she had more support from your grandparents?

External Structure

External structure includes two subcategories:

1. Extended family
2. Larger systems

Extended Family

The subcategory of extended family includes the family of origin and the family of procreation as well as the present generation and stepfamily members. Multiple loyalty ties to extended family members can be invisible but may be very influential forces in the family structure. Special relationships and support can exist at great geographical distances. Also, conflictual and painful relationships can seem fresh and close at hand despite the extended family living far away or not in frequent contact. How each member sees himself or herself as a separate individual yet part of the "family ego mass" (Bowen, 1978) is a critical structural area for assessment.

Levac, Wright, and Leahey (2002) recommend assessment of the quantity and type of contact with extended family to provide information about the quality and quantity of support. For example, Weingarten (2000) recounts the benefits of website interaction experienced by the extended family of a young man paralyzed following a sports injury. The young person stated, "The website has had amazing effects on me. It was a great way for me and my family to communicate...The website helped people understand what happened to me, people I don't talk with daily, without it becoming complicated for me...It's linked people from all areas of my life not just to me but to each other" (p. 159). Weingarten (2000) offers the idea that such connective interaction "does hope," a notion we support and find healing.

In our clinical work we consider whether there are many references to the extended family. How significant is the extended family to the functioning of this particular family? Are they available for support in times of need? If so, how? By mobile or land phones, e-mail, webcam, Skype, ichat, and internet chat groups? Are they in close physical proximity?

Questions to Ask the Family. Where do your parents live, Shafiq? How often do you have contact with them? What about your brothers, sisters, step-relatives? Which family members do you never see? Which of your relatives are you closest to? Who phones who? With what frequency? Who do you ask for help when problems arise in your family, Zabin? What kind of help do you ask for? Would your family in Ireland be available if you needed their help? Would you feel more comfortable contacting them by e-mail or in a chat room?

Larger Systems

The subcategory larger systems refers to the larger social agencies and personnel with whom the family has meaningful contact. Larger systems generally include work systems, and for some families, they include public welfare, child welfare, foster care, courts, and outpatient clinics. There are also larger systems designed for special populations, such as agencies mandated to provide services to the mentally or physically handicapped or the frail elderly. For many families, engagement with such larger systems is not problematic and can be life-affirming. We believe that larger professional systems can be an appreciative audience that supports families' narratives of hope and preferred new lives. We encourage nurses to watch their language in discussing clients with larger system helpers so as to support family stories of courage, growth, and persistence instead of perpetuating stories of hopelessness and problems. Having family group conferences such as those begun as a legal process in New Zealand can be another way of fostering a participatory model of decision making with families in child protection (Connolly, 2006). Such a practice strengthens families. We are particularly drawn to the work of Fraenkel (2006), who engages families as experts and creates community-based programs for families using a collaborative family program development model. He advocates that professionals adopt the stance of being respectful learners and forming collaborative professional relationships with families.

Some families and larger systems, however, may develop difficult relationships that exert a toll on normative development for family members. Some health-care professionals in larger systems contribute to families being labeled "multiproblem," "resistant," "noncompliant," or "uncooperative." These health-care professionals limit their perspective using these labels. In their study evaluating the quality of care coordination provided for children with developmental disabilites, Nolan, Orlando, and Liptak (2007) found that 50% of the 83 families said that medical personnel never or rarely communicated with schools and 27% never or rarely involved families in decision-making. Communication about care across systems was key to satisfaction with service.

Another larger system relationship that nurses should consider is the computer network. Electronic bulletin boards, chat rooms, text messaging, and discussion groups abound. The subject of internet infidelity and cybersex as a prelude to affairs and often sexual addiction, is a hot topic of conversation for many couples and nurses. We believe that infidelity consists of taking energy of any sort (thoughts, feelings, and behavior) outside of the committed relationship in such a way that it damages the relationship. Internet romance may begin outside any real-life context, but it quickly can escalate to a context all its own.

The internet can offer families valuable assistance in terms of information, validation, empathy, advice, and encouragement. Some have used e-mail to augment, extend, deepen, inform, enrich, and prepare for in-person psychotherapy. We have found, however, that online dialogues can sometimes be more sustaining than transformative—in other words, these dialogues tend to support the status quo rather than stimulate change.

Vigorous attention should be given to ways that professional expertise and electronic connectivity can be combined. Telenursing is one such example. Questions for consideration in providing family-centered Telehealth care include how do health professionals ensure that the voices of *all* family members are part of the discussion between the nurse and the family? Using videoconferencing to gather all the larger system helpers in one space with the family to discuss, plan, and evaluate care can be a solution.

In our clinical supervision with nurses, we encourage them to discover whether the *meaningful system* is the family alone or the family *and* its larger system helpers. Nurses can ask themselves questions such as: Who are the health-care professionals involved? What is the relationship between the family and the larger system? How regularly do they interact? Is their relationship symmetrical or complementary? Are the larger systems overconcerned? Overinvolved? Underconcerned? Underinvolved? Does the larger system blame the family for its problems? What do the helpers desire for the family? Is the nurse being asked to take responsibility for another system's task? How do the family and helpers define the problem? One young woman suffering from metastases from breast cancer, when asked, "Who do you think of like family?" answered, "I have three families: my own family, my church family, and my 'family' at the cancer center."

Questions to Ask the Family. What agency professionals are involved with your family, Mr. Rajwani? How many agencies regularly interact with you? Has your family moved from one health-care system to another? Who most thinks that your family needs to be involved with these systems? Who most thinks the opposite? Would there be agreement between your definition of the problem and the system's definition of the problem? How about between the definitions of the solution? What has been the best or worst advice you have been given by professionals for this issue, Atul? How is our working relationship going so far, Laura? If it were not going well, would you tell me?

Context

Context is explained as the whole situation or background relevant to some event or personality. Each family system is itself nested within broader systems, such as neighborhood, class, region, and country, and is influenced by these systems. The connectivity experienced by persons using the internet is another context to be considered. Because the context permeates and circumscribes both the individual and the family, its consequences are pervasive. Context includes but is not limited to these five subcategories:

1. Ethnicity
2. Race

3. Social class

4. Spirituality and/or religion

5. Environment

Ethnicity

Ethnicity refers to the concept of a family's "peoplehood" and is derived from a combination of its history, race, social class, and religion. It describes a commonality of overt and subtle processes transmitted by the family over generations and usually reinforced by the surrounding community. Ethnicity is an important factor that influences family interaction. We believe that nurses must be aware of the great variety within as well as between ethnic groups. Some people are second-, third-, or fourth-generation immigrants, with ancestors who were born in a foreign country. Others may be from "recently arrived" immigrant families, either legally arrived or undocumented, of whom some are refugees. Another category is "immigrant-American" families, in which the parents were born in a foreign country but their children were born in the United States.

According to the 2000 census, the foreign-born population of the United States numbered 31.1 million, representing a 57 percent increase over 1990 and the continuation of an upward trend that began in the 1970s (United States Census Bureau, 2002). Approximately one fifth of children in the United States are growing up in immigrant homes, and many have been separated from one or both parents for extended periods. Suarez-Orozco, Todorova, and Louie (2002) report that results from their study of 385 early adolescents originating from China, Central America, the Dominican Republic, Haiti, and Mexico indicate that "children who were separated from their parents were more likely to report depressive symptoms than children who had not been separated" (p. 625). The immigration experience is central, not incidental, to health care.

For some immigrant families, the impact of cultural adjustment can be seen as a transitional difficulty, with issues such as economic survival, racism, and changes in extended family and support systems needing to be addressed. Specific life experiences, such as a trade school or college education, financial success in business, or family intermarriage, can encourage assimilation into a dominant culture, whereas isolation in a rural area or an urban ghetto tends to foster continuity of ethnic patterns. It is important, though, to recognize that these views of assimilation and isolation are from our "observer perspective." What matters is the family's cultural narrative, how it is deconstructed and co-constructed.

Ethnic differences in family structure and their implications for intervention have often been highlighted in a stereotypical manner. For example, Italians in North America usually have strong extended family connections and loyalties. African-American families tend to have flexible family boundaries, and some may include the grandmother in child rearing. Members of some Latin American cultures encourage emotionality between relatives and between generations, whereas the Irish in North America tend to have more strictly defined boundaries between generations.

Some researchers have tried to move beyond stereotypes. For example, Lonczak et al (2007) conducted a preliminary study examining relationships between both family structure and living with extended family and substance use among 97 American Indian/Alaskan Native (AI/AN) adolescents. Although their work is preliminary, they suggest that living in an original two-parent home may be an important protective mechanism among this group of AI/AN youth. They found a positive association between cohabiting extended family and youth tobacco initiation.

In our clinical work, we have found it essential to recognize the infinite variety and lack of stereotypes among families from various ethnic groups. This is particularly important as internet dating sites are introducing more diverse singles than ever before. Cultural diversity is a matter of balance between validating the differences among us and appreciating the forces of our common humanity. We believe our own cultural narratives help us to organize our thinking and anchor our lives, but they can also blind us to the unfamiliar and unrecognizable and can foster injustice. For example, the importance of listening to history and context in caring for refugee immigrant women cannot be overestimated.

Nurses should sensitize themselves to differences in family beliefs and values and be willing to alter their "ethnic filters." We believe it is important for nurses to recognize their own ethnic blind spots and adjust their interventions accordingly. We are never "expert," "right," or in full possession of the "truth" about a family's ethnicity. Also, if we engage a translator to assist us with family work, we should not assume that the translator is an "expert" on this particular family's ethnicity. Rather, both we and the translator should strive to be informed and curious about ourselves and others' diversity as we collaborate in health care. The importance of participatory models of knowledge transfer and exchange cannot be underestimated whether in working with Aboriginal communities or with other ethnic groups. For example, the findings from the study by Hiott et al (2006) of gender differences in anxiety and depression among immigrant Latinos suggest that clinicians should ask questions about social isolation and separation from family. Answers to such questions may provide insights into stress and its contribution to significant anxiety and depression; these should also be considered when devising a treatment plan.

Some questions that we have found useful to ask ourselves include: What is the family's ethnicity? Have the children and parents had periods of separation in their immigration experience? If so, with what impact? Is their social network from the same ethnic group? Do they find that helpful or not? If the available economic, educational, health, legal, and recreational services were similar to the family's ethnic values, how would our conversation be different? Are the assessment and testing instruments we use in our clinic relevant for this ethnic group? Do they match the values and beliefs of this particular family?

Questions to Ask the Family. Could you tell me about your Japanese cultural practices or traditions regarding illness? How does being an immigrant from Afghanistan influence your beliefs about when to consult with health professionals? What does health mean to you? How would you know that you are healthy? How would I know that you are healthy? As a second-generation Chilean family, how are your health-care practices similar to or different from those of your grandparents? Which practices seem most useful to you at this point in your family's life?

Race

The subcategory of race is a basic construct and not an intermediate variable. Race influences core individual and group identification. For example, in a study conducted by Hill and Thomas (2002), female participants in black–white heterosexual partner relationships described both constraining and empowering identities. Contributors to an empowering identity included the participants having multiple reference group orientations, being strong, and refusing to take sides with blacks or whites. Race intersects with mediating variables such as class, religion, and ethnicity. Racial attitudes, stereotyping, and discrimination are powerful influences on family interaction and, if left unaddressed, can be negative constraints on the relationship between the family and the nurse. The "myth of sameness" (Hardy, 1990) has been challenged and the uniqueness of various family forms emphasized more so in the last decade, especially with increased use of the internet.

Family clinicians appreciate that the variations in family structure and development of African-Americans, Asians, Hispanics, whites, and others are potential strengths in helping these families to function under various economic and social conditions. There is a dearth of literature on potential relationship strengths in intercultural and interracial relationships. We encourage nurses to elicit strengths rather than challenges in working with these couples.

The rapid change in racial patterns in the U.S. is important to note. About one of every two people added to the nation's population between July 1, 2005, and July 1, 2006 was Hispanic (United States Census Bureau, 2007b). People of Hispanic origin are the nation's largest ethnic or race minority and constitute 15% of the nation's total population. Within Hispanic-American households, 64% of families are Mexican, 9% Puerto Rican, 3.5% Cuban, 3% Salvadoran, and 2.7% Dominican (United States Census Bureau, 2007b). The percentage of black residents in the United States is estimated at 13.4% as of July 1, 2005; this includes those of more than one race (United States Census Bureau, 2007a).

Racial differences, whether intracultural or intercultural, are not problems per se. Rather, prejudice, discrimination, and other types of intercultural aggression based on these differences are problems. With the number of interracial families continuing to rise in the United States, we believe race will become less divisive than it was. Penn (2007) reports that "in 2002, 20 percent of 18-19 year olds said they were dating someone of a different race, up from under 10 percent just a decade before. Of members of Match.com, 70 percent say they are willing to date someone of a different race" (p. 63). Interrracial families are quietly eroding many assumptions that have guided America's politics, customs, and habits for many decades.

For some persons whether of the majority or minority race, the word "race" is very distasteful as we are all members of the human race. They feel that the word itself implies harsh borders between groups of people in the human race and is therefore not very constructive in binding us together.

It is important for nurses to understand family health beliefs and behaviors influenced by racial identity, privilege, or oppression. In our clinical work with families, we have found it very useful to critically reflect on our own ideas about our race, marginalization, invisible and visible minorities, and "the myth of sameness" and to vigorously pursue the differences between and within various racial groups. For example, we ask ourselves how a Jamaican-American family might differ from an African-American family in their beliefs about hospitalization or how a Vietnamese couple might differ from a Japanese couple in their beliefs about whether to institutionalize an aging grandmother.

We believe health professionals should be racially and culturally competent. For example, non–African-Americans working with African-American families should not assume familiarity but should address issues of racism, intervene multisystemically, use a problem-solving focus, involve religious leaders as indicated, incorporate fathers, and acknowledge strengths. Many of these guidelines apply equally well for all races working with each other.

Questions to Ask the Family. What differences do you notice between, for example, your Hong Kong relatives' child-rearing practices and your own? If you and I were the same race, would our conversation be different? How? Would our different type of conversation be more or less likely to assist you in regaining your health? Could you help me to understand what I need to know to be most helpful to you?

Social Class

Social class shapes educational attainment, income, and occupation. Each class, whether upper-upper, lower-upper, upper-middle, lower-middle, upper-lower, or lower-lower, has its own clustering of values, lifestyles, and behavior that influences family interaction and health-care practices. Social class affects how family members define themselves and are defined; what they cherish; how they organize their day-to-day living; and how they meet challenges, struggles, and crises. For example, middle-class seniors are likely to help their adult children, whereas working-class older adults are more likely to receive help.

Social class has been referred to as one of the prime molders of the family value and belief system. Much of the sociological and psychological research has been confounded by social class differences among ethnic groups. We believe that, in a racist and classist society, class and race are not inseparable. Because poverty is disproportionately concentrated among racial minorities, many professionals have considered the African-American statistical subgroup to represent the lower-income class and the white statistical subgroup to represent the middle- or upper-income class group. Furthermore, although Hispanics, including Mexicans, Puerto Ricans, Cubans, and people from South and Central America, have increased substantially in number to become a sizable group within the United States, until recently data about marriage and family have excluded them. Such data have generally been limited to blacks (African-Americans) and whites, without taking into account Hispanics or Asians. Much of the literature confounds the effects of race and class, not to mention the "myth of sameness" about families within each race or class.

Just as nursing has often been presented as intercultural, it has also been presented as interclass and nonpolitical. We believe that many nurses have pursued sickness in families to the exclusion of obtaining the *meaning* people give to events; their day-to-day living standards; and their access to employment, income, and housing. Social class issues have often been considered to be of little consequence to the "serious talk" about illness. This viewpoint has enabled nurses to sidestep many class issues associated with inequality and injustice. However, treatment must take into account the cultural, social, and economic context of the people seeking help. From factory workers to farmers to business executives, families are trying to cope with higher health-care costs and threats of losing insurance coverage. They continually make decisions based on which health care they can afford. With higher prescription drug costs and a growth in the aging population, many families are anxious about their long-term care and ability to provide for their loved ones. Economic uncertainty, the war, fears of terrorism and the aftereffects of the September 11 attacks have created increased difficulties for the working poor.

The findings from the study conducted by Tubbs, Roy, and Burton (2005) shed some light on how low-income families construct family time. Four categories of activities provided the context for parent–child interaction: talk time, mealtime, playtime, and sharing treats (e.g., candies, cookies). Family time was embedded in other activities and not in leisure activities or time "off the clock" from mundane daily caretaking of children.

Assessment of social class helps the nurse understand in a new way the family's stressors and resources. Generally speaking, women move down in social class following a divorce, whereas men do not. Recognizing differences in social class beliefs between themselves and families may encourage nurses to utilize new health promotion and intervention strategies. It is important for health-care delivery that nurses be aware of such influences as the "glass ceiling" and part-time temporary work versus full-time permanent work with benefits. The upward mobility risks of harassment faced by women entering some male-dominated work environments, such as the military, should also be known to health-care professionals.

In our clinical work we have often asked ourselves how a family's social class might influence their health-care beliefs, values, utilization of services, and interaction with us. Serious illness can intensify financial problems, diminish the capacity to deal with them, and call for solutions at odds with conventional financial wisdom. We have wondered about the intrafamilial differences with respect to class and how these might help or hinder a family coping with, for example, chronic illness.

Questions to Ask the Family. How many times have you moved within the past 5 years? Have these moves had a positive or negative influence on your ability to deal with your son's acquired immunodeficiency syndrome (AIDS)? How many schools has your daughter, Frishta, attended? How does your money situation influence your use of health-care resources? What impact does Nuar's shift work have on your family's stress level?

Spirituality and/or Religion

Family members' spiritual and religious beliefs, rituals, and practices can have a positive or negative influence on their ability to cope with or manage an illness or health concern. Therefore, nurses must explore this previously neglected area. Emotions such as fear, guilt, anger, peace, and hope can be nurtured or tempered by one's spiritual or religious beliefs. Wright (2005) encourages distinguishing between spirituality and religion for the purposes of assessment and believes that doing so has the potential to invite more openness by family members regarding this potentially sensitive domain of inquiry. *Spirituality* is defined as whatever or whoever gives ultimate meaning and purpose in one's life and invites particular ways of being in the world toward others, oneself, and the universe (Wright, 2005). Religion is defined as an affiliation or a membership in a particular faith community that shares a set of beliefs, rituals, morals, and sometimes a health code centered on a defined higher or transcendent power most frequently referred to as God (Wright, 2005).

Levac, Wright, and Leahey (2002) recommend that assessment of the influence of religion is most critical at the time of diagnosis of a chronic or life-threatening illness. Assessment is especially important and relevant when crises have occurred that may cause extreme suffering, such as a traumatic death caused by a motor vehicle accident; sudden death due to illness, violence, or abuse; or a life-threatening diagnosis. In these situations, it is critical that the nurse ascertain what meaning the family gives to their suffering due to these tragic events and ultimately how family members make sense of their suffering (Wright, 2005). We think that beliefs, spirituality, and transcendence are keys to family resilience.

Spirituality and religion also influence family values, size, health care, and socialization practices. For example, individualism is intricately related to the Protestant work ethic. Community and family support, on the other hand, is evident in the Mormon and Jewish religions, which foster intergenerational and intragenerational support. Folk-healing traditions that combine health and religious practices are quite common in some ethnic groups. In some spiritualistic practices, a medium, or counselor, helps to exorcise the spirits causing illness. For example, *espiritistas*, or healers, can be found in many Cuban and other Latino communities. Such healers, religious leaders, shamans, and clergy can be invaluable resources for families dealing with crises and with long-term needs such as caregiver support.

Spirituality and religion are hidden and commonly underused resources in family work. They involve "streams of experience that flow through all aspects of our lives, from family heritage to personal belief systems, rituals and practices, and congregational affiliations" (Walsh, 1999, p. 3). The striking success of Alcoholics Anonymous is one example of the power of a program that incorporates spirituality.

We encourage nurses visiting families' homes to note the presence of signs of religious influence in the home—for example, statues, candles, flags, and religious texts, such as the Bible, Torah, or Koran. We have been curious about dietary restrictions and habits as well as traditional or alternative health practices influenced by religious beliefs. We have been cautious, however, not to assume that strong spiritual or religious beliefs enhance marital happiness or interaction, although they may diminish the possibility of divorce.

Our clinical work with families has taught us that the experience of suffering frequently becomes transposed to one of spirituality as family members try to find meaning in their suffering (Wright, 2005). If nurses are to be helpful, they must acknowledge that suffering, and in many cases the senselessness of it, is ultimately a spiritual issue. Therefore, in our clinical work we have asked ourselves about the influence of religion and spirituality on the family's health-care practices. For a more in-depth discussion of clinical ideas and examples addressing the connection between spirituality and suffering, as well as how to assess and intervene, we encourage readers to peruse the 2005 text *Spirituality, Suffering, and Illness: Ideas for Healing* by Lorraine M. Wright.

Questions to Ask the Family. What meaning does spirituality or religion have for you in your everyday life? Are you involved with a mosque, temple, or synagogue? Would talking with anyone in your church help you cope with Pierre's illness? Are your spiritual beliefs a source of support for you in coping with your illness? A source of stress for you? For other family members? Who among your family members would most encourage your use of spiritual beliefs to cope with Perminder's cancer? What are your sources of hope? Have you found that prayer or other religious practices help you cope with your son Surinder's schizophrenia? If so, may I ask what you pray for? Have your prayers been answered? What does your religion say about gender roles? Ethnicity? Sexual orientation? How have these beliefs affected you, Davinderpal?

Environment

The subcategory environment encompasses aspects of the larger community, the neighborhood, and the home. Environmental factors such as adequacy of space and privacy and accessibility of schools, day care, recreation, and public transportation influence family functioning. These are especially relevant for older adults, who are more likely to remain in a poor environment even if it has become dangerous to live there. Epstein (2003) raises a disturbing issue about the environment: "In America's rundown urban neighborhoods, the diseases associated with old age are afflicting the young. Could it be that simply living there is enough to make you sick?" Some of these neighborhoods have the highest mortality rates in the country owing to the prevalence of chronic diseases rather than gunshot wounds or drugs. Epstein comments that "the grinding everyday stress of living in poverty in America is 'weathering,' a condition not unlike the effect of exposure to wind and rain on houses" (p. 76). We have adjusted our perceptions of homelessness and come to grips with the idea that families with children are the fastest-growing homeless group. Homelessness is neither an urban nor a regional problem but rather one that is pervasive in North America.

In our clinical work with families, we have asked ourselves and the nurses with whom we work to consider whether the home is adequate for the number of people living there. Does our perception differ from the family's? What health and other basic services are available within the home? Within the neighborhood? How accessible in terms of distance, convenience, and so forth are transportation and recreation services? How safe is the area? By asking in an open-ended way what other contextual forces may influence the family, it is possible to obtain a much broader range of responses. These can vary from "belief in politics" to "shopping at the mall" to "music" to CNN.

Questions to Ask the Family. What community services does your family use? Are there community services you would like to learn about but do not know how to contact? On a scale of 1 to 10, with 10 being most comfortable, how comfortable are you in your neighborhood? What would make you more comfortable so that you can continue to function independently at home?

Structural Assessment Tools

The genogram and the ecomap are two tools that are particularly helpful in outlining a family's internal and external structures. Each is simple to use and requires only a piece of paper and a pen. The genograph designed by Duhamel and Campagna (2000) can also be used to draw the genogram. Alternatively, some computer programs have genograms as a feature.

The *genogram* is a diagram of the family constellation. The *ecomap*, on the other hand, is a diagram of the family's contact with others outside the immediate family. It pictures the important connections between the family and the world. We are aware of the arbitrariness of the distinction for some cultural groups between a genogram and an ecomap. For example, the standard genogram may be inadequate for African-Americans because of its underlying assumption that family is strictly a biological entity. We encourage nurses to develop a fit between these tools to depict specific family compositions.

These tools have been developed as family assessment, planning, and intervention devices. They can be used to reframe behaviors, relationships, and time connections within families, as well as to detoxify and normalize families' perceptions of themselves. By pointing to the future as well as to the past and the present, genograms facilitate alternative interpretations of family experience. They can help both the nurse and the family see the larger picture and view problems in both a historical and current context. Genograms can also be used to foster the training of culturally competent clinicians and for nurses to increase their self-awareness. Rempel, Neufeld, and Kushner (2007) advocate the interactive use of genograms and ecomaps as a data-generation method based on their experience in a study of male caregivers' experiences of supportive and nonsupportive interactions. They found that these tools provided a rich contextual foundation that enhanced the researchers' understanding of family experiences.

We agree with McGoldrick, Gerson, and Petry (2008) that although much can be said about expanding genograms to include issues from larger social contexts (the sexual, cultural, religious, or spiritual genogram), realistically such mapping is extremely difficult to accomplish. Gendergrams have been developed to map gender relationships over the life cycle. At best, we can probably explore only a few dimensions at a time and we recommend that these dimensions be directly connected to the purpose of the family's encounter with the nurse. For example, a nurse meeting with a couple in a rehabilitation treatment center for sexual addiction might reasonably explore a family's sexual and addiction history on a genogram. This content area would likely not be appropriate for a nurse meeting with a family in an intensive care unit. McGoldrick, Gerson, and Petry (2008) have outlined important issues that are difficult to capture on genograms:

- Family members involved in family business
- Family members' relationships to the health-care system
- Cultural genogram issues
- Family secrets
- Particular family-relationship nuances including power, patterns of avoidance, etc.
- Patterns of friendship

- Relationships with work colleagues
- Spiritual genograms
- Community genograms
- Tracking medical and psychological stressors

Genograms don't typically show the emotional connections among family members, present or past. The complex relationships of those who have warmed our hearts, mentored and nurtured us, aggravated us, or caused us severe trauma are not generally depicted. This is both a limitation of genograms and an asset; genograms tend to be a quick snapshot of the present.

With the help of computers, we can make three-dimensional maps that enable us to track complex genogram patterns. Our caution for practicing nurses is to use the genogram as a clinically relevant tool, not as a map or data-collection sheet. Computerized genograms enable us to explore specific family patterns, resiliencies, and symptom constellations. Gathering, mapping, and tracking family history is much easier using a computer database. We urge nurses to ask themselves: What is the purpose of collecting vast amounts of information about this family's history, and how will this information be helpful for the purpose of my work with this family? Using computers and genogram information will provide rich data for family research, but it is unknown how useful this will be for immediate family care. Of course, by using computer genogram software there will be many more possibilities for depicting family issues at different moments in family history. Clinicians and family members will have the opportunity to choose what aspects of a genogram they want to display for a particular purpose and at the same time create a database of a family's whole history.

Genogram

Genograms convey a great deal of information in the form of a visual gestalt. When one considers the number of words it would take to portray the facts thus represented, it becomes clear how simple and useful these tools are. Genograms, when placed on patients' charts, act as constant visual reminders for nurses to "think family." As an engagement tool, it is helpful to use during the first meeting with the family. It provides rich data about relationships over time and may also include small amounts of data about health, occupation, religion, ethnicity, and migrations. The genogram can be used to elicit information helpful to both the family and the nurse about development and other areas of family functioning. It is a tool that enables clinicians to develop hypotheses for additional evaluation in a family assessment.

The skeleton of the genogram tends to follow conventional genetic and genealogic charts. It is a family tree depicting the internal family structure. It is usual practice to include at least three generations. Family members are placed on horizontal rows that signify generational lines. For example, a marriage or common-law relationship is denoted by a horizontal line. Children are denoted by vertical lines. Children are rank-ordered from left to right beginning with the eldest child. Each individual is represented. A blank genogram is shown in Figure 3-2.

Some authors differ slightly in the symbols they use to denote the details of the genogram. The symbols in Figure 3-3, however, are generally agreed on. With increased use of computer genograms, symbols and color coding will become standardized.

The person's name and age should be noted inside the square or circle. Outside the symbol, significant data gathered from the family (e.g., travels a lot, depressed, overinvolved in work) should be noted. If a family member has died, the year of his or her death is indicated above the square or circle. When the symbol for miscarriage is used, the sex of the child should be identified if it is known. A small square is used to denote a sperm donor (McGoldrick, Gerson, & Petry, 2008). It is helpful to draw a circle around the different households. We find that when children have lived in several contexts (e.g., immediate biological family, foster family, grandparents, adoptive family), separate genograms can help to show the child's multiple families over time.

An example of a nuclear and extended family genogram is given in Figure 3-4 for the Lamensa family. Raffaele, age 47, has been married to Silvana, age 35, since 1995. They lived common-law for 2 years prior to their marriage. They have two children: Gemma, age 14, who is in grade 8, and Antonio, age 7, who is repeating grade 1. Raffaele is employed as a machinist, and Silvana refers to him as "alcoholic." Silvana is a homemaker and states that she has been "depressed" for several years. Both of

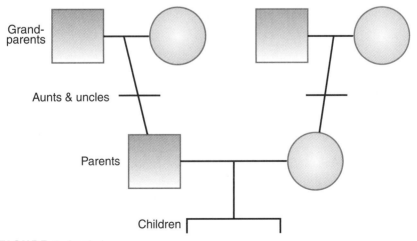

FIGURE 3-2: Blank genogram.

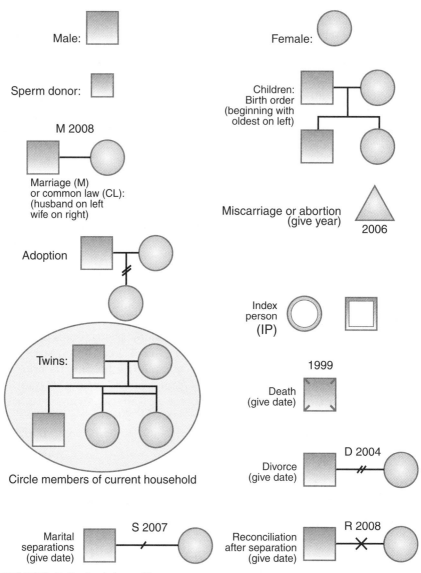

FIGURE 3-3: Symbols used in genograms.

Raffaele's parents are deceased. His father died in 2005, and his mother died in 2003 of a stroke. Raffaele's older brother also has a drinking problem. Young Antonio was named for his grandfather. Silvana's mother, Nunziata, age 54, has arthritis, which has been getting progressively worse since her husband died in 2002. Silvana has two older sisters and a brother.

Figure 3-5 illustrates a lesbian couple with a child born to one of them, Loree (age 30), and adopted by the other, Sarah (age 28). Loree and Sarah have lived as a couple since 2006 and have been married since 2008. Loree's

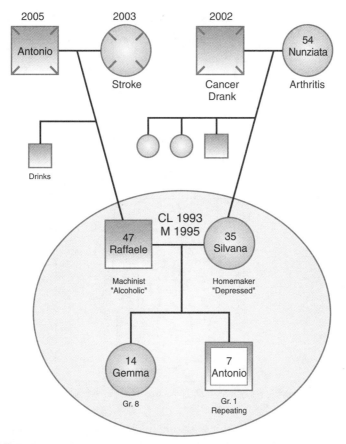

FIGURE 3-4: Sample genogram: The Lamensa family.

biological son, Griffin (age 8), was conceived by artificial insemination. The unknown sperm donor is depicted as a small square. Loree's mother, Adrienne, a Jamaican retired nurse (age 65), divorced Loree's father in 1981, remarried in 1982, had another daughter Mitzi by her second husband and became a widow when he died in 1988. Mitzi is considering transgender surgery. Sarah's parents are separated, and her father is living common-law with Dan, his business partner. Sarah has no siblings. Loree has a younger brother, Spencer (age 28), and her half-sister, Mitzi (age 25).

How to Use a Genogram
At the beginning of the interview, the nurse engages the family by informing them that they will be having a conversation so that the nurse can gain an overview of who is in the family and their situation. The nurse can then use the structure of the genogram to discern the family's internal and external structures as well as context. Thus, the nurse gains an understanding of the family's composition and boundaries.

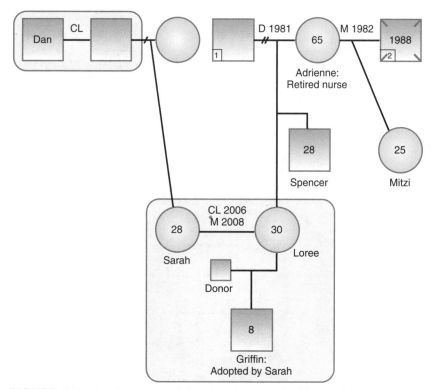

FIGURE 3-5: Sample genogram: Artifical insemination and lesbian couple.

Initially, the nurse starts out with a blank sheet of paper and draws a line or circle for the first person in the family to whom a question is directed. Following is a sample interview with the Manuyag family.

> **Nurse:** Elena, you said you were 23, and Matias, how old are you?
>
> **Matias:** Thirty-four.
>
> **Nurse:** How long have you been married?
>
> **Matias:** This time or the first time?
>
> **Nurse:** This time. And then the first time.
>
> **Matias:** Just 2 years for Elena and me.
>
> **Nurse:** And the first time?
>
> **Matias:** Ten years for the first one.
>
> **Nurse:** And Elena, have you been married before?
>
> **Elena:** (*Laughs nervously*) I'm only 23.
>
> **Nurse:** Sure, it's just that many people have lived together in common-law marriages or married when they were very young.

Elena: No. I lived with my parents till I met Matias.

Nurse: Do either of you have children from prior relationships? (*Turns to both Matias and Elena*)

Matias: Yes, I have two sons.

Elena: No.

Nurse: In addition to Teresita here (*Looks at infant on couch*), do the two of you have any other children?

Elena: Yes, there's Manandro.

Matias: Old stinko, you mean.

Nurse: Old stinko?

Matias: He isn't toilet trained yet.

Nurse: Oh, I see. And he's how old?

Elena: He's almost 3. I've been trying to train him since I knew I was pregnant with Teresita but he just doesn't seem to want to be trained.

Nurse: (*Nods*) Mm.

Matias: Yeah, old stinko!

Nurse: And Teresita is how many weeks now?

Elena: She'll be 21 days tomorrow (*Smiles at infant*).

Nurse: Does anyone else live with you?

Matias: No. Her parents live next door.

The nurse now has a rudimentary genogram of the Manuyag family (Fig. 3-6) and has gathered information that may or may not be significant, depending on the way in which the family has responded to various events in the history of their family, such as:

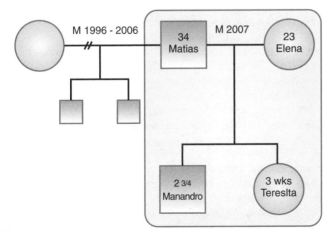

FIGURE 3-6: Genogram of the Manuyag family.

- Manandro was conceived before the marriage.
- Manandro is unaffectionately called "old stinko" by his father.
- Elena has been trying to toilet train Manandro since he was 24 months old.
- Elena lived with her family of origin before the marriage. They live next door.
- Matias has been married before and has two other sons.

After inquiring about the nuclear family, the nurse can continue to inquire about the extended family. It is generally not very important to go into great detail about these relatives, but clinical judgment should prevail. If, for example, the grandparents are involved in a child's colostomy care, then a three-generational genogram should be constructed. On the other hand, if a child has a sprained wrist, then a two-generational genogram is sufficient. After asking questions about the husband's parents and siblings, the nurse should then inquire about the wife's family of origin. It is important for the nurse to gain an overview of the family structure without getting sidetracked or inundated by a large volume of information. Box 3-1 contains helpful hints for constructing genograms.

Box 3-1 Helpful Hints for Constructing Genograms

- Determine priorities for genogram construction based on the family situation.
- A three-generational genogram may be useful when the child's health problem (physical or emotional) is influenced by or affects the third generation.
- A brief two-generational genogram is generally most useful initially, especially for a family that has preventive health-care needs (immunizations) or minor health concerns (sports injury). The nurse can always expand to the third generation if needed.
- Invite as many family members to the initial meeting or visit as possible to obtain each family member's view and to observe family interaction.
- Engage the family in an exercise to complete the genogram.
- Use the genogram to "break the ice," provide structure, and introduce purposeful conversation.
- Ask family members how an absent significant family member might answer a question.
- Avoid discussion that is hurtful or blameful, especially of absent family members.
- Take an interest in each family member, and be sensitive to developmental differences.
- Tailor questions to children's developmental stages so that they become active contributors.
- Notice children's nonverbal and verbal comments.
- If some members are shy or seem uninterested in participating directly (such as adolescents), ask other family members about them.
- Begin by asking "easy" questions of individuals followed by exploration of subsystems.

| **Box 3-1** | Helpful Hints for Constructing Genograms—*Cont'd* |

• Ask concrete, easy-to-answer questions of individuals (especially children) about ages, occupations, interests, health status, school grades, and teachers to increase their comfort levels.
• Move the discussion about individuals to subsystems to elicit family relational data. Inquire about parent–child or sibling relationships, depending on parenting concerns.
• With stepfamilies, ask questions about contact with the noncustodial parent, custody, the children's satisfaction with visits, and stepfamily relationships.
• Observe family interactions.
• During genogram construction, note the content (what is said) and the process (how it is said).
• Move from discussion about present family situation to questions about the extended family if it seems relevant (for example, "Are Ruhi's parents able to help with the baby's tracheostomy care? What about babysitting?")
• When discussing generations, the nurse may find it useful to ask about psychosocial family health history (for example, "Is there a history of alcohol abuse [or violence, learning problems, or mental illness] in your family?") Questions should be tailored to the family's particular area of concern rather than generic exploration.

Levac, A.M., Wright, L.M., & Leahey, M. (2002). Children and families: Models for assessment and intervention. In J. Fox (Ed.), *Primary healthcare of infants, children and adolescents* (p. 14). St. Louis: Mosby. Copyright 2002. Adapted with permission.

The same question format used for nuclear families is used for stepfamilies, with one exception. It is generally easier to ask one spouse about his or her previous relationships before going on to ask the other spouse the same questions. This idea holds true especially in working with complex family situations involving multiple parenting figures and siblings. Again, it is unnecessary to gather specific information on all extended family members. It is useful to draw a circle around the current family members to distinguish among the various households. Usually it is easiest to indicate the year of a divorce rather than the number of years ago that it happened.

Figure 3-7 illustrates a sample genogram of a stepfamily. In this stepfamily, Michael (age 35), has been living in a common-law marriage since 2007 with Melanie (age 33), who is a part-time waitress. Also in the household are Melanie's two children by her first marriage, Kathy (age 11) and Jacob (age 9), who has ADHD and is in a special class in grade 3. Michael married his first wife, Laura, in 1997. They were divorced in 2001. Michael and Laura had one son, who is now age 8. Michael is an only child. His father committed suicide in 2004. His mother is still alive. Melanie is the youngest of three daughters, and both of her parents are living. Melanie married David in 1997, separated in 2004, and divorced in 2007. David, age 36, is a mechanic who is presently living in a common-law marriage with Camille and her three sons. Camille and her first husband, Rob, divorced in 2000, reconciled in 2002, and then divorced in 2003.

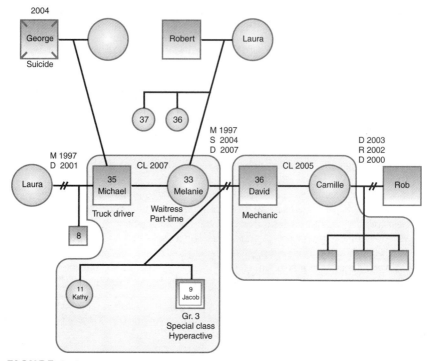

FIGURE 3-7: Sample genogram of a stepfamily.

There are no specific guidelines for drawing genograms illustrating complex stepfamily situations. Generally, however, what works best is for the nurse to start by gathering information about the immediate household. After this, the nurse draws each family's constellation. Whenever possible, it is best to show children from different marriages in their correct birth order, oldest on the left and youngest on the right. We agree with McGoldrick, Gerson, and Petry (2008) that the rule of thumb is, when feasible, that different marriages follow in chronological order from left to right. We have sometimes found it helpful to indicate the number of the relationship or marriage in the lower hand corner when there have been several relationships. See Figure 3-5, where Adrienne's husbands are indicated as #1 and #2. It can be useful to draw a circle around each separate household. If one member of a couple is involved in an affair, then their relationship is depicted with a dotted rather than a solid line. Additional pertinent information, such as children moving between two households, can be written to the side of the genogram. It is important for the nurse to remember that the purpose of drawing the genogram is to obtain a visual overview of the family. The genogram is not meant to be an exact chart for genetics.

Other problems arise when there are multiple marriages, intermarriages, and remarriages within the family. For example, when cousins or stepsiblings marry, the clinician should use separate pages to clarify intricacies. With complex family situations, the nurse needs to choose between clarity and level of detail. When computers are used to diagram genograms, complexity can be reduced by zooming in on relevant significant information. We advise nurses to let practicality and possibility be their guide.

Develop a genogram that is useful rather than one that is overly inclusive and too confusing. Sometimes the only feasible way for pediatric nurses to clarify where children were raised is to take chronological notes on each child and draw multiple genograms through time to show the various family constellations the child experienced. With software, specific genograms can be created for specific moments in a person's life. When discrepancies exist in information shared by various family members, we advise nurses to note this on the genogram but not to take on an investigative role. There can be multiple truths and rememberings of information.

Another perhaps more typical stepfamily genogram is depicted in Figure 3-8. In this genogram, the Faris family is composed of David (age 42), a software designer who has been living common-law since 2005 with Patti (age 40), a part-time retail associate. They have a daughter, Madison (age 1), who was recently diagnosed with juvenile diabetes. David's twin

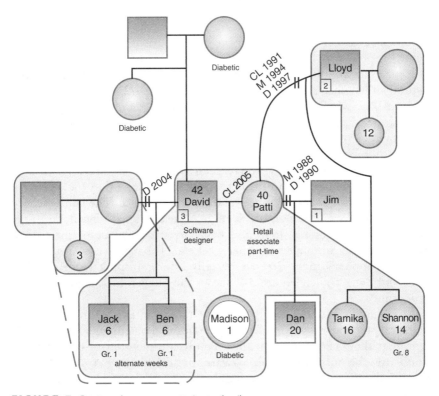

FIGURE 3-8: Sample genogram: Faris stepfamily.

sons, Jack and Ben (age 6), spend alternate weeks at their mom's townhouse and at their dad's apartment. David was divorced in 2004; his former wife has a daughter, age 3. Patti has a son, Dan (age 20), by her first husband, Jim, whom she divorced in 1990. Dan lives alone and works several part-time jobs in bars. Patti also has two other daughters: Tamika (age 16), who recently dropped out of school, and Shannon (age 14), who is in grade 8. They are from her second marriage, to Lloyd, which ended in divorce in 1997. The teenage girls live with their mom and visit Lloyd and his family for 2 weeks most summers. The current health concern is Madison's juvenile diabetes; the current household consists of David, Patti, the three girls, and on alternate weeks the twins. David's mom has diabetes, as does his older sister.

Another sample family situation is the Fitzgerald-Kucewicz family, in which a child lives with the grandmother and her husband. The identified patient, 8-year-old Sophia Kucewicz, lives with her grandmother, 45-year-old Patricia Fitzgerald; Vincent, Patricia's common-law partner of 10 years; and Sophia's 19-year-old aunt, Susan. Patricia was previously married to Steven Fitzgerald for 14 years. Patricia and Steven had three children: 19-year-old Susan, 23-year-old Douglas, and 25-year-old Joan, who is Sophia's mother. Joan became pregnant with Sophia when she was 16. Sophia's father, Michael Kucewicz, and her mother Joan had a brief relationship, through which she was conceived. Although Michael was aware of the pregnancy, he left the city shortly before Sophia was born, never meeting her. When Sophia was 2 years old, Joan had another child, Kayla, who subsequently went to live with her natural father when she was 4. When Sophia was 2 1/2, her mother moved in with Ben, whom Sophia came to know as her father. Joan and Ben had difficulty providing a stable environment for Sophia and Kayla and, from time to time, moved in with Patricia and Vincent. Patricia reports that both Joan and Ben used drugs and alcohol and were often unemployed. Ben was physically and verbally abusive to Joan and, after a particularly frightening episode between Joan and Ben that took place in the basement of Patricia's home, Joan called the police. The child welfare department became involved, leading Patricia and Vincent to take guardianship of Sophia. Joan and Ben moved to a place of their own, agreeing to take Sophia every other weekend. The health concern for this family is Sophia's nightmares, especially after returning from visits to Joan and Ben's trailer. Figure 3-9 shows the Fitzgerald-Kucewicz family genogram.

Most families are extremely receptive to and interested in collaborating with the nurse to complete a genogram. For some, it is the first time that they have ever seen their family life pictured in this manner. Therefore, the nurse needs to be aware that the family may have a reaction to significant events. One family, for example, may express some sensitive material in a very blasé fashion. If divorce is common in

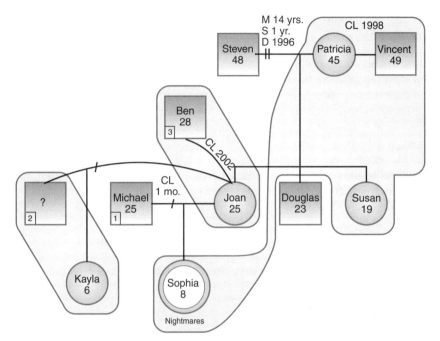

FIGURE 3-9: Genogram of the Fitzgerald-Kucewicz family.

their families of origin, they may not hesitate to discuss their several marriages and those of their siblings. On the other hand, a devout Catholic family may be exquisitely sensitive to seeing the nurse write the word "divorce."

Ecomap
As with the genogram, the primary value of the ecomap is in its visual impact. The purpose of the ecomap is to depict the family members' contact with larger systems. Hartman (1978) notes:

> The eco-map [*sic*] portrays an overview of the family in their situation; it pictures the important nurturant or conflict-laden connections between the family and the world. It demonstrates the flow of resources, or the lack of and deprivations. This mapping procedure highlights the nature of the interfaces and points to conflicts to be mediated, bridges to be built, and resources to be sought and mobilized. (p. 467).

Ecomaps shift the emphasis away from the historical genogram to the current functioning of the family and its environmental context. This focus on the present is an important message in our outcome-based health-care climate. The ecomap depicts reciprocal relationships between family members and broader community institutions such as schools, courts, health-care facilities, and so forth.

How to Use an Ecomap

As with the genogram, family members can actively participate in working on the ecomap during the assessment process.

The family genogram is placed in the center circle, labeled "Family or household." The outer circles represent significant people, agencies, or institutions in the family's context. The size of the circles is not important. Lines are drawn between the family and the outer circles to indicate the nature of the connections that exist. Straight lines indicate strong connections, dotted lines indicate tenuous connections, and slashed lines indicate stressful relations. The wider the line, the stronger the tie. Arrows can be drawn alongside the lines to indicate the flow of energy and resources. Additional circles may be drawn as necessary, depending on the number of significant contacts the family has.

An ecomap for the Lamensa family is illustrated in Figure 3-10. In this family, Raffaele, Silvana, Gemma, and Antonio are placed in the center

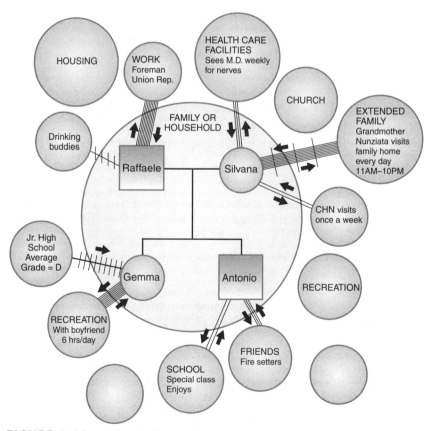

FIGURE 3-10: Lamensa family ecomap.

Box 3-2	Helpful Hints for Drawing Ecomaps

- Pose questions that explore the family's connections to other individuals or groups outside the family, such as:
  - What community agencies are you involved with now? Which are most and least helpful?
  - How would you describe your relationship with school staff?
  - How did you first become involved with Child Protective Services? What is the nature of your current relationship with them?

Levac, A.M., Wright, L.M., & Leahey, M. (2002). Children and families: Models for assessment and intervention. In J. Fox (Ed.), *Primary healthcare of infants, children and adolescents* (p. 14). St. Louis: Mosby. Copyright 2002. Adapted with permission.

circle. Raffaele has strong connections with his workplace, where he is foreman and a union representative. He has moderately strong bonds with his "drinking buddies." These relationships, however, are stressful for him. Silvana's connections are mainly with her mother and the health-care system. She sees her family physician every week "for nerves" and sees a community health nurse (CHN) once a week. Silvana's mother, Nunziata, visits Silvana every day from 11 AM to 10 PM. There is a strong connection between Silvana and her mother, but Silvana says she really "doesn't like Mom coming over so often." Antonio has a few friends, most of whom set fires. He is in a special class for his learning disability and enjoys both the teacher and the school. Gemma is in junior high school, where she maintains an average grade of D. She frequently does not attend school, and when she does attend, she participates little. She spends about 6 hours a day with her boyfriend.

When the CHN completed the ecomap with the Lamensa family, Mrs. Lamensa (Silvana) commented, "I seem to spend all my time with medical or health people." Mr. Lamensa (Raffaele) then said, "You're also so busy with your mother that you don't have time for anybody else." The nurse was able to use this information from the ecomap to discuss further with the family the types of relationships they wanted both with those inside their household and with those outside the immediate family.

In summary, the genogram and the ecomap can be used in *all* health-care settings, especially in primary care, to increase the nurse's awareness of the whole family and the family's interactions with larger systems and their extended family. Box 3-2 gives helpful hints for drawing ecomaps.

DEVELOPMENTAL ASSESSMENT

In addition to understanding the family structure, the nurse must understand the developmental life cycle for each family. Most nurses are familiar with the stages of child development and the literature in the area of adult development. Many are becoming interested in the burgeoning literature about development in the senior years, an interest that has been fostered by the aging of the Baby Boomer generation. But what of family development? It is more than the concurrent development at different phases of children, adults, and seniors who happen to call themselves "family." We believe families are people who have a shared history and a shared future.

Family development is an over-arching concept, but each family has its own developmental path, influenced by its past and present context and its future aspirations. McGoldrick, Gerson, and Petry (2008, p. 14) define family "as those who are tied together through their common biological, legal, physical, social, and emotional history and by their implied future together."

There is no single family developmental life cycle or model. This is especially evident as our population ages. The natural sequential phases of generational boundaries are not as clear as in the past with for example, children maturing at earlier ages but living at home longer, the trend toward later marriages, and seniors continuing to work well into their 60s. This blurring of boundaries can sometimes lead to tension and confusion within families.

In keeping with postmodernist ideas, we believe that there are limits to describing family development in precise, absolute, universal ways. Postmodernists differ from modernists in that exceptions interest them more than rules; specific, contextualized details more than grand generalizations; difference rather than similarity. We are not concerned with authoritative truth, facts, and rules, but rather with the meaning a family gives to its particular story of development over time.

In our clinical supervision with nurses, we have found it useful to distinguish between "family development" and "family life cycle." *Family development* emphasizes the *unique* path constructed by a family. It is shaped by predictable and unpredictable events, such as illness, catastrophes (e.g., terrorist attacks, fires, earthquakes, hurricanes, floods), and societal trends (e.g., internet and cell phone usage, stock market fluctuations, company mergers, changes in crime and birth rates). *Family life cycle* refers to the *typical* path most families go through. The typical life cycle events are connected to the comings and goings of family members. For example, most families experience in their life cycle the events of birth, child rearing, departure of children from the household, retirement, and death. Such events generate changes requiring formal reorganization of roles and rules within the family. The life cycle course of families evolves through a generally predictable sequence of stages, despite cultural and ethnic variations. Although individual variations, timing, and coping strategies exist, biological time clocks and societal expectations for events such as entrance into elementary school and retirement from work are relatively typical in North America.

Given our keen interest in a particular family's specific development over time, it might be questioned why we include a family developmental section in CFAM at all. We take the position that an informed "not-knowing" stance is useful when working with families. That is, we seek to be informed by the literature, research, and other families' stories of development. Yet, we are "not knowing" but curious about this particular family's developmental story in terms of how they progressed through time.

A rich history about family development still pervades clinicians' thinking. We believe that it is useful for nurses to have some understanding of this history. The early proponents of the family life cycle (Duvall, 1977) developed a four-stage model that was subsequently expanded into an eight-stage model featuring successive stages in the progression of primary marriages. With the increase in various family forms, more complex designs were created (Carter & McGoldrick, 1988, 1998, 1999a; McGoldrick & Carter, 2003). Most early analyses of the family life cycle began with a discussion of the first marriage, but also considered activities that preceded the first marriage, such as cohabitation. In 2000, more than 3 million unmarried couples cohabited (Fields & Casper, 2001). The median age of first marriage has been rising since 1970 to 27.1 years for men and 25.3 years for women in the United States in 2003 (United States Census Bureau, 2007c).

In the field of family therapy, there were "pioneers" in applying the family development framework. Much was written about the interface among family development, functioning, and therapy. Carter and McGoldrick (1988) believed that the family life cycle perspective viewed symptoms in relation to normal functioning over time and that "therapy" helped to reestablish the family's developmental momentum. Family therapists such as Haley (1977), Minuchin (1974), and the Milan Group (Selvini et al.,1980) noted the frequency of symptom appearance with the addition or loss of a family member. These therapists worked with families that did not move smoothly or automatically from one stage in the family life cycle to another, and they focused on the stressful transition points between stages. In doing an assessment and in planning interventions, these therapists paid considerable attention to life-cycle events as markers of change. Although their approaches differed, these therapists similarly sought to understand the relationship between psychopathology and the family's developmental life cycle stage. For example, Minuchin took normative expectations into account when validating goals, whereas the Milan systemic group purposefully avoided a normative direction (Wright & Watson, 1988). Carter and McGoldrick (1988, 1998) included the impact of transgenerational stress intersecting with family developmental transitions. They believed that if vertical (transgenerational) stress was too high, a small amount of horizontal (current) stress would lead to great disruption and symptom formation.

Over the last decade there have been a great many changes in the family life cycle. First, there has been an increase in literature discussing families and their developmental phases (e.g., divorce, remarriage, foster families, impact of immigration, chronic illness, terrorism). Second, there has been an increased consciousness of differences in male and female development and a rethinking of the trajectory of various ethnic groups in North American society. Third, there has been a lower birth rate, a longer life expectancy, a change in the roles of women and men, an awareness of microtrends (Penn, 2007), and increasing divorce and remarriage rates. Fourth, the conception of history as an "objective" ordering of the "facts" of the past has changed. Family development is now seen as an interactive process in which the historian influences which stories of development are told and emphasized. All of these changes have required a critical rethinking of our assumptions about "normality" and the idea of "family" development. The relationship between demographic changes and alterations in the prevalence, timing, and sequencing of some key family transitions must also be noted.

In our clinical work with families presenting in various forms and at all stages of development, we have found it useful to adopt Falicov's (2003, 2007) ideas about family development. She emphasizes culture and gender relativity rather than universality, transitions rather than stages, dimensions and processes rather than markers, and a resource rather than a deficit orientation. We concur with her idea that a systems approach to family development calls for a dialectical integration of two tendencies: stability and change. The emphasis is on both tendencies rather than one or the other. Change and stability must be addressed simultaneously. We do not find it clinically useful to think of families as "stuck" and unable to bring about change. Rather, we find it clinically useful to look for patterns of continuity, identity, and stability that can be maintained while new behavioral patterns are changing.

We believe that there is much evidence to support the position that nurses will find heuristic value in the family development category of CFAM. They should be aware, however, of some of the problems in its indiscriminate adoption and application. We find it indefensible for some nurses to make sweeping generalizations such as, "The family life cycle is genetically determined," or, "The family life cycle is culturally universal." We urge nurses to carefully consider the implication of a family's ethnicity, race, and social class in applying the family development category.

We also caution nurses against *indiscriminately* applying the family development category and overemphasizing *smooth progression*. Contradictions and difficulties inherent in progressing through the life cycle are normal. Families are complex systems that need to deal with many different progressions at once—that is, there are biological, psychological, sociological, and cultural progressions. Tensions and continuing change brought about by contradiction between these progressions are normal. Family life is seldom smooth or bland; rather, it is zestful and active. We therefore encourage nurses, when using the family development category, to have families discuss their joys and satisfactions as well as their tensions and stresses. The family developmental story told by one family member is from that member's "observer perspective" (Maturana & Varela, 1992).

In addition to delineating stages and tasks implicit in the family life cycle, we have found it useful to notice the attachments between family members. *Attachment* refers to a relatively enduring, unique emotional tie between two specific persons. Each person has the need for emotional connection while also remaining secure in his or her own individuality. There is the need to balance two life forces: (1) togetherness and the capacity for intense intimacy in relationships and individuality, and (2) the capacity for independent thinking and goal-oriented action (Rovers, 2006). Bowlby (1977) notes:

> Affectional bonds and subjective states of a strong emotion tend to go together...Thus many of the most intensive of all emotions arise during the formation, the maintenance, the disruption and renewal of affectional bonds which for that reason are sometimes called emotional bonds. In terms of subjective experience the formation of a bond is described as falling in love, maintaining a bond as loving someone, and losing a partner as grieving over someone. Similarly the threat of loss arouses anxiety and actual loss causes sorrow, while both situations are likely to arouse anger. Finally the unchallenged maintenance of a bond is experienced as a source of security and renewal of a bond as a source of joy. (p. 203)

Although the terms "bonding" and "attachment" are sometimes used to describe different relationships, we have chosen in this book and in our clinical work to make no distinction between these terms. We recognize the complexity of relationships that arise from international connections between family members, the relationship stresses and the hard choices economic and social immigrants face with separations and reunions of parents, young children, and elderly family members. We agree with Falicov (2007) that difficult gender and generational transformations need to be considered when discussing attachments. When working with a family, we tend to pay the most attention to the reciprocal nature of an attachment and the quality of the affectional tie. We illustrate these bonds between family members by drawing attachment diagrams. The symbols used in these diagrams (Fig. 3-11) are similar to those used in the structural assessment diagrams. Again, it is important for us to emphasize that there is no one right level of attachment or best attachment configuration.

We are partial to the idea of the network paradigm as a useful base to integrate attachment and family systems theories. Such a paradigm integrates dyadic and family systems as simultaneously distinct and yet interconnected. The clinician holds multiple perspectives in mind, considers each system level as both a part and a whole, and shifts the focus between levels as required. We like this concept because it expands attachment to include multiple system levels and networks, which is especially important as the Baby Boomer cohort increases in age. Attachment theory is relevant to more than just parent–infant bonding; it is important for all ages. We

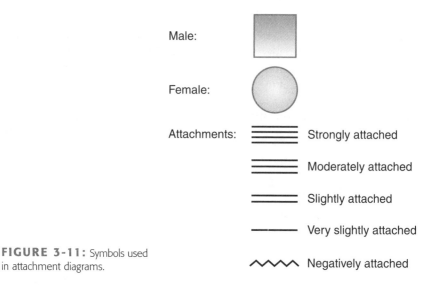

Male:

Female:

Attachments: ══════ Strongly attached

═════ Moderately attached

════ Slightly attached

─────── Very slightly attached

FIGURE 3-11: Symbols used in attachment diagrams.

∿∿∿ Negatively attached

believe that the key elements of attachment processes (affect regulation, interpersonal understanding, information processing, and the provision of comfort within intimate relationships) are as applicable to family systems as they are to individual development.

In the CFAM developmental category, we discuss family life cycle stages, the emotional process of transition (namely, key principles), and second-order changes—the issues dealt with and tasks often accomplished during each stage. In an effort to emphasize the variability of family development, we discuss six sample types of family life cycles:

1. Middle-class North American family life cycle

2. Divorce and postdivorce family life cycle

3. Remarried family life cycle

4. Professional and low-income family life cycles

5. Adoptive family life cycle

6. Lesbian, gay, bisexual, queer, intersexed, transgendered and twin-spirited family life cycles

Middle Class North American Family Life

We are grateful to Carter and McGoldrick (1988, 1999b) for delineating six stages in the North American middle-class family life cycle (Table 3-1). We highlight the expansion, contraction, and realignment of relationships as entries, exits, and development of family members occur. Although the relationship patterns and family themes may sound familiar, we wish to emphasize that the structure and form of the North American family is changing radically. We believe that it is important for nurses to have a

Table 3-1	The Stages of the Family Life Cycle		
STAGE	**EMOTIONAL PROCESS OF TRANSITION: KEY PRINCIPLES**	**SECOND-ORDER CHANGES IN FAMILY STATUS REQUIRED TO PROCEED DEVELOPMENTALLY**
1. Leaving home: Single young adults	Accepting emotional and financial responsibility for self	1. Differentiation of self in relation to family of origin 2. Development of intimate peer relationships 3. Establishment of self related to work and financial independence
2. The joining of families through marriage: The new couple	Commitment to new system	1. Formation of marital system 2. Realignment of relationships with extended families and friends to include spouse
3. Families with young children	Accepting new members into system	1. Adjusting marital system to make space for child(ren) 2. Joining in childrearing, financial, and household tasks 3. Realignment of relationships with extended family to include parenting and grandparenting roles
4. Families with adolescents	Increasing flexibility of family boundaries to include children's independence and grandparents' frailties	1. Shifting of parent–child relationships to permit adolescent to move in and out of system 2. Refocus on midlife marital and career issues 3. Beginning shift toward joint caring for older generation
5. Launching children and moving on	Accepting a multitude of exits from and entries into the family system	1. Renegotiation of marital system as a dyad 2. Development of adult-to-adult relationships between grown children and their parents 3. Realignment of relationships to include in-laws and grandchildren 4. Dealing with disabilities and death of parents (grandparents)
6. Families in later life	Accepting the shifting of generational roles	1. Maintaining own and couple functioning and interests in face of physiological decline; exploration of new familial and social role options 2. Support for a more central role of middle generation 3. Making room in the system for the wisdom and experience of elderly people, supporting the older generation without overfunctioning for them 4. Dealing with loss of spouse, siblings, and other peers and preparation for own death; life review and integration

Carter, B., & McGoldrick, M. (1999) Overview: The expanded family life cycle: Individual, family and social perspectives. In B. Carter & M. McGoldrick (Eds.), *The expanded family life cycle: Individual, family and social perspectives* (3rd ed.) (p. 2). Boston: Allyn & Bacon. Copyright 1999 by Allyn & Bacon. Reprinted by permission.

positive conceptual framework for what *is*: dual-career families, permanent single-parent households, unmarried couples, homosexual couples, remarried couples, and sole-parent adoptions. Transitional crises should not be thought of as permanent traumas. We believe it is imperative that the use of language that links us to previous stereotypes be dropped. For example, we try to eliminate such phrases as "children of divorce," "working mother," "out-of-wedlock child," "fatherless home," and so forth, from the language we use about families. Also, we urge nurses to critically reflect on how culture, ethnicity, gender, race, and sexual orientation influence a family's developmental stages and tasks as well as attachments.

Stage One: The Launching of the Single Young Adult

In outlining the stages of the middle-class North American family life cycle, we have chosen to start with the stage of young adults. The primary task of young adults is to come to terms with their family of origin by remaining connected and yet separate, without cutting off or fleeing reactively to a substitute emotional source. The family of origin has a profound influence on who, when, how, and whether the young adult will marry. There have been sharp increases in the proportion of never married, primarily among men and women in their late 20s and early 30s who continue to live in the family home. These increases are noted for Hispanics, blacks, and whites. In 2004 in the United States, 86.4% of men aged 20 to 24 years and 56.6% aged 25 to 29 years were never married, while 75.4% of women aged 20 to 24 years and 40.8% aged 25 to 29 years were never married (United States Census Bureau, 2007d). Furthermore, the median age of first marriage is increasing. More than 50% of young men and 46% of young women (ages 18 to 24) lived with their parents in the United States in 2000 (Fields & Casper, 2001).

This stage may last for several years in a family's development. It is an opportunity for young adults to sort out emotionally what they will take along from the family of origin, what they will leave behind, and what they will establish for themselves as they progress through succeeding stages of the family life cycle. For both men and women, this is a particularly critical phase. During this stage, men sometimes have difficulty committing themselves to relationships and form a pseudoindependent identity centered around work. Women may choose to define themselves in relation to a male and postpone or forgo establishing an independent identity.

We find it helpful to be curious in our clinical work and try to understand the client's views and legacies regarding marital status and the flexibility of the young person's expectations about pathways to adulthood. With approximately one in four single Americans looking for a romantic partner using the 1,000 or more dating websites, the previous venues for social networking are being replaced by the internet and chat rooms (Penn, 2007). Internet marriage is becoming increasingly common, and this will likely lead to more diverse pairings across race, ethnicity, and nationality.

Tasks

1. **Differentiation of self in relation to family of origin.** The young adult's shift toward adult status involves the development of a mutually respectful form of relating with his or her parents in which the young adult's parents can be appreciated for who they are. The young adult adjusts the view of the parents by neither making them into what they are not nor blaming them for what they could not be. The complexity of this task is not to be underestimated. Each ethnic and racial group has norms and expectations regarding acceptable ways to be attached and connected to family and about issues of dependence versus independence.

2. **Development of intimate peer relationships.** The emphasis is on the young adult's passing from an individual orientation to an interdependent orientation of self. There is no single mold of social experience for young adults to follow as they develop intimate relationships. During this task, young adults strive to bridge the gap between autonomy and attachment as they share themselves with others rather than using others as the source of self. With the increased use of internet dating sites, Facebook, and chat rooms, the young adult will be exposed to a wide variety of personal styles and personalities.

3. **Establishment of self in relation to work and financial independence.** In a young adult's 20s and 30s, the "trying on" of various identities to test or refine career skills and interest is typical. The young adult who is committed to a career path or occupational choice by his or her late 20s or early 30s is less vulnerable to self-doubt or decreased self-esteem than the young adult without direction. Issues of competitiveness, expectations, and differences regarding work and financial goals require sorting through by the young adult and his or her family of origin.

Attachments

There are no right or wrong attachments for young adults in stage one. Rather, it is important for the nurse to draw forth from family members their beliefs about attachment to one other and how they regard these attachments. These beliefs are influenced by culture, gender, race, sexual orientation, and social class as well as by whether the young adult lives at home. Some sample attachments for stage one are given in Figure 3-12. The first diagram illustrates a young adult who is bonded equally with her father and mother. The second diagram illustrates a young adult who is more closely attached to each parent than the parents are to each other; the parents are negatively bonded. Of significance in the second diagram is that there was a death during the childhood of the young adult. It could be hypothesized that his difficulties in establishing his own identity are related to the family's hesitancy to come to grips with his deceased sister and the parents' living alone without children.

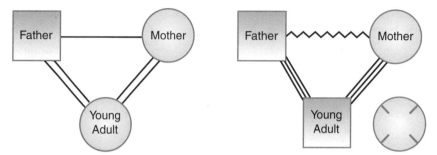

FIGURE 3-12: Sample attachments in stage 1.

Questions to Ask the Family. Which of your parents is most accepting of your career plans? How does he or she show this? What does your sister, Manal, think of your parents' reaction to your career plans? If your father were more accepting of your desire to move into an independent living situation with people not of the Muslim faith, how do you think your mother would react? If you continue to wear hijab because it is integral to your religious beliefs, would this reassure your parents?

Stage Two: Marriage: The Joining of Families

Many couples believe that when they marry, it is just two individuals who are joining together. However, both spouses have grown up in families that have now become interconnected through marriage. Both spouses, although in some ways differentiated from their families of origin in an emotional, financial, and functional way, carry their whole family into the relationship. This is particularly relevant if the marriage is an arranged one. Marriage is a two-generational relationship with a minimum of three families coming together: his family of origin, her family of origin, and the new couple. Given the current prevalence of stepfamilies, the likelihood of several families coming together is increased exponentially. Also, the certainty that the couple will be heterosexual is not evident because, in both the United States and in Canada, gay marriages and civil unions have increasingly been formally recognized.

Tasks

1. **Establishment of couple identity.** The new couple must establish itself as an identifiable unit. This requires negotiation of many issues that were previously defined on an individual level. These issues include routine matters such as eating and sleeping patterns, sexual contact, and use of space and time. The couple must decide about which traditions and rules to retain from each family and which ones they will develop for themselves. They must develop acceptable closeness-distance styles and recognize individual differences in adult attachment styles. Although the majority of studies on the quality and stability of marriage focus on couple communication, we believe that love is the decisive factor for quality and stability. For some cultures,

however, the concept of a "love marriage" as compared to an arranged marriage is quite different.

2. **Realignment of relationships with extended families to include spouse.** A renegotiation of relationships with each spouse's family of origin has to take place to accommodate the new spouse. This places no small stress on both the couple and each family of origin to open itself to new ways of being. Some couples deal with their parents by cutting off the relationship in a bid for independence. Other couples choose to handle this task of realignment by absorbing the new spouse into the family of origin. The third common pattern involves a balance between some contact and some distance. LaSala (2002) points out the great variability in attachment styles. For example, "gay men emphasized the importance of independence from their parents while lesbians sought harmonious intergenerational connections" (p. 327).

3. **Decisions about parenthood.** For most couples, happiness is highest at the beginning of the life cycle stage of marriage. Although a small but increasing number of married couples are deciding not to have children, most still plan on becoming parents. The question of *when* to conceive is becoming increasingly complex, especially with the changed role of women, the widespread use of contraceptives, the availability of a wide range of fertilization strategies, and the trend toward later marriages. Couples who have evolved more competent marital structures prenatally are more likely to successfully incorporate a child into the family.

Attachments

Figure 3-13 illustrates a sample attachment for a couple in stage two: the development of close emotional ties between the spouses. The first diagram illustrates how they do not have to break ties with their families of origin, but rather maintain and adjust ties with them. A different type of attachment (illustrated in the second diagram) can occur if both members of a couple do not align themselves together. The wife is more heavily bonded to her family of origin than she is to her husband. The husband is more tied to outside interests (such as work and friends) than to his wife. We have found that negative attachment-related events occurring early in the marriage are especially distressing for the couple. These and other attachment injuries can be characterized by a betrayal of trust during a critical moment of need.

Questions to Ask the Family. Which family, Sabeen, was most in favor of your marriage to Hashim? How did you incorporate Pakistani and American traditions in your marriage? How did your siblings show that they supported your marriage? What does your spouse think of your parents' marital relationship? If you two as a couple were to model your marriage on your parents' marriage, what would you incorporate into

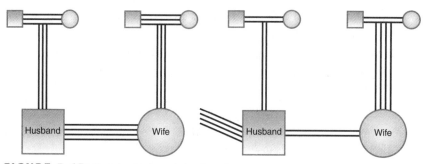

FIGURE 3-13: Sample attachments in stage 2.

your marriage? How did the diagnosis of multiple sclerosis influence your bonding as a couple?

Stage Three: Families with Young Children

During this stage, the adults now become caregivers to a younger generation. Family-of-origin experiences can influence the forming of a new family as the study by Perren, et al. (2005) showed. They found that study participants who recollected negative qualities in their parents' relationship reported more negative changes in the quality of their own marriages during their first year of transition to parenthood.

The birth and rearing of a baby present varying challenges. Moreover, taking responsibility and dealing with the demands of dependent children are challenging for most families when financial resources are stretched and the parents are heavily involved in career development. The disposition of childcare responsibilities and household chores in dual-career households is a particular struggle. We have found that men and women often differ in the coping strategies they use to deal with this issue. Women with young children tend to use cognitive restructuring, delegating, limiting avocational activities, and using social support significantly more often than do men.

We believe the work-family issue of juggling childcare and other household accountabilities is a social problem to be dealt with by the couple, not a "woman's problem" for her to struggle with alone. How the increase in "old new Dads" in the United States will impact this struggle is unknown. What is evident is that the birth rate between 1980 and 2002 increased 32% among fathers in the United States aged 40 to 44 and increased 21% among fathers aged 45 to 49 (Penn, 2007). It went up almost 10% for dads 50 to 54. This trend means that the joys of family life go on well into many dads' 60s. Generational boundaries quickly become blurred with "old new Dads" being concerned simultaneously about children's schools and sports and their own retirement finances.

Tasks

1. **Adjusting marital system to make space for child.** The couple must continue to meet each other's personal needs as well as their

parental responsibilities. With the introduction of the first child, challenges for personal space, sexual and emotional intimacy, and socializing exist. Both mothers and fathers are increasingly aware of the need for emotional integration of the child into the family. Children can be brought into three types of environments: (1) there is no space for them, (2) there is space for them, or (3) there is a vacuum that they are expected to fill. If the child has a handicap, the couple faces more stress as they adjust their expectations and deal with their emotional reactions. We have found that normal family processes in couples becoming parents include shifts in the sense of self, shifts in relationships with families of origin, shifts in relation to the child, changes in stress and social support, and changes in the couple.

2. **Joining in childbearing, financial, and household tasks.** The couple must find a mutually satisfying way to deal with childcare responsibility and household chores that does not overburden one partner. Balancing the budget and juggling family and other responsibilities is a major task. The emotional and financial cost of solutions to deal with child-care responsibilities must be addressed. Both mothers and fathers contribute to the child's development and can do so in different or similar ways. Physical and playful stimulation of the child complements verbal interaction. Parents can either support or hinder their children's success in developing peer relationships and achieving at school. Some middle-class families, responding to intense pressure from the school system, tend to stress the values of achievement and productivity, whereas some working-class families may respond to this pressure by feelings of alienation. Recent immigration experiences and whether the children are documented or undocumented can also influence peer and school interaction.

3. **Realignment of relationships with extended family to include parenting and grandparenting roles.** The couple must design and develop the new roles of father and mother in addition to the marital role rather than replacing it. Members of each family of origin also take on new roles, for example, grandfather or aunt. In some cases, grandparents who perhaps were opposed to the marriage in the beginning become very interested in the young children. For many older adults, this is an especially gratifying time because it allows them to have intimacy with their grandchildren without the responsibilities of parenting. It also permits them to develop a new type of adult–adult relationship with their children. Opportunities for intergenerational support or conflict abound as expectations about child-rearing and health-care practices are expressed. Smith (2000) reports that, in 1995, "fifty percent of preschoolers (in the United States) were cared for by a relative, with grandparents being the single most frequently mentioned care provider (30 percent)" (p. 2).

Attachments

Parents need to maintain a marital bond and continue personal, adult-centered conversations in addition to child-centered conversations. Space for privacy and time spent together are important needs. Gottman and Notarius (2002) report that for 40% to 70% of couples, marital quality drops following the transition to parenthood, with people commonly reverting to stereotypic gender roles as they become overwhelmed by the complexity of housework, childcare, and work. Marital conversation and sex sharply decrease. However, joy and pleasure with the baby increase.

Children require security and warm attachments to adults, as well as opportunities to develop positive sibling relationships. We believe teaching interdependence is a central goal of parenting, helping children see themselves as part of a community and living cooperatively with others.

In Figure 3-14, sample attachment diagrams are given for this stage. A competitive, negative relationship (illustrated by the wavy line) exists between the children and spouses in the second diagram. The mother is overbonded to the daughter, and the father is underinvolved with the daughter. The father is overattached to the son, and the mother is underinvolved with the son. This is an example of same-sex coalitions existing cross-generationally.

Questions to Ask the Family. What percentage of your time do you spend taking care of your children? What percentage do you spend taking care of your marriage? Is this a comfortable balance for the two of you? What effect does this pattern have on your children? If your children thought that you should be closer, how might they tell you this? What impact did the miscarriages have on your marriage?

Stage Four: Families with Adolescents

This period has often been characterized as one of intense upheaval and transition, in which biological, emotional, and sociocultural changes occur with great and ever-increasing rapidity. Peers, internet technology such as instant messaging and Facebook, pornography, sports, and other activities all compete for the adolescent's attention. This stage is highly influenced by

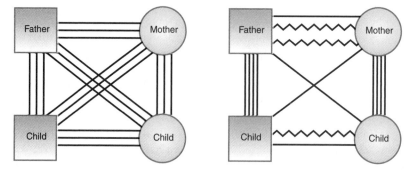

FIGURE 3-14: Sample attachments in stage 3.

class. Adolescence can begin early within poor, inner-city communities when, at a very young age, children are often faced with pressures related to sexuality, household responsibility, drugs, and alcohol use. In many middle-class families, adolescence can last well into the young adult's 20s and 30s, with the young person being financially dependent on the parents and continuing to live in the family home.

Tasks

1. **Shift in parent–child relationships to permit adolescents to move in or out of the system.** The family must move from the dependency relationship previously established with a young child to an increasingly independent relationship with the adolescent. Growing psychological independence is frequently not recognized because of continuing physical dependence. Conflict often surfaces when a teenager's independence threatens the family. For example, teenagers may precipitate marital conflict when they question who makes the family rules about the car: Mom or Dad? Families frequently respond to an adolescent's request for increasing autonomy in two ways: (1) they abruptly define rigid rules and recreate an earlier stage of dependency, or (2) they establish premature independence. In the second scenario, the family supports only independence and ignores dependent needs. This may result in premature separation when the teenager is not really ready to be fully autonomous. The teenager may thus return home defeated. Parents need to shift from the parental role of "protector" to that of "preparer" for the challenges of adulthood.

   The challenge for parents to shift responsibility in a balanced way to their teens is often complicated if there are health problems. For example, Fulkerson, et al. (2007) found that general family connectedness, priority of family meals, and positive mealtime environment were significantly positively associated with psychosocial well-being in overweight adolescents. These authors also noted that weight-based teasing and parental encouragement to diet were associated with poor psychological health in the 7th to 12th graders they studied. For parents to find a balance between encouraging healthy eating and avoiding encouraging dieting with at-risk-for-overweight or overweight teens is a challenge.

2. **Refocus on midlife marital and career issues.** During this stage, parents are often struggling with what Erickson (1963) calls *generativity*, the need to be useful as a human being, partner, and mentor to another generation. The socially and sexually maturing teenager's frequent questioning and conflict about values, lifestyles, career plans, and so forth can thrust the parents into an examination of their own marital and career issues. Depending on many factors, including cultural and gender expectations, this may be a period of positive growth or painful struggle for men and women.

3. Beginning shift toward joint caring for older generation. As parents are aging, so too are the grandparents. Parents (especially women) sometimes feel that they are besieged on both sides: teenagers are asking for more freedom, and grandparents are asking for more support. With the trend of women having children later in life and seniors living longer, this double demand for attention and resources most likely will intensify. Celebrating the wisdom of seniors and intergenerational reciprocity are key tasks.

Attachments

All family members continue to have their relationships within the family, while teenagers become increasingly more involved with their friends than with family members. These transitions through the family life cycle can be stressful because they challenge attachment bonds among family members. We advocate open communication and the addressing of primary emotions. A decrease in parental attachment is normative and developmentally appropriate for adolescents. The young person's widening social network, however, does not preclude strong family relationships, although family relationships are altered. The husband and wife need to reinvest in the marital relationship while this is taking place.

An example of an attachment pattern is illustrated in Figure 3-15. In the second diagram, the mother is overinvolved with the eldest son and has a negative relationship with the husband. The father tends to be minimally involved with all family members. There is conflict between the two sons.

Questions to Ask the Family. What privileges do your teenagers have now that they did not have when they were younger? *Ask the adolescents:* How do you think your parents will handle it when your younger sister, Nenita, wants to date? Will it be different from when you wanted to date? On a scale of 1 to 10, with 10 being the highest, how much confidence do your parents have in your ability to say no to crystal meth?

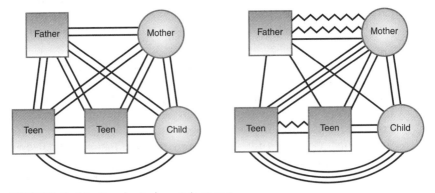

FIGURE 3-15: Sample attachments in stage 4.

Stage Five: Launching Children and Moving On

Many middle-class North Americans whose children are grown up used to assume they would have an empty nest. However, this expectation is in the process of change. Rising housing costs and beginning pay rates that have not risen as fast as those of more experienced workers have been singled out as some of the causes of this trend. A different explanation is that young North Americans are having difficulty growing up and are unwilling to go out on their own and settle for less affluence than their parents afford them.

Tasks

1. **Renegotiation of marital system as a dyad.** In many cases, a thrust to alter some of the basic tenets of the marital relationship occurs. This is especially true if both partners are working and the children have left home. The couple bond can take on a more prominent position. The balance between dependency, independency, and interdependency must be re-examined.

2. **Development of adult–adult relationships between grown children and their parents.** The family of origin must relinquish the primary roles of parent and child. They must adapt to the new roles of parent and adult child. This involves renegotiation of emotional and financial commitments. The key emotional process during this stage is for family members to deal with a multitude of exits from and entries into the family system.

3. **Realignment of relationships to include in-laws and grown children.** The parents adjust family ties and expectations to include their child's spouse or partner. This can sometimes be particularly challenging if the parents' expectation is for a heterosexual son-in-law or daughter-in-law of the family's race, religion and ethnicity and the child chooses someone different. The once-prevalent idea that the time after a grown child marries is a lonely, sad time, especially for women, has been replaced. Increases in marital satisfaction have frequently been noted.

4. **Dealing with disabilities and death of grandparents.** Many families regard the disability or death of an elderly parent as a natural occurrence. It can be a time of relishing and finding comfort in the happy memories, wisdom, and contributions of the elder. If, however, the couple and the elderly parents have unfinished business between them, there may be serious repercussions, not only for the children but also for the new third generation. The type of disability afflicting the seniors determines the effects on the immediate family. For example, caregivers who do not understand Alzheimer's dementia and its effects on cognitive function and behavior often attempt to deal with inappropriate or disruptive behavior in ineffective and counterproductive ways. Thus, they inadvertently intensify their own stress. Fruhauf and Aberle (2007) note that many times female caregivers seek support for depression that often stems from the multiple roles, losses, and guilt they are experiencing.

We recommend that health professionals, in addition to attending to the family's multigenerational legacies of illness, loss, and crisis, also note intergenerational strengths and wisdom. Tracking key events, transitions, and coping strategies helps elicit resiliencies.

Attachments

Each family member continues to have outside interests and establish new roles appropriate to this stage. Sample attachment patterns are illustrated in Figure 3-16. A problem may arise when both husband and wife hold onto their last child. They may avoid conflict by allowing the eldest child to leave home and then focusing on the next child.

Questions to Ask the Family. How did your parents help you to leave home? What is the difference between how you left home and how your son, Zubin, is leaving home? Will your parents get along better, worse, or the same with each other once you have left home? Who, between Mom and Dad, will miss the children the most? As you see your child moving on with a new relationship, what would you like your child to do differently than you did? If your parents are still alive, are there any issues you would like to discuss with them?

Stage Six: Families in Later Life

This stage can begin with retirement and last until the death of both spouses. It is hard to say, however, when the stage actually begins for each family, considering that "today there are 5 million people 65 and older in the US labor force, almost twice what there were in the early 1980s and that number is about to explode" (Penn, 2007, p.29). Potentially, this stage can last 20 to 30 years for many couples. Key emotional processes in this stage are to flexibly adjust to the shift of generational roles and to foster an appreciation of the wisdom of the elders.

Tasks

1. **Maintaining own or couple functioning and interest in the face of physiological decline: exploration of new familial and social role options.** Marital relationships continue to be important, and marital

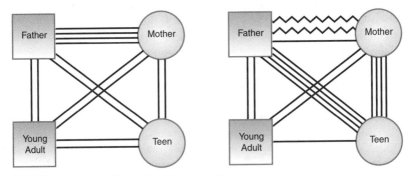

FIGURE 3-16: Sample attachments in stage 5.

satisfaction contributes to both the morale and ongoing activity of both spouses. We have noted that the husband's morale is often strongly associated with health, socioeconomic status, income and, to a lesser extent, family functioning. The wife's morale is most strongly associated with family functioning and, to a lesser extent, with health and socioeconomic status.

As the couple in later life find themselves in new roles as grandparents and mother-in-law and father-in-law, they must adjust to their children's spouses and open space for the new grandchildren. Difficulty in making the status changes required can be reflected in an older family member refusing to relinquish some of his or her power, for example, refusing to turn over a company or making plans for succession in a family business. The shift in status between the senior family members and the middle-aged family members is a reciprocal one. Difficulties and confusion may occur in several ways. Older adults may give up and become totally dependent on the next generation; the next generation may not accept the seniors' diminishing powers and may continue to treat them as totally competent, or the next generation may see only the seniors' frailties and may treat them as totally incompetent.

2. **Making room in the system for the wisdom and experience of the seniors.** The task of supporting the older generation without overfunctioning for them is particularly salient because, in general, people are living longer. It is not uncommon for a 90-year-old woman to be cared for by her 70-year-old daughter, with both of them living in close proximity to a 50-year-old son and grandson. The parents of the Baby Boomers are the current generation of "young-old." They are highly motivated to participate in self-help groups and are interested in improving their quality of life through counseling, traditional and alternative health activities, and education. Many have found "new" family connections through the use of e-mail and cell phones. They do not live by the aging myths of the past. Rather, as consumers, they expect and demand a good quality of life. Many grandparents continue to be involved in childrearing. According to the U.S. Census Bureau (2002), in 2000, 42% of grandparents who lived with any of their grandchildren under age 18 were responsible for most of the basic needs of one or more of these grandchildren.

3. **Dealing with loss of spouse, siblings, and other peers and preparation for death.** This is a time for life review and taking care of unfinished business with family as well as with business and social contacts. Many people find it helpful to discuss their life, review it, and enjoy the opportunity of passing this information along to succeeding generations.

Attachments
The couple reinvests and modifies the marital relationship based on the level of functioning of both partners. In 2000 in the United States, the vast

majority of adults over age 65 did not live alone but lived with other family members; less than 5% lived in institutions. Among the population aged 75 years and older, 67% of men lived with their spouses. Forty-nine percent of women lived alone, and another 22% were not currently married but lived with either relatives or nonrelatives (Fields & Casper, 2001).

This stage is characterized by an appropriate interdependence with the next generation. The concept of interdependence is particularly important for nurses to understand in working with families with adult daughters and their parents. Middle-class older men and women seem equally likely to aid and support their children, especially daughters. Frequency of contact, however, tends to be higher with daughters than with sons. Thus, the possibility of strong intergenerational attachments between a daughter and her parents exists. In the attachment pattern illustrated in Figures 3-16 and 3-17, the couple project their conflicts onto the extended family. This causes difficulty for the succeeding generations.

Questions to Ask the Family. When you look back over your life, what aspects have you enjoyed the most? What has given you the most happiness? About what aspects do you feel the most regret? What would you hope that your children would do differently than you did? Similarly to what you did? As your health is declining, what plans have you and your daughter, Aminah, made for her because of her schizophrenia?

Divorce and Postdivorce Family Life Cycle

Many changes in marital status and living arrangements are prevalent in North America today. Noteworthy is the high level of divorce. In the United States in 1996, divorced people represented 10% of adults age 18 and older, an increase from 3% in 1970 (Saluter & Lugaila, 1998).

In 2005, the divorce rate in the United States was 3.6 per 1,000 population, down from 4.2 in 2000 and 4.4 in 1995 (Daily Almanac, 2007). Whether the divorce rate will level off, climb, or decline is a matter of speculation that can be backed up by various theories. Unstable economic conditions, the AIDS

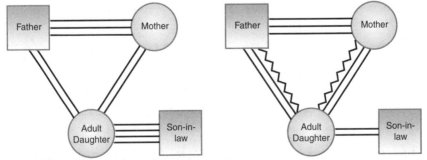

FIGURE 3-17: Sample attachments in stage 6.

epidemic, fear of terrorism, and increased faith-based initiatives may cause divorce rates to decline. Single-parent families are on the rise. The number of single-mother families increased from 3 million (12%) in 1970 to 10 million (26%) in 2000 in the United States. Similarly, single-father families grew from 393,000 (1%) to 2 million (5%) in 2000 (Fields & Casper, 2001).

Families experiencing divorce are often under enormous pressure. Single-parent families must accomplish most of the same developmental tasks as two-parent families, but without all the resources. This places extra burden on the remaining family members, who must compensate with increased effort to accomplish family tasks such as physical maintenance, social control, and tension management. We caution nurses, however, not to assume that single-parent status alone will influence family functioning. We have found that family composition alone is too broad a variable to predict health outcomes, and we recommend a focus on more specific variables such as parental cooperation in parenting following divorce.

Single-parent houeholds generally experience challenges in managing shortages of time, money, and energy. Some parents voice serious concerns about failure to meet perceived family and societal expectations for living "in a normal family" with two parents. Some women feel they must display behaviors that are contradictory to those they assume they should exhibit if they were to remarry. They perceive ongoing pressure from family, friends, and church to marry again to give their children a "normal" family. These women report being caught in a double-bind, trying to demonstrate behaviors such as submissiveness that might attract a new husband while trying to use seemingly opposing behaviors such as assertiveness to successfully manage their lives. We encourage nurses working with single-parent families to explore the parent's feelings about opposing expectations. This is a way of helping these parents plan their responses to various paradoxical situations.

It is also important for nurses engaged in relational family nursing practice to focus on the positive changes experienced by many separated spouses. Separated women often use growth-oriented coping, such as becoming more autonomous and furthering their education, and experience positive changes, such as increased confidence and feelings of control in the post-separation phase.

Resilience in the postdivorce period is another focus for nurses. Resilience commonly depends on the ability of parents and children to build close, constructive, mutually supportive relationships that play a significant role in buffering families from the effects of related adversity. Factors that promote resiliency and positive adjustment to divorce include those associated with children's living arrangements. Kelly's review (2007) of the large empirical research findings indicates that "children's contacts with their nonresident parent should not be based on every-other-weekend guidelines but should reflect the diversity of parental interest, capability, and the quality of the parent-child relationship" (p. 47). She recommends that children, depending on their age and developmental capacity, should have input into the living arrangements but not be asked to choose between parents.

It should be noted that approximately 75% of children involved in divorce are resilient and able to move on with their lives; only about 25% experience more lasting problems in adjustment (Greene, et al. 2003). Findings from Baum's (2003) study of former couples in Israel showed that the longer and more conflictual the legal proceedings, the worse the coparental relationship in the view of both parents. Interestingly, Baum also found that the more responsibility the father took for the divorce and the more he viewed himself as the initiator, the more he fulfilled his parental functions. The findings from Ahrons' longitudinal study (2007) of children 20 years after their parents' divorce showed that children who reported their parents as being cooperative also reported better relationships with their parents, grandparents, step-parents, and siblings. Whether family relationships postdivorce improve, remain stable, or get worse is dependent on a complex interweaving of many factors. Many of the problems previously attributed to "the divorce" are now seen to be located in the pre-divorce family situation; divorce is a long-term process that begins prior to separation and lasts long after the legal event of divorce (Ahrons, 2006).

In our clinical supervision with nurses, we encourage focusing on the siblings, a subsystem that generally remains undisrupted during the process of family reorganization. Siblings are often the unit of continuity. We also try to notice and support cooperative postdivorce parenting environments such as mutual parental support; teamwork; clear, flexible boundaries; high information exchange; constructive problem solving; and knowledgeable, experienced, involved, and authoritative parenting. Because many fathers are not used to taking care of their children without their wives orchestrating things, fathers often fade out of their children's lives. They want to avoid ex-wives and conflict and may feel uncomfortable if they have an unclear role of authority in their children's lives. Ahrons found (2007) that when children's relationships with their fathers deteriorated after divorce, their relationships with their paternal grandparents, stepmothers and stepsiblings were distant, negative, or nonexistent (p. 53). Nurses can be extremely helpful in intervening in these situations and fostering mutually agreeable postdivorce arrangements for the benefit of the children. Nurses can help fathers redefine their parental roles and identity in distinction from their spousal role and identity, as Baum (2006) recommends. For families locked in intractable disputes, we encourage them to develop a good-enough climate in which parents maintain distance from one another and conflict and triangulation is minimized.

Divorce may occur at any stage of the family life cycle and with any family, irrespective of class or race. However, it has a different impact on family functioning depending on its timing and the diversity of individuals involved in the process. The marital breakdown may be sudden, or it may be long and drawn out. In either case, emotional work is required so that the family may deal with the shifts, gains, and losses in family membership. Some sample phases involved in divorce and postdivorce are depicted in Table 3-2. Carter and McGoldrick (1999) found a clinical usefulness in the distinctions made between the three columns given in the table. Column 1 lists the phase. Column 2 gives the prerequisite attitudes that will assist family members to make the transition and come through the developmental issues listed in column 3 en route to the next phase. We believe that clinical work directed at column 3 will not succeed if the family is having difficulty dealing with the issues in column 2.

Questions to Ask the Family. How do you explain to yourself the reasons for your divorce? Who initiated the idea of divorce? Who left who? Who was

Table 3-2	Stages of Divorce Family Life Cycle	
PHASE	**EMOTIONAL PROCESS OF TRANSITION, PREREQUISITE ATTITUDE**	**DEVELOPMENTAL ISSUES**
Divorce		
1. Deciding to divorce	Accepting inability to resolve marital tensions sufficiently to continue relationship	Accepting one's own part in the failure of the marriage
2. Planning the break-up of the system	Supporting viable arrangements for all parts of the system	Working cooperatively on problems of custody, visitation, and finances Dealing with extended family about the divorce
3. Separation	Being willing to continue cooperative coparental relationship and joint financial support of children Working on resolution of attachment to spouse	Mourning loss of nuclear family Restructuring, marital and parent–child relationships and finances; adaptation to living apart Realigning relationships with extended family; staying connected with spouse's extended family
4. Divorce	More work on emotional divorce: overcoming hurt, anger, guilt, and so forth	Retrieving hopes, dreams, and expectations from the marriage
Postdivorce		
1. Single-parent (custodial household or primary residence)	Being willing to maintain financial responsibilities, continue parental contact with ex-spouse, and support contact of children with ex-spouse and his or her family	Making flexible visitation arrangements with ex-spouse and his or her family Rebuilding own financial resources Rebuilding own social network
2. Single-parent (noncustodial)	Being willing to maintain parental contact with ex-spouse and support custodial parent's relationship with children	Finding ways to continue effective parenting relationship with children Maintaining financial responsibilities to ex-spouse and children Rebuilding own social network

Carter, B., & McGoldrick, M. (1999). The divorce cycle: A major variation in the American family life cycle. In B. Carter & M. McGoldrick (Eds.), *The expanded family life cycle: Individual, family, and social perspectives* (3rd ed.) (pp. 373–380). Boston: Allyn & Bacon. Copyright 1999 by Allyn & Bacon. Reprinted by permission.

most supportive of developing viable arrangements for *everyone* in the family? How did your ex-husband, Luis, show his willingness to continue a cooperative co-parental relationship with you? How did you respond to this? As you changed your attachment to Luis, what changes did you notice in your children? What would your in-laws say about how you have fostered your children's relationship with them? What would your children say? What methods have you found most successful in resolving conflicting issues with Luis? What advice would you give to other divorced parents on how to resolve conflictual issues with their ex-partners? How have your children helped you and your ex-spouse to maintain a supportive environment for them?

Remarried Family Life Cycle

"Stepfamilies are families emerging out of hope" (Visher, Visher, & Pasley, 2003, p. 171). The rise of remarriage and the stepfamily in North America in recent decades has been striking. According to the Stepfamily Association of America (2003), estimates from 1988 to 1990 suggest that:

- 52% to 62% of all first marriages will eventually end in legal divorce
- about 75% of all divorced people will eventually remarry
- about 43% of all marriages are remarriages by at least one of the adults
- about 65% of remarriages involve children from the prior marriage and from stepfamilies
- 60% of all remarriages eventually end in legal divorce.

Berger (1998) reports that one in three Americans is a member of a stepfamily as either a stepchild, step-parent, remarried parent, or step-grandparent. Ahrons' longitudinal study (2007) of children 20 years after parental divorce found that most of the children experienced the remarriage of one or both parents, and one-third of her sample remembered the remarriage as more stressful than the divorce. Two-thirds reported their father's remarriage as more stressful than their mother's.

The family emotional process at the transition to remarriage consists of struggling with fears about investment in new relationships: one's own fears, the new spouse's fears, and the fears of the children (of either or both spouses). It also consists of dealing with hostile or upset reactions of the children, extended families, and ex-spouse. Unlike biological families, in which family membership is defined by bloodlines, legal contracts, and spatial arrangements and is characterized by explicit boundaries, the structure of a stepfamily is less clear. Nurses must address the ambiguity of the new family organization, including roles and relationships. Visher, Visher, and Pasley (2003) point out the following major dynamic issues for stepfamily households (p. 160):

- Outsiders versus insiders
- Boundary disputes
- Power issues
- Conflicting loyalties
- Rigid, unproductive triangles
- Unity versus fragmentation of the new couple relationship

We have found it helpful to use attachment theory as a framework for conceptualizing the impact of structural change and loss on stepfamily adjustment. Furrow and Palmer (2007) think of the stepfamily as an emerging family system; problem patterns are understood in this context where bids for connection may be missed or misinterpreted. We believe nurses can assist stepfamilies in increasing emotional connectivity and stability.

In many cases, parental guilt and concerns about the children are increased, and a positive or negative rearousal of the old attachment to the ex-spouse may occur (Carter & McGoldrick, 1999b). Table 3-3 summarizes Carter and McGoldrick's developmental outline for stepfamily formation.

Ahrons and Rodgers (1987) have advocated for models of healthy, well-functioning binuclear families. Having been angered by a predominant emphasis on pathology in the divorce literature, Ahrons began to study what she calls "binuclear families." This term not only refers to joint-custody families or to families in which the relationship between ex-spouses is friendly but indicates a different familial structure, without inferring anything about the nature or quality of the ex-spouses' relationship. Ahrons and Rodgers (1987), who worked with 98 divorced couples over a 5-year period, produced some interesting relationship types, including "perfect pals," a small group of divorced spouses whose previous marriage had not overshadowed their longstanding friendship. The second group, "cooperative colleagues," was a considerably larger and more typical group found by Ahrons and Rodgers. Although not good friends, they worked well together on issues concerning their children. The third group was the "angry associates," and the fourth group was "fiery foes," who felt nothing but fury for their ex-spouses. Ahrons and Rodgers termed the fifth group "dissolved duos," who after the separation or divorce discontinued any contact with each other. Ahrons (1999) advocates for a normative process model of divorce rather than focusing on evidence of pathology or dysfunction. We agree with this stance, mindful though that approximately 25% of children involved in divorce do seem to have longer-lasting adjustment difficulties (Greene, et al. 2003).

We encourage nurses working with divorced and remarried families to bring to their patients research knowledge of what works and does not work to foster continuing family relationships. Nurses should be cautious,

Table 3-3	Remarried Family Formation: A Development Outline	
STEPS	PREREQUISITE ATTITUDE	DEVELOPMENTAL ISSUES
1. Entering the new relationship	Recovery from loss of first marriage (adequate "emotional divorce")	1. Recommitting to marriage and to forming a family with readiness to deal with the complexity and ambiguity
2. Conceptualizing and planning the new marriage and family	Accepting one's own fears and those of new spouse and children about remarriage and forming a stepfamily Accepting need for time and patience for adjustment to complexity and ambiguity of: 1. Multiple new roles 2. Boundaries: space, time, membership, authority 3. Affective issues: guilt, loyalty conflicts, desire for mutuality, unresolvable past hurts	1. Working on openness in the new relationships to avoid pseudo-mutuality 2. Planning for maintenance of cooper-ative financial and co-parental relationships with ex-spouses 3. Planning to help children deal with fears, loyalty conflicts, and member-ship in two systems 4. Realigning relationships with extended family to include new spouse and children 5. Planning maintenance of connections for children with extended family of ex-spouse(s)
3. Remarriage and reconstruction of family	Final resolution of attachment to previous spouse and ideal of "intact" family Accepting a different model of family with permeable boundaries	1. Restructuring family boundaries to allow inclusion of new spouse–step-parent 2. Realignment of relationships and financial arrangements throughout subsystems to permit interweaving of several systems 3. Making room for relationships of all children with biological (noncusto-dial) parents, grandparents, and other extended family 4. Sharing memories and histories to enhance stepfamily integration

Carter, B., & McGoldrick, M. (1999). The divorce cycle: A major variation in the American family life cycle. In B. Carter & M. McGoldrick (Eds.), *The expanded family life cycle: Individual, family, and social perspectives* (3rd ed.) (pp. 373–380). Boston: Allyn & Bacon. Copyright 1999 by Allyn & Bacon. Reprinted by permission.

however, because complex problems seldom have simple answers. For example, predictors such as a child's age and gender, the frequency and regularity of father/mother–child visitation, father/mother–child closeness, and the effect of parental legal conflict on the child's self-esteem have different implications for different groups of 6- to 12-year-old children and for children in different situations.

We also encourage nurses working with stepfamilies to increase their knowledge about stepfamily issues and respect the uniqueness of complex stepfamily life. Clawson and Ganong (2002), for example, found in their research that adult stepchildren and step-parents agreed that stepchildren have few obligations to assist step-parents. However, the key in deciding whether a responsibility to assist existed was how the relationship was defined. Nurses could assist stepfamilies to discuss topics such as these. We encourage nurses to educate themselves about the beliefs of a particular stepfamily because uninformed clinicians may unwittingly increase rather than decrease family tensions if they communicate to stepfamilies that they should be like biological families.

Questions to Ask the Family. Reeves, what were the differences between you and your wife, Lily, in how you each successfully recovered from your first marriage? What most helped each of you deal with your own fears about remarriage? About forming a stepfamily? How did Lily invite your children to adjust to her? What do your children think was the most useful thing you did in helping them deal with loyalty conflicts? What advice do you have for other stepfamilies on how to create a new family? What are you most proud of in how you have helped your stepfamily successfully make the transition from what they were before to what they are now?

Comparison of Professional and Low-Income Family Life Cycle Stages

The family life cycle of the poor commonly does not match the middle-class paradigm so often used to conceptualize their situations. Anderson (2003) points out that when poverty is factored out, the differences between the adjustment of children in one- and two-parent families almost disappear. Low-income single parents who are also minorities face special issues. Currently, close to 75% of all single-parent families are minorities (Anderson, 2003). The family life cycle of the poor can be divided into three phases: the unattached young adult (perhaps younger than 12 years old), who is virtually unaccountable to any adults; families with children—a phase occupying most of the life span and including three- and four-generational households; and the final phase of the grandmother who continues to be involved in central childrearing in her senior years. Fields (2003) reports that in 2002, "ten percent of children who lived with a single mother were grandchildren of the householder...When children lived in households without either of their parents very often (44% of children) they were living in their grandparent's household" (p. 3). We encourage nurses to consider the effects of ethnicity and religion, socioeconomic status, race, and environment on when and how a family makes transitions in its life cycle. This is especially important in relational family nursing practice in primary care.

Adoptive Family Life Cycle

In adoption, the family boundaries of all those involved are expanded. Reitz and Watson (1992) define adoption as:

> A means of providing some children with security and meeting their developmental needs by legally transferring ongoing parental responsibilities from their birth parents to their adoptive parents;

recognizing that in so doing we have created a new kinship network that forever links those two families together through the child, who is shared by both. (p. 11)

We agree with this definition. As with marriage, the new legal status of the adoptive family does not automatically sever the psychological ties to the earlier family. Rather, family boundaries are expanded and realigned. Multiple statistical systems make it difficult to find concrete data on the number of children adopted each year. Fein (1998) found that 127,441 children were adopted in the United States in 1992, a slight increase from 118,000 children 5 years earlier. Approximately 42% of those adoptions involved step-parents and relatives. The biggest increase, according to Fein, has been children adopted from other countries. "Because they require visas, there are up to date statistics for these adoptions and since 1990, their numbers have nearly doubled from 7,093 to 13,620 in 1997" (Fein, 1998, p. 1). This has resulted in increased visibility for the adoption process and the issues involved for parents and children. In their study of 20 families who adopted children from Russian and Romanian institutions, Linville and Lyness (2007) reported that the families described having gone through a metamorphosis particularly in the areas of roles, emotional strain, parenting techniques, resilience and connection to the children's country of origin. They suggest, and we agree, that the way the story of international adoption is told and retold in the family can have lasting positive or negative consequences for the child's adjustment and emotional well-being. This is an area in which nurses can have a tremendous positive impact in assisting families.

We believe that nurses should be aware of the trends and special circumstances in forming adoptive families. For example, most agencies offer adoption services along a continuum of openness. Some potential benefits of open adoption for birth parents, include increased empathy for adoptive parents, reassurance that the child is safe and loved, and a reduction of shame and guilt. For adoptive parents, benefits include increased empathy for the birth parents, reduced stress imposed by secrecy and the unknown, and an embracing from the start of an affirmative acceptance of the child's cultural heritage. For the child, benefits include increased empathy for the adoptive parents, enriched connections with them, and reduced stress of disconnection. Simultaneously, the child experiences increased empathy for the birth parents, a reduction in fantasies about them, and—with clear, consistent information— increased control in dealing with adoptive issues. We believe that these potential benefits are very significant, especially for families adopting babies from different cultures and races. Adoptive families can include divorced, single-parent, married, or remarried families as well as extended families and families with various forms of open dual parentage.

The adoption process, including the decision, application, and final adoption, can be a stressful as well as joyful experience for many couples. During the preschool developmental phase, the family must acknowledge the adoption as a fact of family life. The question of the permanency of the relationship sometimes arises from both the child and the parents. Clark, Thigpen, and Yates' study (2006) of 11 families who reported having successfully integrated into their family unit at least one older/special needs adoptive child poignantly shows the process these families underwent. Parental perceptions that facilitated the successful process included finding strengths in the children overlooked by previous caregivers, viewing behavior in context, reframing negative behavior, and attributing improvement in behavior to parenting efforts.

In our clinical work with adoptive families, we have found it useful to consider many aspects of the adoption including:

1. Genetic, hereditary factors in the child

2. Deficiencies in the child's prenatal and perinatal care

3. Adverse circumstances of adoption, including the child's having had multiple disruptions in early life

4. Conditions in the adoptive home, including pre-existing and current family resiliencies, problems, and strengths

5. Temperamental similarities and differences between the adoptee and the adoptive parents or family

6. Fantasy system and communication regarding adoption, including parental attitudes about adoption

7. Difficulties establishing a firm sense of identity during adolescence

8. Greater age difference than usual between parents and adoptees

We believe that it is important in relational family nursing practice to recognize adoptive families' strengths and resources as they deal with challenging issues. During the adolescent stage of family development, a major task is to increase the flexibility of family boundaries. In adoptive families, altercations may give rise to threats of desertion or rejection. During the young adult or launching phase, the young adult may "adopt" the parents in a recontracting phase.

As the adopted child proceeds to develop his or her own family of procreation, the integration of the adoptee's biological progeny can be a developmental challenge for everyone. Adoptive parents may be delighted with the psychological and social continuity. Simultaneously, they may mourn the loss of biological grandchildren and the pain of genealogical discontinuity. For the adoptee, reproduction includes the thrill of a biological relationship and possibly some fears of the unknowns in their own genetic history.

We believe that nurses can play an important role in helping families navigate the complexities of the adoption process and life cycle. When complexity is accepted, when the losses are acknowledged and resolved, when parents and their children feel satisfied with adoption as a legitimate route to becoming a family, and when the community of family, friends, and professionals who surround them is affirming, then the outcomes for adoptive families are very positive.

Lesbian, Gay, Bisexual, Queer, Intersexed, Transgendered, Twin-Spirited Family Life Cycles

Until recently, popular culture has ignored LGBQITT people in couple or family relationships or has portrayed them as part of an invisible subculture. Much of what we see, read, and hear in the media and society at large express a patriarchal, Anglo-Saxon, white, Christian, male, middle-class, ableist, and heterosexual view of the world. More recently, with open discussion about same-sex marriage or union, more attention is being focused on these relationships, their structures, developmental life cycles, challenges, strengths, and issues. Long and Andrews (2007) point out that for same-sex couples, the family functions of formation and membership, nurturance and socialization, and protection of vulnerable members are particularly important. We believe that the popular family life cycle model does not apply to lesbians and gays because it is based on the notions that child-rearing is fundamental to family and that blood and legal ties constitute criteria for definition as a family.

Furthermore, the transmission of norms, rituals, folk wisdom, and values from generation to generation is not typically associated with lesbian and gay life. In many cases, the family of origin may not know what name to call their daughter's partner. For example, the term "girlfriend" doesn't connote the significance of the relationship.

We believe, however, that more differences exist *within* traditionally defined families than *between* LGBQITT families and those families designated as traditional. There are also many differing beliefs *within* diverse couples. For example, Shernoff (2006) points out—and we agree—that male couples need to negotiate their views on monogamy. For many clinicians, sexual nonexclusivity challenges fundamental beliefs. Our view of family life is socially constructed, as is the view held by each nurse. Managing multiple views of relationships is an important task for nurses working with families.

The stages of the traditional family life cycle can be applied to lesbians and gays, with some unique differences. During adolescence, which can be a tumultuous time for most families, gays and lesbians face similar identity and individuation tasks as heterosexuals but often without the support of such rituals as proms or "going steady." Parents frequently struggle more with parenting to "protect" than to "prepare" the young person to live in a homophobic social environment.

The stages of leaving home, single young adulthood, and coupling present challenges for the young person who needs to learn from the gay/lesbian world about dating and cannot rely on the family of origin for modeling in this area. Couch-surfing and seeking hospitality from friends' parents, LGBQITT-friendly shelters, and transitional living programs are examples of the living arrangement options for what some have called "throwaway" youth (i.e., LGBQITT youth in crisis). These are young people who have "come out" to their families and were then pushed out of the family home.

In discussing their homosexual relationship with their parents, many lesbian and gay couples have found it useful to focus on the strengths of their homosexual relationship. When parents see that the relationship has such strengths and can be beneficial for their son or daughter, they often adjust more easily. Dealing with the core issues of coupling—money, work, and sex—involves addressing gender scripts. Sample issues unique to parenting by lesbian and gay couples include the limited options available for getting pregnant by such means as artificial insemination owing to biases by fertility clinics, difficulties with health insurance, the reaction of the family of origin and relatives to the news about parenting, and the often blurred role of the nonbiological parent.

During mid and later life, the LGBQITT family continues to adapt and renegotiate with their families of origin. These relationships may be influenced by illness within either the aging family or the midlife chosen family. Intergenerational responsibility for caregiving and legacy issues may need to be addressed. We believe nurses engaged in relational practice can be helpful in providing a context for these conversations between family members.

We recommend an oppression-sensitive approach to working with LGBQITT families. This approach invites a stance of respectful curiosity for exploring domains of convergence and difference. For nurses working with these couples, some questions that might be useful to ask include:

- In what area do you feel privileged? Oppressed? How do you as a couple deal with these similarities and differences? How does the more privileged one respond to the other's sense of oppression?

- How does each member of the couple deal with heterosexism? With your families of origin? With the dominant gay culture?

- What are your strengths as a couple? How does spirituality influence your relationship?

We encourage nurses to avoid the alpha bias of exaggerating differences between groups of people and the beta bias of ignoring differences that do exist. In their privileged role working with families who are dealing with health issues, nurses can play a significant part in modeling inclusivity and respect for diversity.

In this CFAM developmental category, we have presented six sample types of family life cycles. Nursing is beginning to recognize the special characteristics of diverse family forms, such as lesbian and gay couples. We encourage nurses to broaden their perspectives when interacting with various family forms. What we do know is that great variety exists: the poor and homeless family, the lesbian or gay couple, the single parent, the adopted child with parent, the stepfamily, the divorced family, the separated family, the foster family, the nuclear family, the extended family, the household of children raising children without a parent present, and so forth.

FUNCTIONAL ASSESSMENT

The family functional assessment deals with how individuals *actually* behave in relation to one another. It is the here-and-now aspect of a family's life that is observed and that the family presents. There are two basic aspects of family functioning: instrumental and expressive. Each will be dealt with separately.

Instrumental Functioning

The instrumental aspect of family functioning refers to routine activities of daily living, such as eating, sleeping, preparing meals, giving injections, changing dressings, and so forth. For families with health problems, this area is particularly important. The instrumental activities of daily life are generally more numerous and more frequent and take on a greater significance because of a family member's illness. A quadriplegic, for example, requires assistance with almost every instrumental task. If a baby is attached to an apnea monitor, the parents almost always alter the manner in which they take care of instrumental tasks. For example, one parent will leave the apartment to do a load of wash only if the other parent is sufficiently awake to attend to the infant. If a senior family member is unable to distinguish what medication to take at a specific time, other family members often alter their daily routines to telephone or drop in on the senior.

The interaction between instrumental and psychosocial processes in clients' lives is an important consideration for nurses. For example, nurses can pay attention to a family's routines around eating and bedtime rituals and incorporate new health-care practices into the family's routine rather than "adding on" to the family's already busy schedule. Knafl and Deatrick (2006) have tried to develop an instrument to quantify family management style to assess the family's response to a child's chronic illness. This has proved to be a challenging task because families respond in unique ways. Much depends on how they view the situation and their active behavioral response to the illness. We recommend that health professionals understand that caregiving to a spouse who has cancer by an elderly spouse constitutes a major challenge in late-life adaptation. These spouses often rate the overall burden of caregiving as well as personal strain (the subjective component) as heavier than do their children and the cancer patients themselves. The importance of *family* nursing care is thus highlighted.

We believe nurses will find it useful to think of possible stages of health and illness together with family interaction. Friedman, Bowden, and Jones (2003) outlined six such stages: (1) family efforts at health promotion, (2) family appraisal of symptoms, (3) care seeking, (4) referral and obtaining care, (5) acute response to illness by client and family, and (6) adaptation to illness and recovery. The concept of time phases and stages has expanded, however, with predictive, presymtomatic, or carrier genetic testing to include the time before a genomic disease appears clinically. Phases before the clinical onset of genomic disease include the (1) nonsymptomatic/awareness phase, (2) crisis I pretesting phase, (3) crisis II test/postesting phase, and (4) long-term adaptation phase. Rolland and Williams (2005) point out that these stages are distinguished by questions of living with uncertainty.

As the nurse hypothesizes about the family's possible stage of health and illness and inquires into their ordinary routines of living alongside illness, the nurse and family will discover resiliencies and areas for possible assistance. Effective assistance consists of a series of events rather than single interactions. The trajectory of cardiac illness suggests that interventions may be most effective when provided during all stages of illness and may best be tailored to meet the specific needs of individuals and families in each stage.

Expressive Functioning

The expressive aspect of functioning refers to nine categories:

1. Emotional communication
2. Verbal communication
3. Nonverbal communication
4. Circular communication
5. Problem solving
6. Roles
7. Influence and power
8. Beliefs
9. Alliances and coalitions

These nine subcategories are derived in part from the Family Categories Schema developed by Epstein, Sigal, and Rakoff (1968) and later published by Epstein, Bishop, and Levin (1978). These categories were expanded by Tomm (1977) and later published by Tomm and Sanders (1983). Early work (Westley & Epstein, 1969) suggested that several of these categories distinguished emotionally healthy families from those that were experiencing more than the usual emotional distress. A more recent study by Aarons, et al. (2007) noted that the Family Assessment Device is less applicable for Hispanic Americans than for Caucasian Americans. They suggest, for example, that Hispanic American families often operate according to more stable hierarchical roles, more often encourage the avoidance of interpersonal conflict, and more often stress family collectivism compared to Caucasian American families. The importance of cultural variability is highlighted.

We have expanded on these works in our earlier editions of *Nurses and Families* to include nonverbal and circular communication, beliefs, and power. However, we do not use any of these categories as determinants of whether a family is emotionally healthy. Rather, it is the family's judgment of whether they are functioning well that is most salient. With the exception, of course, of issues such as violence and abuse, we encourage nurses to find ways to support the family's definition of health versus imposing their own definition on the family.

Before discussing each subcategory, we would like to point out that most families must deal with a combination of instrumental and expressive issues. For example, an older woman has a burn. The instrumental issues revolve around dressing changes and an exercise program. The expressive or affective issues might center on roles or problem solving. The family might be considering the following questions:

- Whose role is it to change Gram's dressing?
- Are women better "nurses" than men?
- Whose turn is it to call the physical therapist?
- Why is it that Jasdev never gets involved in Gram's care?
- How can we get Jasdev to drive Gram to her doctor's visit?

If a family is not coping well with instrumental issues, expressive issues almost always exist. However, a family can deal well with instrumental issues and still have expressive or emotional difficulties. Therefore, it is useful for the nurse and the family together to delineate the instrumental from the expressive issues. Both need to be explored when the nurse and family have a conversation about family functioning. Robinson (1998) points out the importance of nurses attending to what she calls "illness work" and "illness burden." Making arrangements for managing chronic or life-threatening illness does not just happen. The ordinary context of women generally shouldering the larger burden of housework than men do is the one in which additional illness arrangements are made.

Although both past behaviors and future goals are taken into consideration in the functional assessment, the primary focus is on the here and now. It is helpful for both the nurse and family to identify a family's strengths and limitations in each of the aforementioned subcategories. We find it helpful to remember that the very conversation the nurse and family have about the family system shapes that system. People continually and actively reauthor their lives and stories. Our commitment to families is to show curiosity, delight, interest, and appreciation for their resiliency. Naturally, this does not mean that we condone family violence or abuse. Rather, it means that we recognize that families are trying to make sense of their lives and stories. Our job is to witness this.

Patterns of interaction are the main thrust of the expressive part of the functional assessment category. Families are obviously composed of individuals, but the focus of a family assessment is less on the individual and more on the interaction *among* all of the individuals within the family. Thus, the family is viewed as a system of interacting members. In conducting this part of the family assessment, the nurse operates under the assumption that individuals are best understood within their immediate social context. The nurse conceives of the individual as defining and being defined by that context. Each individual's relationships with family members and other meaningful members of the larger social environment are thus very important. If we do not attend to ideas and practices at play in the larger social context, we run the risk of focusing too narrowly on small, rather tight, recursive feedback loops. We have found this to be especially important since we have witnessed September 11, random acts of terrorism, and mass slayings and we and families have struggled to adapt to a changed social and political context.

By interviewing family members together, the nurse can observe how they spontaneously interact with and influence each other. Furthermore, the nurse can ask questions about the impact family members have on one another and on the health problem. Reciprocally, the nurse can inquire about the impact of the health problem on the family. If the nurse thinks "interactionally" rather than "individually," each individual family member's behavior will not be considered in isolation but rather will be understood in context.

It is important for nurses to remember that, if they embrace a postmodernist worldview, they will not be able to conduct an objective family evaluation. Rather, the nurse and the family, in talking about the family's patterns of interacting, will bring forth a new story, rich in contextualized details. Particular attention is paid to the ways that even the small and the ordinary—single words, single gestures, minor asides, trivial actions—can provide opportunities for generating new meanings. Unlike modernist nurses who define themselves as separate from the family with whom they are working, nurses with postmodernist views assume that each participant in the family interview—wife, husband, partner, nurse—makes an equal and often different contribution to the process. It is the nurse's task to help family members engage in conversations to make sense of their lives rather than to explain their behavior.

Real-life clinical examples using the functional categories of CFAM are given in Chapters 4, 7, 8, 9, and 10.

Emotional Communication

This subcategory refers to the range and types of emotions or feelings that families express or the practitioner observes. Families generally express a wide spectrum of feelings, from happiness to sadness to anger, whereas families with difficulties commonly have quite rigid patterns within a narrow range of emotional expression. For example, some families experiencing difficulties almost always argue and rarely show affection. In other families, parents may express anger but children may not, or the family may have no difficulty with women expressing tenderness but feel that men are not permitted to express it.

Lyken (2006) suggests from his studies of middle-aged twins, both monozygotic and dizygotic, reared together and apart, that "the heritability of the set-point, or mean happiness level is about 80%" (p. 19). The feelings of subjective well-being, he asserts, are unrelated to socioeconomic status, income, levels of education, gender, or race. Rather, they are related to the genetic lottery and fortune's favors, good or bad. The influence of biology on emotional communication is an intriguing developing area and families will, no doubt, have many beliefs about this.

Questions to Ask the Family. Who in the family tends to start conversations about feelings? How can you tell when your dad is feeling happy? Angry? Sad? How about your mom? What effect does your anger have on your son Noah? What does your mom do when your dad is angry? If your grandmother were to express sadness about her upcoming chemotherapy to your parents, how do you think your parents would react? When your brother Hiesem was killed in the accident, what most helped your family to cope with the grief?

Verbal Communication

This subcategory focuses on the meaning of an oral (or written) message between those involved in the interaction. That is, the focus is on the meaning of the words in terms of the relationship.

Direct communication implies that the message is sent to the intended recipient. An elderly woman may be upset by what her husband is saying but corrects her grandson's inconsequential fidgeting with the comment, "Stop doing that to me." This could represent a displaced message, whereas the same statement directed at her husband would be considered direct.

Another way of looking at verbal communication is to distinguish between clear versus masked messages. In a clear message, there is a lack of distortion in the message. A father's statement to his child, "Children who cry when they get needles are babies," may be masked criticism if the child is fighting back tears at the time of his injection. The old child management strategy of "say what you mean and mean what you say" is a good guideline for clear, direct communication.

Questions to Ask the Family. Who among your family members is the most clear and direct when communicating verbally? When you state clearly to your young adult son that he has to pay rent to you, what effect does that have on him? When your teenagers talk directly to each other about the use of condoms, what do you notice? If your adolescents were to talk more with you and your husband about safer sex, what do you think your husband's reaction might be? What ways have you found for you and Manuel to have good, direct conversations? In person? On the cell phone? By e-mail? Through text messaging?

Nonverbal Communication

This subcategory focuses on the various nonverbal and paraverbal messages that family members communicate. Nonverbal messages include body posture (slumped, fidgeting, open, closed), eye contact (intense, minimal), touch (soft, rough), gestures, facial movements (grimaces, stares, yawns), and so forth. Personal space, the proximity or distance between family members, is also an important part of nonverbal communication. Paraverbal communication includes tonality, guttural sounds, crying, stammering, and so forth.

Nurses must remember that nonverbal communication is highly influenced by culture. For example, Lewinsohn and Werner (1997) suggest that, in Taiwanese-Chinese couples, indirect, nonverbal means of communicating and relating serve a positive function but are viewed among Euro-Caucasian groups in the United States as an indicator of intrusiveness or overinvolvement. Kaufman (2002) points out that gestures such as hand signs, shrugs, and posture shifts are specific to different cultures, noting that as many as 200 of these gestures may exist among all cultures.

Nurses should note the sequence of nonverbal messages as well as their timing. For example, when an older man starts to talk about his terminal illness and his adult daughter turns her head and casts her tear-filled eyes toward the floor, the nurse can infer that the daughter is sad about her father's impending death. Her sequence of nonverbal behavior is congruent with sadness and the topic of conversation. Note, however, that this behavior sequence may not necessarily be the most supportive for her father.

Nonverbal communication is closely linked to emotional communication. We encourage nurses to inquire about the meaning of nonverbal communication when it is inconsistent with verbal communication.

Questions to Ask the Family. Who in your family shows the most distress when your foster father is drinking? How does Sheldon show it? What does your foster mother do when your foster father is drinking? When your sister Seema turns her head and stares out the window as your stepfather is talking, what effect does it have on you? If your dad were to stop talking at the same time as your stepmother, would you think she might move closer to him?

Circular Communication

Circular communication refers to reciprocal communication between people (Watzlawick, Beavin, & Jackson, 1967). A pattern exists to most relationship issues. For example, a common circular pattern occurs when a wife feels angry and criticizes her husband; in return, the husband feels angry and avoids both the issues and her. The more he avoids, the angrier she becomes. The wife tends to see the problem only as her husband's, whereas the husband identifies the wife's criticism as the only problem. This type of pattern is often called the demand/withdraw pattern. The circularity of this pattern is the most important aspect in understanding interaction in dyads. Each person influences the behavior of the other. More information about this topic is available in Chapter 2.

Circular communication patterns can also be adaptive. For example, an older parent feels competent and negotiates well with the landlord; the adult son feels proud and praises his parent. The more reinforcement the adult son gives, the more confident and self-assured the senior feels. This pattern is diagrammed in Figure 3-18.

Circular pattern diagrams (CPDs) concretize and simplify repetitive sequences noted in a relationship. This method of diagramming interaction patterns, first developed by Tomm in 1980, may be applied to relationships between family members or between the nurse and the family. Because the nurse and the family also mutually influence each other, the nurse is encouraged to think interactionally about situations and offer the family an opportunity to think interactionally.

The simplest CPD includes two behaviors and two inferences of meaning. The inferences can be cognitive, affective, or both. Inferences about cognition refer to ideas, concepts, or beliefs, whereas inferences about affect refer to emotional states. Affect and/or cognition propels the behavior. Figure 3-19 illustrates the relationship between these elements. "The inference is entered inside the enclosure and represents some internal process (what is going on inside each interactant). The connecting arrows represent information conveyed from each person to the other through behavior. The circular linkage implies an interaction pattern that is repetitive, stable, and self-regulatory" (Tomm, 1980, p. 8). CPDs encourage a position of curiosity rather than a passion for particular values and a stand against others.

Although CPDs can be used to foster circular thinking, one must be mindful of their limitations. CPDs can tempt us to look within families for collaborative causation of problems. This may distract from personal responsibility for unacceptable behavior such as violence. Small, tight feedback loops may be highlighted and the "big picture" of the negative influence of particular values, institutions, and cultural practices may be forgotten. Another limitation of CPDs is that they may encourage nurses to believe that they are outside the family system. As a participant observer in

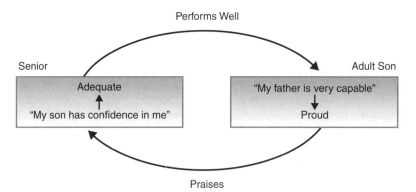

FIGURE 3-18: Adaptive circular pattern diagram.

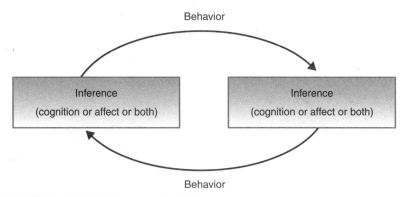

FIGURE 3-19: Basic elements of a CPD.

the larger system, the nurse is shown and hears about circular patterns reflecting family functioning. The interdependence of the nurse interviewer and family must be recognized. Both the nurse and family members cannot be decontextualized from their social and historical surroundings.

In what has come to be called the "feminist critique" of systems, several writers (Goldner, 1985; Ault-Rich', 1986) have taken exception to the simplistic causation ideas advanced by a circular perspective. CPDs, by virtue of their neutral context, ignore power differentials and imply a discourse or relationship between equals. These writers criticize circularity for not being transparent about responsibility and minimizing power differentials in relationships. Of particular concern are such issues as incest, abuse, violence, intimidation, and battering.

Despite these valid criticisms, we believe that it is still useful in clinical work with families to subscribe to the notion of circularity but simultaneously hold to the idea of personal responsibility. Fekete, et al. (2007) point out the importance of circularity in their study of 243 women experiencing lupus flare-ups and their husbands. They found that more spousal emotional (empathic) support was interpreted as the husband's being more emotionally responsive, which in turn was associated with the wife's greater sense of well-being. In contrast, more problematic (minimizing) spousal support was interpreted as the husband's being less emotionally responsive, which in turn was associated with the wife's poorer sense of well-being. These findings have large implications for helping couples adjust and cope with chronic illness.

An example of a circular argument is illustrated in Figure 3-20. Each party blames and threatens the other. An example of a supportive relationship is illustrated in Figure 3-21. The husband trusts his wife and reveals his needs and fears. She is concerned and, in turn, sustains and supports him. This leads him to trust her more, and the relationship progresses.

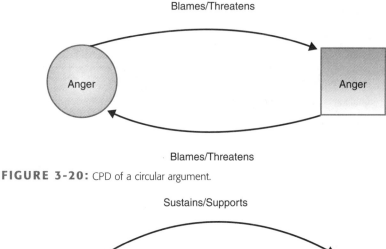

FIGURE 3-20: CPD of a circular argument.

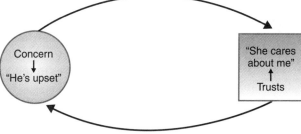

FIGURE 3-21: CPD of a supportive relationship.

Sample Conversation with the Family

Nurse: You say your wife "always" criticizes you. (Nurse conceptualizes Figure 3-22). What do you do then? (Nurse tries to fill in the husband's behavior in Figure 3-23.)

Husband: I don't like to discuss things. I avoid conflict. I leave. I go in the other room. What else can I do? She is always telling me what I did wrong. I go to the computer.

Nurse: So she expresses her needs and you leave. How do you think that makes her feel? (Nurse tries to fill in the inferred emotion in the wife's circle in Figure 3-24.)

Wife: I'll tell you. I get annoyed. I feel ignored, rejected.

Nurse: So you're annoyed when he leaves and ignores you. And then you become more critical. Is that right?

Wife: Well I don't really criticize, I just...

Husband: Yeah, you got it, nurse.

Nurse: So, when you try to express your concerns, how do you think it makes him feel? (Nurse tries to fill in the inference in the square in Figure 3-24.)

Criticizes

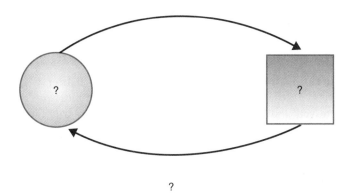

?

FIGURE 3-22: Beginning conceptualization of CPD.

Criticizes

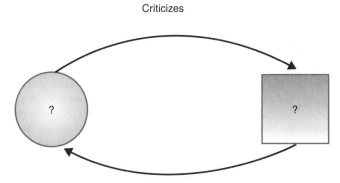

Avoids/Ignores

FIGURE 3-23: CPD illustrating husband's and wife's behaviors.

Criticizes

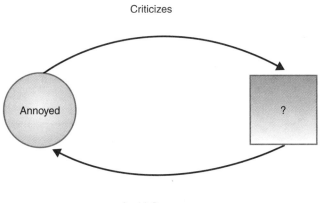

Avoids/Ignores

FIGURE 3-24: CPD illustrating wife's emotion.

Wife: I don't know.

Nurse: If he thinks you're lecturing and avoids the issues by leaving the room and going to the computer, what effect do you think your talking might be having on him?

Wife: Well, I suppose he could be feeling frustrated. He sulks.

Nurse: So the pattern seems to be that, no matter who starts it, the circle completes itself: Sometimes you're annoyed and you criticize. Your husband feels frustrated and ignores you. He sulks in the garage. Other times he avoids issues, and this arouses your frustration and criticism. (Nurse explains Figure 3-25.)

Wife: It's a vicious circle.

Husband: I don't want it to go on this way any more. We both get too upset.

Once the nurse has elicited a CPD, he or she should ask the family members to contextualize their discussion. One context might be that the wife is exhausted by her factory job and all the housework and childcare. The husband does not see why he should change his life because his wife has a stressful job and works long hours. They may engage in this particular negative circular interaction pattern every night while caring for their 3-year-old child with asthma.

Problem Solving

This subcategory refers to the family's ability to solve its own problems effectively. Family problem solving is strongly influenced by the family's beliefs about its abilities and past successes. How much influence the family believes it has on the problem or illness is useful to know. Who identifies the problems is important. Is it characteristically someone from outside the family or from inside the family?

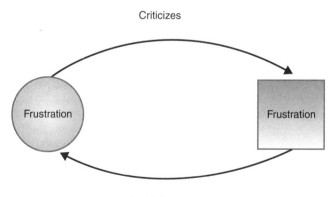

FIGURE 3-25: Nurse's conceptualization of this couple's communication pattern.

Once the problems are identified, are they mainly instrumental (routine, day-to-day logistics) or emotional problems? Families sometimes encounter difficulties when they identify an emotional problem as an instrumental one. For example, a mother who states that she cannot get her child who has food allergies to maintain the diet is really discussing an emotional issue rather than an instrumental one; she has difficulty influencing her child. As more families cope with issues such as childhood obesity, this is a particularly important distinction for nurses to notice. Is the obesity an instrumental or emotional problem? An individual, family, or societal problem?

What are the family's solution patterns? Are they proactive in planning for issues that might arise? For example, a couple dealing with the wife's myeloma might decide to harvest stem cells as a proactive measure. Many close-knit extended families rely on relatives for assistance in time of need. Others tend to seek help from professionals. Knowing a family's usual solution style can give the nurse insight into why this family may seem to be "stuck" at this particular time with this particular issue. For example, older parents move to a retirement community. The wife breaks her hip. The husband is used to being self-reliant or, in a pinch, depending on his middle-aged daughter. The older couple know few people in their new community. The husband is reluctant to accept help from the visiting nurse. He states that he can manage all his wife's care despite the fact that he is losing weight and getting insufficient rest. The husband's solution pattern conflicts with that of the nurse.

Knowledge of whether a family evaluates the cost of its solutions can be helpful to the nurse. For example, a 68-year-old grandmother tells Kiran, the nurse, "I can't afford to let myself cry about the death of my son's infant. I have to go on for the sake of my other children." Kiran was able to evaluate with the grandmother the cost of her solution pattern. Neither the grandmother nor the son discussed the infant's death with each other. The grandchildren's questions about why the baby did not come home from the hospital were left unanswered. There was considerable tension between the son and the grandmother, and the son was particularly overprotective with his 4-year-old boy (the only surviving male child). By gently exploring the cost of the solution (tension and overprotection), the nurse was able to suggest other solution patterns (e.g., shared grieving).

Questions to Ask the Family. Who first noticed the problem? Are you the one who usually notices such things? What most helped you to take the first step toward eliminating the addiction and violence pattern? What effect did it have when Toya also took steps to stop the cycle of violence in your family? How did the relationship between your son Jeremiah and your husband change when the violence stopped? When the addiction stopped? If a violent episode were to occur again, how do you think you and your daughter would deal with it? If his cocaine addiction were to flare up again, what steps would you take to protect your family?

Roles

This subcategory refers to the established patterns of behavior for family members. A role is consistent behavior in a particular situation. Roles, however, are not static but are developed through an individual's interactions with others. Roles are thus influenced by culture, race, and others' sanctions and norms. In Hispanic families, for example, *machismo* can be very significant for the hierarchical male role and *simpatia* or the avoidance of conflict and the ability to get along well is often highly valued. Haddock, Zimmerman, and Lyness (2003) point out that the idea that women have a life cycle apart from their roles as wife and mother is a relatively recent one and is still not widely accepted in our culture. The expectation for women has been that they would take care of the needs of others, first men, then children, then the older generation.

The psychological cost of providing care for a parent with Alzheimer's disease is often anxiety, depression, guilt, and resentment in the caregiver. The fact that women dominate as adult caregivers reflects a North American pattern. The gender differences clearly profile women's more frequent, intensive, affective involvement with the caregiver role.

Women's roles have changed in recent years and are now less defined by the men in their lives. The birth rate has fallen below replacement levels, and many more women are concentrating on jobs and education. Nevertheless, on average, women still make less than men do for the same job (Haddock, Zimmerman, & Lyness, 2003). In many cases, a husband's income is negatively related to role sharing and a wife's education is positively related to role sharing.

Although role change is increasingly prevalent for both men and women in today's society, what is important for nurses to assess is how family members cope with their roles. Does role conflict or cooperation exist? Are roles determined solely by age, rank order, or gender? Do additional criteria, such as social class and culture, influence roles? Are the women in the family more involved with a wider network of people for whom they feel responsible? Do the men hear less than the women in the family about stress in their family network?

Formal roles are those for which the community has broadly agreed on a norm. Examples include the roles of mother, husband, and friend. Informal roles refer to the established patterns of behavior that are idiosyncratic to particular individuals in certain settings. Examples include the roles of "bad kid," "angel," and "class clown." These serve a specific function in a particular family. If Dad is the "softie," most likely Mom is the "heavy." If Giffy is the "good daughter," Kweisi is probably the "black sheep." The roles of "parentified child," "good child," and "symptomatic child" have been identified in many families. Auxiliary roles of "child advocate," "analyst," "peacemaker," and "therapist" have also been described.

It is helpful for the nurse to learn how family roles evolved, their impact on family functioning, and whether the family believes they need to be altered. The findings from the study (Stein, Rotheram-Borus, & Lester, 2007) of adolescents whose parents had HIV/AIDS show that there can be positive effects to what typically might be perceived as a negative role of a "parentified adolescent." Early parentification predicted better adaptive coping skills and less alcohol and tobacco use 6 years later. The authors hypothesized that parentification skills were adaptive in the long run, especially with adolescents who had dying or ill parents, impoverished environments, and family instability.

It is important for nurses to conceptualize the functional assessment category of roles in a family-oriented rather than an individual-oriented way. According to Hoffman (1981):

> The individual-oriented approach badly misrepresents the subject. For instance, to speak of the "role of the scapegoat" is to present the deviant as a person with fixed characteristics rather than a person involved in a process. "Scapegoating" technically applies to only one stage of a shifting scenario—the stage where the person is metaphorically cast out of the village. After all, the term originates from an ancient Hebrew ritual in which a goat was turned loose in the desert after the sins of the people had been symbolically laid on its head. The deviant can begin like a hero and go out like a villain, or vice versa. There is a positive-negative continuum on which he can be rated depending on which stage of the deviation process we are looking at, which sequence the process follows, and the degree to which the social system is stressed.
>
> At the time, the character of the deviant may vary in another direction, depending on the way his particular group does its type-casting. Which symptoms crop up in members of a group is itself a kind of typecasting. Thus the deviant may appear in many guises: the mascot, the clown, the sad sack, the erratic genius, the black sheep, the wise guy, the saint, the idiot, the fool, the imposter, the malingerer, the boaster, the villain, and so on. Literature and folklore abound with such figures. (p. 58)

Questions to Ask the Family. To whom do most of you go when you need someone to talk to? What effect does it have on Maxine when Ken helps with the baby's care? When Maxine and Ken collaborate instead of competing, who would be the first to notice? If Ken were to be more responsible for initiating contact with the relatives around Cherie's day-care arrangements and baby sitting, how do you think Maxine would feel?

Influence and Power

This subcategory refers to behavior used by one person to affect another's behavior. Power is the ability of a person to regulate the criteria by which differing views of 'reality' are judged and resources apportioned. Power addresses hierarchical and egalitarian positions in relationships. In a hierarchical relationship, a person can be in a one-up or a one-down position in the relationship and can be dominant in one context and subordinate in another. In an egalitarian relationship, there is equality in the relationship. Silverstein, et al. (2006) describe a hierarchical position-directed relationship as "focussing on the needs of the dominant person, expecting the subordinate person to stifle own thoughts and feelings and know those of the dominant person, approaching decisions from a one-up/one-down position, and perceiving own needs in the context of what is good for the dominant person" (p. 394). In an egalitarian relationship, they describe a give-and-take negotiation of individual needs, goals, and desires with an expectation of reciprocal attunement to the needs of the relationship or each other.

Gender, race, and cultural issues are frequently intermingled with power issues. For example, in many relationships, women tend to raise issues and draw men out in the early phase of a discussion, whereas men tend to control the content and emotional depth of the later discussion phases and largely dominate the outcome. Shifts in power are preceded by changes in "reality," an expansion from a single perspective to a multiverse. We encourage nurses to adopt a postmodernist worldview because it offers useful ideas about how power and "truth" are socially constructed, constituted through language, organized, and maintained in families and larger cultural contexts.

A nurse who is unaware of power differences among family members, in terms of roles, gender, economics, or social class, can inadvertently encourage family members in positions of less power to accept goals that decrease their power and constrain their choices. Haddock, Zimmerman, and MacPhee (2000) suggest using the Power Equity Guide to discuss with family members areas of power and influence such as decision-making, work, life goals and activities, housework, finances, and sex.

Whether all family members contribute equally to problems and share responsibility for resolution is something that the nurse can pose for consideration. We believe that the most clinically useful stance to take with regard to the idea of power is to say, "Power is..." It can be used positively or negatively, overtly or covertly, to enhance or constrain options. Power relations exist among family members, their health-care providers, and institutions. McGoldrick, Gerson, and Petry (2008, p. 78) have depicted a negative power and control pyramid that includes eight levels and combines racism, heterosexism, and sexism:

1. "isolation, controlling whom she can see and when and where

2. sexual abuse, abusive touching, sexual acts against her will, having affairs, exposing her to HIV

3. using children, being abusive, controlling, guilt-inducing or under-responsible regarding visitation, etc.

4. physical abuse, hitting, shoving, choking, kicking, grabbing, etc.

5. economic abuse, controlling her financially, not sharing financial information or resources, challenging her every purchase

6. threats and intimidation, threatening to hurt her physically, to commit suicide, have an affair, divorce, report her to welfare, take away children or cut off her emotional support system, putting her in fear by looks, actions, destroying property, stalking, driving car too fast

7. using immigration status, using her undocumented status to threaten deportation, loss of children, job, healthcare, etc.

8. emotional abuse and use of male privilege, putting her down, name calling, making her think she's crazy, playing mind games, stonewalling, treating her like a servant, assuming right to make all major decisions or to neglect "2nd shift" home responsibilities such as housework and childcare."

Instrumental influence, power, or control refers to the use of objects or privileges (e.g., money; television watching; computer, car, or cellphone use; candy; vacations; and so forth) as reinforcers. Psychological influence or power refers to the use of communication and feelings to influence behavior. Examples include directives, praise, criticism, threats, and guilt induction. Corporal control refers to actual body contact, such as hugging, spanking, and so forth. It is important to note the positive and negative influences used in the family, especially with infants and seniors. Abuse of seniors by informal and sometimes formal caregivers is not infrequent.

We have found the most important positive predictors of compliance for children is consistency of enforcement of rules, encouragement of mature action, use of psychological rewards such as praise and approval, and play with the child. The most important negative one is the amount of physical punishment. The use of praise is positively related to success, whereas physical punishment and verbal, psychological punishment are constraining influences.

Questions to Ask the Family. Which of your parents is best at getting Nirmala to take her medication? When Delvecchio dominates the conversation, what effect does that have on Jamilett? What does your mother feel about how your stepfather disciplines your sister? If your stepfather were to be more positive with your sister Tiffany, how might his relationship with your mother change? Whose interests are most reflected in major decisions in the Veliz family? Who is more likely to accommodate to the other person, Gustavo or Fines?

Beliefs
This subcategory refers to fundamental attitudes, premises, values, and assumptions held by individuals and families. Beliefs are the blueprint from which people construct their lives and intermingle them with the lives of others. Families co-evolve an ecology of beliefs that arise from interactional, social, and cultural contexts (Wright & Bell, in press). When illness arises, our beliefs about health are challenged, threatened, or affirmed. During times of illness, nurses may assess patients', family members', or even their own beliefs to be constraining or facilitating. Constraining beliefs can enhance suffering and decrease solution options,

whereas facilitating beliefs can soften illness suffering and increase solution options to managing an illnesss (Wright & Bell, in press). Which illness beliefs are determined to be constraining or facilitating is determined by the clinical judgment of the nurse in collaboration with the family. Any healing transaction involves at least three sets of beliefs: those of the ill patient, those of other family members, and those of the nurse (Hougher Limacher & Wright, 2006; Moules, 1998; Moules, Thirsk, & Bell, 2006; Watson & Lee, 1993; Wright & Nagy, 1993; Wright & Simpson, 1991; Wright & Watson, 1988; Wright & Bell, in press). Cousins (1979) offered the poignant idea that what we believe is the most powerful option of all.

Beliefs and behavior are intricately connected. Every action and every choice that families and individuals make evolves from their beliefs. Consequently, beliefs shape the way in which families adapt to chronic and life-threatening illness. For example, if a family believes that the best treatment for colon cancer is a nontraditional approach, it makes good sense for the family to pursue acupuncture. Because North American culture tends to use a paradigm of control about symptoms (it is good to be in control and bad to be out of control), nurses might find it useful to explore family members' beliefs about control and mastery over their symptoms.

Beliefs are intricately intertwined with familial and socioeconomic contexts. The research of Corbet-Owen and Kruger (2001) found that the meaning pregnancy had for the women in their study not only determined the meaning of their pregnancy loss but also impacted their emotional needs at the time of the loss. For example, if a mother was very happy about being pregnant and felt devastated by her miscarriage, then her emotional needs would differ dramatically from those of another mother who didn't want to be pregnant and felt relieved by her miscarriage. Feelings about pregnancy loss ranged from feelings of devastation to relief.

In another example, a 51-year-old father of two teenage girls wrote to a nurse about his beliefs about his chronic pain:

> I think each person has a different threshold of pain. Every day I try to disassociate the pain…I try to "get into" my work and life. I am not always successful…but I try as hard as I can. The why, is because of my family, friends, and faith (gushy, eh?, but it's true). I think you have to find out what is important in your life and let it motivate you, as terrible as this will be to say, there are always thoughts of "ending it all"…but then you think about the sadness you would leave with the ones you love…it keeps you going. I really think the key is to find one important thing as a start, and let that be the fuel that keeps you motivated to do the things you would like to do. I wish there were more I could say…It's a day to day struggle.

Wright and Bell (in press) have suggested that the most relevant beliefs to explore with patients and their families are: beliefs about etiology, diagnosis, prognosis, healing, and treatment; spirituality and religion; mastery and control; role of family members; and role of health-care providers.

Box 3-3 provides a list of areas for nurses to explore when assessing family beliefs about the health problem.

Questions to Ask the Family. What do you believe is the cause of your sexual addiction? How much control do you believe your family has over chronic pain? How much control does chronic pain have over your family? What do you believe the effect, if any, would be on chronic pain if you and your wife agreed on treatment? Who do you believe is suffering the most in your family because of the changes in your family life due to your multiple sclerosis? What do you believe has been the most useful thing health professionals have offered to help you cope with your suffering from fibromyalgia? What has been the least helpful? Have any of your Buddhist beliefs helped you to cope with the tragic loss of your son?

Box 3-3 Beliefs about the Health Problem

A. Beliefs about:
   1. Diagnosis
   2. Etiology
   3. Prognosis
   4. Healing and treatment
   5. Mastery, control, and influence
   6. Religion and spirituality
   7. Place of illness in lives and relationships
   8. Role of family members
   9. Role of health-care professionals

B. Influence of the family on the health problem
   1. Resource utilization
      a. Internal (to family)
      b. External
   2. Medication and treatment

C. Influence of the health problem on the family
   1. Client response to the illness
   2. Family members' responses to illness
   3. Perceived difficulties and changes related to the health problem

D. Strengths related to the health problem at present

E. Concerns related to the health problem at present

Adapted from Family Nursing Unit records, Faculty of Nursing, University of Calgary, Calgary, Alberta.

Alliances and Coalitions

This subcategory focuses on the directionality, balance, and intensity of relationships between family members or between families and nurses. *Complementary* and *symmetrical* are terms used to describe a two-person relationship (see Chapter 2). A term commonly used to distinguish a three-person relationship is *triangle*, a term first coined by Bowen (1978). Bowen, a psychiatrist and family therapist, explains:

> The two-person relationship is unstable in that it has a low tolerance for anxiety and it is easily disturbed by emotional forces within the twosome and by relationship forces from outside the twosome. When anxiety increases, the emotional flow in a twosome intensifies and the relationship becomes uncomfortable. When the intensity reaches a certain level the twosome predictably and automatically involves a vulnerable third person in the emotional issue. The twosome might "reach out" and pull in the other person, the emotions might "overflow" to the third person, or the third person might be emotionally programmed to initiate the involvement. With involvement of the third person, the anxiety level decreases. It is as if the anxiety is diluted as it shifts from one to another of the three relationships in a triangle. The triangle is more stable and flexible than the twosome. It has a much higher tolerance of anxiety and is capable of handling a fair percentage of life stresses. (p. 400)

Most family relationships are organized around threesomes or triangles. Triangular alliances can be helpful or unhelpful. We have learned that, in families of combat veterans experiencing post-traumatic stress disorder, the veteran can sometimes become triangulated with a dead buddy without the spouse's knowledge. With soldiers returning from the Iraq or Afghanistan war, the ongoing impact of their military alliances may be a useful area for the nurse to explore if the family is having difficulty realigning as a unit. Restless days, fractured relationships, and vials of pills that help with some types of pain, but not all types, have commonly been reported by these families. Relationships are not unidirectional, even if one member of the triangle is an infant, an older person, or a person who has a handicap. The intensity of each relationship and the total amount of interaction is often fairly balanced. If one relationship becomes more intense, another one or two become less intense. Also, if one member of a threesome withdraws, the other two become closer.

We believe that it is important for the nurse to note the degree of flexibility and fluidity within the family as they adjust to new arrivals, death, or illness. Findings from the study conducted by Fivaz-Depeursinge and Favez (2006) on triangulation in infancy support this notion and offer ideas for intervention. For example, if the father acts intrusively while playing with his baby, the infant often averts and turns to the mother. The authors found that the regulation of this intrusion-avoidance pattern at the family level depends on the couple alliance. When co-parenting is supportive, the mother validates the infant's bid for help without interfering with the father. Thus, the problematic pattern is contained within the dyad of father–baby. If co-parenting is hostile/competitive, the mother ignores the infant's bid or engages with her in a way that interferes with her play with her father. In this case, triangulation occurs and tension is lessened, but at a cost. The nurse can identify these patterns with the couple and then collaborate with them to design effective interventions.

As nurses address this functional subcategory of alliances and coalitions, they will be aware of its interconnection with structural and developmental categories. The structural subcategory of boundaries is an important part of the alliance or coalition subcategory. The boundary defines who is part of the triangle and who is not. Of course, there are many triangles and many shifting alliances and coalitions within families. What is important for the nurse and family to note, therefore, is whether these are problematic or enriching.

Rolland (1999) offers an example of what can inadvertently occur in a family if a patient's illness is seen as "his problem" versus "our challenge." If the condition becomes defined as the affected patient's problem, a fundamental split occurs between the patient, well partner, and other family members. By introducing the concept of "our challenge" early on, the nurse "provides an opportunity for all family members to examine cultural and multigenerational beliefs about the rights and privileges of ill and well family members" (p. 258). An alternate example of a positive coalition is when family members join together to help another family member stop smoking or stop drinking alcohol. They collectively voice their concerns to the individual and their intent to provide support and help.

We have observed that cross-generational coalitions sometimes coincide with symptomatic behavior. Hoffman (1981) provided an excellent example of a pattern of shifting cross-generational triadic processes. The pattern focuses around the inappropriate behavior of a youngster:

> Stage one: Mother coaxes, child refuses to obey, mother threatens to tell father (father–mother against child). Stage two: when father comes home, mother tells him how bad child has been, and father sends child to his room without supper. Mother sneaks up after father has left the table and brings child a little food on a plate (mother–child against father). Stage three: when child comes down later, father, trying to make up, offers to play a game with him that mother has expressly forbidden because it gets him too excited before bedtime (father–child against mother). Stage four: mother scolds father for this; the child, overexcited indeed, has a tantrum and is sent to bed; and the original triangle comes round again (mother–father against child). (p. 32)

In addition to noting the connection between the structural subcategory of boundaries and the functional subcategory of alliances and coalitions, nurses should be aware of the interconnection with the developmental subcategory of attachments. Family attachments, or underlying emotional bonds that have an enduring or stable quality, are similar to alliances in that they are both unions. Attachments tend to differ from coalitions, however, in that the latter imply an alignment between two members with a third member being split off or opposed.

Questions to Ask the Family. When Demi and Tyson argue, who is most likely to get in the middle of the fight? If the children are playing very well together, who would most likely come along and *start* them fighting? Who would *stop* them from fighting? What impact has Don's brain tumor had on family members coming together or becoming further distanced?

CONCLUSIONS

The CFAM, although a very comprehensive and inclusive family assessment model, need not be overwhelming if viewed as a "map of the family" from the nurse's and the family's observer perspectives. The model provides a framework that can be drawn on as the nurse and the family discuss the issues. The nurse can use three main categories (structural, developmental, and functional) to obtain a macroassessment of family strengths and problems. Depending on his or her confidence and competence level, the nurse may also do a microassessment and explore in detail specific areas of family functioning. In either situation, the nurse needs to be able to draw together all relevant information into an integrated assessment. In doing this, the nurse synthesizes information and is not stymied by complexity. It is insufficient to focus on a family's difficulties with problem solving when the specific family structure is unknown. Also, if the nurse focuses too much on previous developmental history, the nurse may be ignoring important current functioning issues. Naturally, past history cannot be ignored. It should be integrated, however, only insofar as it helps to explain current functioning.

Once a thorough family assessment has been completed, the nurse and the family may now determine whether intervention is needed. However, we wish to emphasize that the completion of a family assessment utilizing CFAM does not mean that the nurse or the family now has the "truth" about the family's functioning related to a health problem or concern. Rather, the nurse and family members each have their own integrated assessment from their "observer perspectives."

References

Aarons, G.A., et al. (2007). Assessment of family functioning in Caucasian and Hispanic Americans: Reliability, validity, and factor structure of the Family Assessment Device. *Family Process, 46*(4), 557–569.

Ahrons, C.R. (1999). Divorce: An unscheduled family transition. In B. Carter & M. McGoldrick (Eds.), *The expanded family life cycle: Individual, family, and social perspectives* (3rd ed.) (pp. 381–98). Boston: Allyn & Bacon.

Ahrons, C.R. (2006). Long-term effects of divorce on children. *Family Therapy Magazine, 5*(1), 24–27.

Ahrons, C.R. (2007). Family ties after divorce: Long-term implications for children. *Family Process, 46*(1), 53–65.

Ahrons, C.R., & Rodgers, R.H. (1987). *Divorced families: A multidisciplinary developmental view.* New York: Norton.

American Academy of Pediatrics (2002). *Technical report: Coparent or second-parent adoption by same-sex parents.* http://www.aap.org/policy/020008t.html

Anderson, C.M. (2003). The diversity, strengths, and challenges of single-parent households. In F. Walsh (Ed.), *Normal family processes: growing diversity and complexity* (3rd ed.) (pp. 121–152). New York: Guilford Press.

Ault-Rich', M. (1986). A feminist critique of five schools of family therapy. *Family Therapy Collections, 16,* 1–15.

Baum, N. (2003). Divorce process variables and the co-parental relationship and parental role fulfilment of divorced parents. *Family Process, 42*(1), 117–131.

Baum, N. (2006). Postdivorce paternal disengagement: Failed mourning and role fusion. *Journal of Marital and Family Therapy, 32*(2), 245–254.

Becvar, D.S. (2001). *In the presence of grief: Helping family members resolve death, dying, and bereavement issues.* New York: Guilford Press.

Becvar, D.S. (2003). Introduction to the special section: Death, dying, and bereavement. *Journal of Marital and Family Therapy, 29*(4), 437–438.

Berger, R. (1998). *Stepfamilies: A multi-dimensional perspective.* New York: Haworth Press.

Boss, P.G. (2002). Ambiguous loss: Working with families of the missing. *Family Process, 41*(1), 14–17.

Bowen, M. (1978). *Family therapy in clinical practice.* Northvale, NJ: Jason Aronson.

Bowlby, J. (1977). The making and breaking of affectional bonds. *British Journal of Psychiatry, 130,* 201–210.

Bowse, B.P., et al. (2003). Death in the family and HIV risk-taking among intravenous drug users. *Family Process, 42*(2), 291–304.

Brown-Standridge, M.D., & Floyd, C.W. (2000). Healing bittersweet legacies: Revisiting contextual family therapy for grandparents raising grandchildren in crisis. *Journal of Marital and Family Therapy, 26*(2), 185–197.

Carter, B., & McGoldrick, M. (Eds.) (1988). *The changing family life cycle: A framework for family therapy* (2nd ed.). New York: Gardner Press.

Carter, B., & McGoldrick, M. (1999). The divorce cycle: A major variation in the American family life cycle. In B. Carter & M. McGoldrick (Eds.), *The expanded family life cycle: Individual, family, and social perspectives* (3rd ed.) (pp. 373–380). Boston: Allyn & Bacon.

Carter, B., & McGoldrick, M. (Eds.) (1999a). *The expanded family life cycle: Individual, family, and social perspectives* (3rd ed.). Boston: Allyn & Bacon.

Carter, B., & McGoldrick, M. (1999b). Overview: The expanded family life cycle: Individual, family, and social perspectives. In B. Carter & M. McGoldrick (Eds.), *The expanded family life cycle: Individual, family, and social perspectives* (3rd ed.) (pp. 1–26). Boston: Allyn & Bacon.

Clark, P., Thigpen, S. & Yates, A.M. (2006). Integrating the older/special needs adoptive child into the family. *Journal of Marital and Family Therapy, 32*(2), 181–194.

Clawson, J., & Ganong, L. (2002). Adult stepchildren's obligations to older stepparents. *Journal of Family Nursing, 8*(1), 50–72.

Connolly, M. (2006). Up front and personal: Confronting dynamics in the family group conference. *Family Process, 45*(3), 345–357.

Corbet-Owen, C., & Kruger, L. (2001). The health system and emotional care: Validating the many meanings of spontaneous pregnancy loss. *Families, Systems & Health, 19*(4), 411–427.

Cousins, N. (1979). *Anatomy of an illness as perceived by the patient: Reflections on healing and regeneration.* New York: Bantam Books.

Daily Almanac (November 22, 2007). *Marriages and divorces, 1900–2005, U.S statistics.* www.infoplease.com/ipa/A0005044.html accessed 11/22/07.

Dolbin-Macnab, M.L., & Rausch, D.T. (2006). Egg and sperm donors: The role of marriage and family therapists in third-party reproduction. *Family Therapy Magazine, 5*(1), 24–29.

Duhamel, F., & Campagna, L. (2000). *Family genograph.* Montreal: Universite de Montreal, Faculty of Nursing. Available from www.familynursingresources.com.

Duvall, E.R. (1977). *Marriage and family development* (5th ed.). Philadelphia: Lippincott.

Egan, J. (2002, March 24). The hidden lives of homeless children. *The New York Times Magazine,* Section 6, pp. 32–37, 58–59.

Epstein, H. (2003, October 12) Enough to make you sick? *The New York Times Magazine,* Section 6, pp.75–81.

Epstein, N., Bishop, D., & Levin, S. (1978). The McMaster model of family functioning. *Journal of Marriage and Family Counseling, 4,* 19–31.

Epstein, N., Sigal, J., & Rakoff, V. (1968). *Family categories schema* [Unpublished manuscript]. Jewish General Hospital, Department of Psychiatry, Montreal.

Erickson, E. (1963). *Childhood and society* (2nd ed.). New York: Norton.

Falicov, C. (2003). Immigrant family processes. In F. Walsh (Ed.), *Normal family processes: Growing diversity and complexity* (3rd ed.) (pp. 280–300). New York: Guilford Press.

Falicov, C.J. (2007). Working with transnational immigrants: Expanding meanings of family, community, and culture. *Family Process, 46,* 157–171.

Fein, E.B. (1998, October 24). Secrecy and stigma no longer clouding adoptions. *The New York Times,* Section 1, p. 1.

Fekete, E.M., et al. (2007). Couples' support provision during illness: The role of perceived emotional responsiveness. *Families, Systems & Health, 25*(2), 204–217.

Fields, J. (2003). *Children's living arrangements and characteristics: March 2002.* U.S. Census Bureau, P20–547.

Fields, J., & Casper, L.M. (2001). *America's families and living arrangements: Population characteristics.* U.S. Dept. of Commerce. U.S. Census Bureau, P20–537.

Fivaz-Depeursinge, E., & Favez, N. (2006). Exploring triangulation in infancy: Two contrasted cases. *Family Process, 45*(1), 3–18.

Fraenkel, P. (2006). Engaging families as experts: Collaborative family program development. *Family Process, 45*(2), 237–257.

Friedman, M.M., Bowden, V.R., & Jones, E.G. (2003). *Family nursing: Research, theory and practice* (5th ed.). Upper Saddle River, NJ: Prentice Hall.

Fruhauf, C.A., & Aberle, J.T. (2007). Women caring for partners with dementia: A contextual model. In *The therapist's notebook for family health care* (pp. 157–165). New York: Hawort Press.

Fulkerson, J.A., et al. (2007). Correlates of psychosocial well-being among overweight adolescents: The role of the family. *Journal of Consulting and Clinical Psychology,* 75(1), 181–186.

Furrow, J., & Palmer, G. (2007). EFFT and blended families: Building bonds from the inside out. *Journal of Systemic Therapies, 26*(4), 44–58.

Goldner, V. (1985). Feminism and family therapy. *Family Process, 24*(1), 31–47.

Greene, S.M., Anderson, E.R., Hetherington, E.M., Forgatch, M.S., & DeGarmo, D.S. (2003). Risk and resilience after divorce. In F. Walsh (Ed.), *Normal family processes. Growing diversity and complexity* (3rd ed.) (pp. 96–120). New York: Guilford Press.

Haddock, S.A., Zimmerman, T.S., & Lyness, K.P. (2003). Changing gender norms. In F. Walsh (Ed.), *Normal family processes: Growing diversity and complexity,* (3rd ed.) (pp. 301–336). New York: Guilford Press.

Haddock, S.A., Zimmerman, T.S., & MacPhee, D. (2000). The Power Equity Guide: Attending to gender in family therapy. *Journal of Marital and Family Therapy, 26*(2), 153–170.

Hagestad, G.O. (1988). Demographic change and the life course: Some emerging trends in the family realm. *Family Relations, 37,* 405–410.

Haglund, K. (2000). Parenting a second time around: An ethnography of African American grandmothers parenting grandchildren amid parental cocaine abuse. *Journal of Family Nursing, 6*(2), 120–135.

Haley, J. (1977). Toward a theory of pathological systems. In P. Watzlawick & J.H. Weakland (Eds.), *The interactional view.* New York: Norton.

Harburg, E., Kaciroti, N., & Gleiberman, L. (2008). Marital pair anger coping types may act as an entity to affect mortality: Preliminary findings from a prospective study. *Journal of Family Communication, 8*(1), 44–61.

Hardy, K.V. (1990). Much more than techniques needed in treating minorities. *Family Therapy News.*

Hartman, A. (1978). Diagrammatic assessment of family relationships. *Social Casework, 59,* 465–476.

Haskell, K. (2003, November 30). When grandparents step into the child care gap, money can be scarce. *The New York Times,* Section 1, p. 29.

Hawley, D.R., & DeHaan, L. (1996). Toward a definition of family resilience: Integrating life-span and family perspectives. *Family Process, 35*(3), 283–298.

Hill, M.R., & Thomas,V. (2002). Racial and gender identity development for black and white women in heterosexual partner relationships. *Journal of Couple and Relationship Therapy, 1*(4), 1–35.

Hiott, A., et al (2006). Gender differences in anxiety and depression among immigrant Latinos. *Families, Systems & Health, 24*(2), 137–146.

Hoff, A.L., et al (2005). An intervention to decrease uncertainty and distress among parents of children newly diagnosed with diabetes: A pilot study. *Families, Systems & Health, 23*(3), 329–342.

Hoffman, L. (1981). *Foundations of family therapy.* New York: Basic Books.

Hougher Limacher, L., & Wright, L.M. (2006) Exploring the therapeutic family intervention of commendations: Insights from research. *Journal of Family Nursing, 12*(3), 307–331.

Kaufman, M.T. (2002, September 8). Face it: Your looks are revealing. *New York Times,* Section IV, p. 3.

Kelly, J.B. (2007). Children's living arrangements following separation and divorce: Insights from empirical and clinical research. *Family Process, 46*(1), 35–52.

Knafl, K.A., & Deatrick, J.A. (2006). Family management style and the challenge of moving from conceptualization to measurement. *Journal of Oncology Nursing, 23*(1), 12–18.

LaSala, M.C. (2002). Walls and bridges: How coupled gay men and lesbians manage their intergenerational relationships. *Journal of Marital and Family Therapy, 28*(3), 327–339.

Levac, A.M.C., Wright, L.M., & Leahey, M. (2002). Children and families: Models for assessment and intervention. In J.A. Fox (Ed.), *Primary Health Care of Infants, Children, and Adolescents* (2nd ed.) (pp. 10–19). St. Louis: Mosby.

Lewinsohn, M.A., & Werner, P.D. (1997). Factors in Chinese marital process: Relationship to marital adjustment. *Family Process, 36*(1), 43–61.

Linville, D., & Lyness, A.P. (2007). Twenty American families' stories of adaptation: Adoption of children from Russian and Romanian institutions. *Journal of Marital and Family Therapy, 33*(1), 77–93.

Lonczak, H.S., et al (2007). Family structure and substance use among American Indian youth: A preliminary study. *Families, Systems & Health, 25*(1),10–22.

Long, J.K., & Andrews, B.V. (2007). Fostering strength and resiliency in same-sex couples: An overview. *Journal of Couple and Relationship Therapy, 6*(1/2), 153–165.

Lyken, D.T. (2006). The heritability of happiness. *Family Therapy Magazine, 5*(6), 18–21.

Maturana, H.R., & Varela, F. (1992). *The tree of knowledge: The biological roots of human understanding.* Boston: Shambhala Publications, Inc.

McGoldrick, M., & Carter, B. (2003). The family life cycle. In F. Walsh (Ed.), *Normal family processes: Growing diversity and complexity* (3rd. ed.) (pp. 375–398). New York: Guilford Press.

McGoldrick, M., Gerson, R., & Petry, S. (2008). *Genograms: assessment and intervention* (3rd ed.). New York, WW Norton & Company.

McNally, R.J., Bryant, R.A., & Ehlers, A. (2003). Does early psychological intervention promote recovery from posttraumatic stress? *Psychological Science in the Public Interest, 4*(2), 45–79.

Minuchin, S. (1974). *Families and family therapy.* Cambridge, MA: Harvard University Press.

Moules, N.J. (1998). Legitimizing grief: Challenging beliefs that constrain. *Journal of Family Nursing, 4*(2), 138–162.

Moules, N.J., Thirsk, L.M., & Bell, J.M. (2006). A Christmas without memories: Beliefs about grief and mothering—A clinical case analysis. *Journal of Family Nursing, 12*(4), 426–441.

Nolan, K.W., Orlando, M., & Liptak, G.S. (2007). Care coordination services for children with special health care needs: Are we family-centered yet? *Families, Systems & Health, 25*(3), 293–306.

Penn, M.J., with Zalesne, E.K. (2007). *Microtrends: The small forces behind tomorrow's big changes.* New York: 12, Hachette Book Group USA.

Perren, S., et al. (2005). Intergenerational transmission of marital quality across the transition to parenthood. *Family Process, 44*, 441–459.

Post, S., & Neimark, J. (2007). *Why good things happen to good people.* New York: Broadway Books.

Reitz, M., & Watson, K.W. (1992). *Adoption and the family system.* New York: Guilford Press.

Rempel, G.R., Neufeld, A., & Kushner, K.E. (2007). Interactive use of genograms and ecomaps in family caregiving research. *Journal of Family Nursing, 13*(4), 403–419.

Robinson, C.A. (1998). Women, families, chronic illness, and nursing interventions: From burden to balance. *Journal of Family Nursing, 4*(3), 271–290.

Rolland, J.S. (1999). Parental illness and disability: A family systems framework. *Journal of Family Therapy, 21*(3), 242–267.

Rolland, J.S., & Williams, J.K. (2005). Toward a biopsychosocial model for 21st century genetics. *Family Process, 44*, 1, 3–24.

Rovers, M.W. (2006). Overview of attachment theory: A continuous thread. *Family Therapy Magazine, 5*(5), 8–11.

Saluter, A.F., & Lugaila, T.A. (1998). *Marital status and living arrangements: March 1996.* U.S. Dept. of Commerce, U.S. Census Bureau, Current Population Reports, Population Characteristics, P20–496, pp. 1–6.

Samir, Y. (2002, October 27). I stand alone. *The New York Times Magazine,* Section 6, p. 98. Frameworks for Practice. Geneva: International Council of Nurses.

Schober, M., & Affara, F. (2001). *The family nurse: Frameworks for practice.* Geneva: International Council of Nurses.

Selvini-Palazzoli, M., et al. (1980). Hypothesizing circularity-neutrality: Three guidelines for the conductor of the session. *Family Process, 19*(3), 3–12.

Shernoff, M. (2006). Negotiated monogamy and male couples. *Family Process, 45*(4), 407–418.

Silverstein, R., et al. (2006). What does it mean to be relational? A framework for assessment and practice. *Family Process, 45*(4), 391–405.

Smith, K. (2000). *Who's minding the kids? Child care arrangements.* Fall 1995. U.S. Census Bureau, P70–70.

Stein, J.A., Rotheram-Borus, M., & Lester, P. (2007). Impact of parentification on long-term outcomes among children of parents with HIV/AIDS. *Family Process, 46*(3), 317–333.

Stepfamily Association of America. (2003). *Stepfamily facts.* Accessed online July 23, 2003, at www.saafamilies.org/faqs/index.htm.

Suarez-Orozco, C., Todorova, I.L., & Louie, J. (2002). Making up for lost time: The experience of separation and reunification among immigrant families. *Family Process, 41*(4), 625–643.

Suro, R. (1991). The new American family: Reality is wearing the pants. *The New York Times,* Section 4, p. 2.

Toman, W. (1976). *Family constellation: Its effects on personality and social behavior* (3rd ed.). New York: Springer.

Toman, W. (1988). Basics of family structure and sibling position. In M.D. Kahn & K.G. Lewis (Eds.), *Siblings in therapy: Life span and clinical issues* (pp. 46–65). New York: Norton.

Tomm, K. (1977). *Tripartite family assessment* [Unpublished manuscript]. University of Calgary, Alberta.

Tomm, K. (1980). Towards a cybernetic-systems approach to family therapy at the University of Calgary. In D.S. Freeman (Ed.), *Perspectives on family therapy* (pp. 3–18). Toronto: Butterworths.

Tomm, K., & Sanders, G. (1983). Family assessment in a problem oriented record. In J.C. Hansen & B.F. Keeney (Eds.), *Diagnosis and assessment in family therapy* (pp. 101–22). London: Aspen Systems Corporation.

Tubbs, C.Y., Roy, K.M., & Burton, L.M. (2005). Family ties: Constructing family time in low-income families. *Family Process, 44*(1), 77–91.

United States Census Bureau (2002). *Number of foreign-born up 57 percent since 1990, according to Census 2000.* U.S. Department of Commerce News, Washington, DC, CB02–CN.117.

United States Census Bureau (2007a). *African Americans by the numbers.* Daily Almanac. www.infoplease.com/spot/bhmcensus1.html accessed 11/22/07.

United States Census Bureau (2007b). *Hispanic Americans by the numbers.* Daily Almanac. www.infoplease.com/spot/hhmcensus1.html accessed 11/22/07

United States Census Bureau (2007c). *Median age at first marriage.* Daily Almanac. www.infoplease.com/ipa/A0005061.html accessed 11/22/ 07.

United States Census Bureau (2007d). *Percent never married.* Daily Almanac. www.infoplease.com/ipa/A0763219.html accessed 11/22/07.

USA Today. (2003, August 5). Gay marriage debate clouds real issue of equal treatment. *USA Today,* p. 10A.

Visher, E.B., Visher, J.S., & Pasley, K. (2003). Remarriage families and stepparenting. In F. Walsh (Ed.), *Normal family processes: Growing diversity and complexity* (3rd ed.) (pp. 153–175). New York: Guilford Press.

Walsh, F. (1999). Religion and spirituality: Wellsprings for healing and resilience. In F. Walsh (Ed.), *Spiritual resources in family therapy* (pp. 3–27). New York: Guilford Press.

Watson, W.L., & Lee, D. (1993). Is there life after suicide? The systemic belief approach for "survivors" of suicide. *Archives of Psychiatric Nursing, 7*(1), 37–43.

Watzlawick, P., Beavin, J.H., & Jackson, D.D. (1967). *Pragmatics of human communication: A study of interactional patterns, pathologies, and paradoxes.* New York: Norton.

Weingarten, K. (2000). Using the internet to build social support: Implications for well-being and hope. *Families, Systems & Health, 18*(2), 157–160.

Westley, W.A., & Epstein, N.B. (1969). *The silent majority: Families of emotionally healthy college students.* San Francisco: Jossey-Bass.

Wright, L.M. (2005). *Spirituality, suffering, and illness: Ideas for healing.* Philadelphia: F.A. Davis.

Wright, L.M., & Bell, J.M. (in press). *Beliefs and illness: A model to invite healing.* Calgary, AB: 4th Floor Press.

Wright, L.M., & Nagy, J. (1993). Death: The most troublesome family secret of all. In E. Imber-Black (Ed.), *Secrets in families and family therapy* (pp. 121–137). New York: Norton.

Wright, L.M., & Simpson, P. (1991). A systemic belief approach to epileptic seizures: A case of being spellbound. *Contemporary Family Therapy: An International Journal, 13*(2), 165–180.

Wright, L.M., & Watson, W.L. (1988). Systemic family therapy and family development. In C.J. Falicov (Ed.), *Family transitions: Continuity and change over the life cycle* (pp. 407–30). New York: Guilford Press.

Wright, L.M., Watson, W.L., & Bell, J.M. (1990). The family nursing unit: A unique integration of research, education, and clinical practice. In L.M. Wright & J.M. Bell (in press). *Beliefs and illness: A model for healing.* Calgary, AB: 4th Floor Press.

Chapter **4**

The Calgary Family
Intervention Model

The Calgary Family Intervention Model (CFIM) is a companion to the Calgary Family Assessment Model (CFAM) (see Chapter 3). To our knowledge, the CFIM is the first family intervention model to emerge within nursing. We also are not aware of any other intervention models that have been developed since we first introduced our model in the second edition of *Nurses and Families* in 1994. However, the importance and effectiveness of family interventions in health care in the treatment of physical illness seem to have received much more recognition in the last five years (Campbell, 2003). In addition, the focus of health-care providers has shifted from deficit- or dysfunction-based family assessments to strengths- and resiliency-based family interventions. For example, the McGill Model of Nursing states that one of its goals is to "help families use the strengths of the individual family members and of the family as a unit, as well as resources external to the family system" (Feeley & Gottlieb, 2000, p. 11). Another example is Rungreangkulkij and Gilliss' (2000) use of the Family Resiliency Model for the study of families that have a member with a severe and persistent mental illness.

The CFIM is a strengths- and resiliency-based model. We believe that this type of shift in emphasis from deficits and dysfunction to strengths and resiliency in family nursing practice greatly influences the types of interventions offered to and chosen by families within our model.

Of course, the interventions offered should depend on the nurse's scope of practice, degree of independence, autonomy, and responsibility associated with his or her role in family care (Schober & Affara, 2001). Nursing care may range from "delegated tasks such as wound care in the home, to complex assessment and curative management in health centres and clinics" (Schober & Affara, 2001, p. 23).

This chapter presents our definition and description of the CFIM, examples of interventions in three domains of family functioning, and actual clinical examples using the CFIM. This chapter concludes with intervention ideas for family situations that nurses commonly encounter.

DEFINITION AND DESCRIPTION

If a comprehensive family assessment has been completed and family intervention is indicated, a nurse must then consider how to intervene to facilitate change. The CFIM is an organizing framework for conceptualizing the intersection between a particular domain of family functioning and the specific intervention offered by the nurse (Fig. 4-1). The elements of the CFIM are interventions, domains of family functioning, and "fit" (i.e., effectiveness). The CFIM visually portrays the fit between a domain of family functioning and a nursing intervention; that is, it answers the question, "In what domain of family functioning does this intervention intend a change? Is it a fit for this family?" The CFIM focuses on promoting, improving, and sustaining effective family functioning in three domains or areas: cognitive, affective, and behavioral.

Interventions can be designed to promote, improve, or sustain family functioning in any or all of the three domains, but a change in one area can affect the other domains. We believe that the most profound and sustaining changes are the ones that occur within the family's beliefs (cognition). In other words, as a family thinks, so *is* it. In many cases, one intervention can actually simultaneously influence all three domains of family functioning.

We believe that nurses can only offer interventions to the family, not instruct, direct, demand, or insist on a particular kind of change or way of family functioning. Whether the family is open to an intervention depends on its genetic makeup and the family's history of interactions among family members and between family members and health professionals (Maturana & Varela, 1992). Openness to certain interventions is also profoundly influenced by the relationship between the nurse and the family (Bohn, Wright, & Moules, 2003; Duhamel & Talbot 2004; Leahey & Harper-Jaques, 1996; Houger Limacher & Wright, 2003, 2006; McLeod & Wright, 2008; Moules, 2002, Moules, et al. 2004, 2007; Robinson & Wright, 1995; Tapp, 2001; Thorne & Robinson, 1989) and the nurse's ability to help the family reflect on their health problems (Wright & Bell, in press; Wright & Levac, 1992). Second-order cybernetics and the biology of

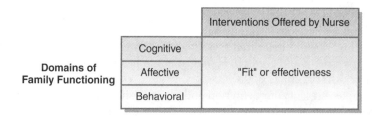

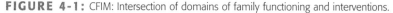

FIGURE 4-1: CFIM: Intersection of domains of family functioning and interventions.

cognition (Maturana & Varela, 1992) have influenced our ideas in this area (see Chapter 2).

Intervening in a family system in a manner that promotes or facilitates change and healing is the most challenging and exciting aspect of clinical work with families. The intervention process represents the core of clinical practice with families. It provides an appropriate context in which the family can make necessary changes that enhance the possibilities of healing. Myriad interventions are possible, but nurses need to tailor their interventions to each family and to the chosen domain of family functioning. An awareness of ethical considerations is necessary. Specific interventions usually vary for each family, although in some instances the same intervention may be used for several families and for different problems. We wish to emphasize, however, that each family is unique and that, although labeling particular interventions is an important part of putting our practice into language, it does not represent a "cookbook" approach. We also wish to emphasize that the interventions we list are examples of interventions that can be used; they are not intended to be all-inclusive. We provide examples of interventions that we have found from our clinical practice and research to be very useful. The interventions that we cite are based on several important theoretical foundations: postmodernism, systems theory, cybernetics, communication theory, change theory, and biology of cognition (see Chapter 2).

In summary, the CFIM is not a list of family functions or a list of nursing interventions. Rather, it provides a means to conceptualize a fit between domains or areas of family functioning and selected interventions offered by the nurse. The CFIM assists in determining the domain of family functioning that predominantly needs changing, usually where there is the greatest suffering, and the most useful intervention to effect change in that domain. Through therapeutic conversations, the family and nurse collaborate and co-evolve to discover the most useful fit (Duhamel & Dupuis, 2004; Holtslander, 2005; McLeod & Wright, 2008; Moules, et al. 2004, 2007; Wright & Bell, in press). We use the qualitative term *fit* because we emphasize whether or not the interventions effect change and/or soften suffering in the presenting problem. Fit involves recognition of reciprocity between the nurse's ideas and opinions and the family's illness experience. Therefore, determining fit may involve some experimentation or trial and error. It also entails a belief by nurses that each family is unique and has particular strengths. In Chapter 7, we outline techniques for enhancing the likelihood that interventions will stimulate change in the desired domain of family functioning.

INTERVENTIVE QUESTIONS

One of the simplest but most powerful nursing interventions for families experiencing health problems is the use of interventive questions. Interventive questions are intended to actively effect change in any or all of the three domains. Nurses conducting family interviews should remember, however, that knowing when, how, and why to pose questions is more important than simply choosing one type of question over another (Wright & Bell, in press).

Linear Versus Circular Questions

Interventive questions are usually of two types: linear and circular (Tomm, 1987, 1988). The important difference between these kinds of questions is their intent. Linear questions are meant to inform the nurse, whereas circular questions are meant to effect change (Tomm, 1985, 1987, 1988).

Linear questions are investigative; they explore a family member's descriptions or perceptions of a problem. For example, when exploring parents' perceptions of their daughter Cheyenne's anorexia nervosa, the nurse could begin with linear questions, such as, "When did you notice that your daughter had changed her eating habits?" or, "What do you think caused your daughter to stop eating as she normally would?" These linear questions not only inform the nurse of the history of the young woman's eating patterns but also help to illuminate family perceptions or beliefs about eating patterns. Linear questions are frequently used to begin gathering information about families' problems, whereas circular questions reveal families' understanding of problems.

Circular questions aim to reveal explanations of problems. For example, with the same family, the nurse could ask, "Who in the family is most worried about Cheyenne's anorexia?" or "How does Mother show that she is the one who worries the most?" Circular questions help the nurse to discover valuable information because they seek out information about relationships between individuals, events, ideas, or beliefs.

The effect of these different question types on families is quite distinct. Linear questions tend to be constraining to any further understanding whereas circular questions are generative and open possibilities for new understandings. Circular questions introduce new cognitive connections or a change in the illness beliefs of families, paving the way for new or different family behaviors. Linear questioning implies that the nurse knows what is best for the family and therefore operating under the "sin of certainty" or objectivity without parentheses (Maturana & Varela, 1992) (see Chapter 2). It also implies that the nurse has become purposive and invested in a particular outcome. Linear questions are intended to correct behavior; circular questions are intended to facilitate behavioral change.

The primary distinction between circular and linear questions lies in the notion that information reveals differences in relationships (Bateson, 1979). With circular questions, a relationship or connection between individuals, events, ideas, or beliefs is always sought and in a context of compassion and curiosity. With linear questions, the focus is on cause and effect. The idea of circular questions evolved from the concept of circularity, and the method of circular interviewing developed by the originators of Milan Systemic Family Therapy (Selvini-Palazzoli, et al. 1980; Tomm, 1984, 1985, 1987) (see Chapters 6 and 7).

Circularity involves the cycle of questions and answers between families and nurses that occurs during the interview process. The nurse's skillful questions are based on thoughtful assessment, conceptualization, and hypotheses that can foster understanding and obtaining information that the family gives in response to the questions the nurse asks, and thus the cycle continues. The family's responses to questions provide information for the nurse and the family. Questions in and of themselves can also provide new information and answers for the family; thus, they become interventions. Interventive questions may encourage family members to see their problems in a new way and subsequently to soften their suffering and see new solutions. Thus, as the family's answers provide information for the nurse, the nurse's questions may provide information for the family.

Circular questions have various applications in family nursing. Loos and Bell (1990) creatively applied the use of circular questions to critical care nursing. Wright and Bell (in press) demonstrated the therapeutic aspect of circular questions with families experiencing chronic illness, life-threatening illness, and psychosocial problems. Utilizing the CFIM, Duhamel and Talbot (2004) found that nurses considered interventive questioning useful because it stimulated discussion on specific topics. "One of the questions was formulated as 'What were the most significant changes that occurred in the family since the onset of the illness?' This question led to the identification of efforts made by the couples to comply with medical recommendations, and of their progress in the rehabilitation process" (Duhamel & Talbot, 2004, p. 23).

Tomm (1987) embellished the types of circular questions used by the Milan Systemic Family Therapy team and identified, defined, and classified various circular questions. The ones we have found most useful in relational clinical practice with families are difference questions, behavioral effect questions, and hypothetical or future-oriented question. We have expanded the use of circular questions by providing examples of questions that can be asked to intervene in the cognitive, affective, and behavioral domains of family functioning.

The question types, definitions, and examples are given in Table 4–1.

We have also written and produced a DVD to demonstrate the use of questions in actual clinical practice as part of The *"How to" Family Nursing Series*. It is titled *How to Use Questions in Family Interviewing* (Wright & Leahey, 2006). In addition, we have also written and produced four other DVDs in The *"How to" Family Nursing Series: How to Intervene with Families with Health Concerns* (Wright & Leahey, 2003); *How To Do A 15 Minute (Or Less) Family Interview* (Wright & Leahey, 2000); *Family Nursing Interviewing Skills: How to Engage, Assess, Intervene, and Terminate With Families* (Wright & Leahey, 2002); and *Calgary Family Assessment Model: How to Apply in Clinical Practice* (Wright & Leahey, 2001). These educational programs demonstrate the use of interventive questions in actual

Table 4-1	Circular Questions to Invite Change in Cognitive, Affective, and Behavioral Domains of Family Functioning

1. TYPE: DIFFERENCE QUESTION

Definition: Explores differences between people, relationships, time, ideas, or beliefs.
Examples of intervening in three domains of family functioning:

COGNITIVE	AFFECTIVE	BEHAVIORAL
• What is the best advice that you have received about managing your son's AIDS? • What is the worst advice?	• Who in the family is most worried about how AIDS is transmitted?	• Who in the family is best at getting your son to take his medication on time?
• What information would be most helpful to you about managing the effects of sexual abuse? • Who in the family would benefit most from the information?	• Who finds your disclosure of sexual abuse most difficult?	• When you first disclosed your sexual abuse, what actions by professionals were most helpful?

2. TYPE: BEHAVIORAL EFFECT QUESTION

Definition: Explores the effect of one family member's behavior on another.
Examples of intervening in three domains of family functioning:

COGNITIVE	AFFECTIVE	BEHAVIORAL
• How do you make sense of your husband not visiting your son in the hospital?	• What do you feel when you see your son crying after his treatments?	• What do you do when your husband does not visit your son in the hospital?
• What do you know about the effect of life-threatening illness on children?	• How does your mother show that she is afraid of dying?	• What could your father do to indicate to your mother that he understands her fears?

3. TYPE: HYPOTHETICAL/FUTURE-ORIENTED QUESTION

Definition: Explores family options and alternative actions or meanings in the future.
Examples of intervening in three domains of family functioning:

COGNITIVE	AFFECTIVE	BEHAVIORAL
• What do you think will happen if these skin grafts continue to be so painful for your son?	• If your son's skin grafts are not successful, what do you think his mood will be? Sad? Angry? Resigned?	• How much longer do you think it will be before your son engages in treatment for his contractures?
• If the worst occurs, how do you think your family will cope? • If you decide to have your grandmother institutionalized, with whom would you discuss the decision?	• If your grandmother's treatment does not go well, who will be most affected?	• How long do you think your grandmother will have to remain in the hospital? • If she stays longer, what new self-care behaviors will she be doing?

clinical interviews. To learn more about these DVDs or to view a sample video clip, visit www.familynursingresources.com.

In summary, difference questions, behavioral effect questions, and hypothetical questions can be used to facilitate change in any or all of the domains of family functioning. Figure 4-2 illustrates the intersection of various types of circular questions and the domains of family functioning. We wish to strongly emphasize that the effectiveness, usefulness, and fit of the question, rather than the specific question itself, are most critical in effecting change.

Other Examples of Interventions

To illustrate the intersection of the three domains or areas of family functioning (cognitive, affective, and behavioral) and various interventions, we have chosen a few examples of interventions that can be used in addition to circular questions. This list is not meant to be exhaustive; rather, it is a selection of interventions that we have found useful and effective in our own clinical practice and research. Examples include:

- Commending family and individual strengths
- Offering information and opinions
- Validating or normalizing emotional responses
- Encouraging the telling of illness narratives
- Drawing forth family support
- Encouraging family members to be caregivers and offering caregiver support
- Encouraging respite
- Devising rituals

These interventions can influence change in any or all of the domains of family functioning. For example, the nurse can offer information to promote change in cognitive, affective, or behavioral family functioning (Fig. 4-3).

		Interventions Offered by Nurse: Circular Questions			
		Difference	Behavioral Effect	Hypothetical	Triadic
	Cognitive				
Domains of Family Functioning	Affective				
	Behavioral				

FIGURE 4-2: Intersection of circular questions and domains of family functioning.

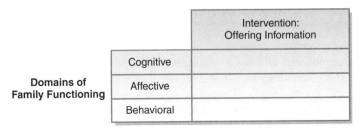

FIGURE 4-3: Intersection of intervention (offering information) and domains of family functioning.

The following section describes each intervention and offers a case example illustrating its application. We have chosen to cluster the sample interventions around a particular domain of family functioning. In doing this, we do not wish to imply that one intervention can be used to facilitate change in only one domain of family functioning or that one intervention is a "cognitive intervention" and another an "affective intervention." Rather, these are examples of the fit between a specific problem or illness, a particular intervention, and a domain of family functioning.

INTERVENTIONS TO CHANGE THE COGNITIVE DOMAIN OF FAMILY FUNCTIONING

Interventions directed at the cognitive domain of family functioning usually offer new ideas, opinions, beliefs, information, or education on a particular health problem or risk. The treatment goal or desired outcome is to change the way in which a particular family perceives its health problems so that members can discover new solutions to these problems. The following interventions are examples of ways to change the cognitive domain of family functioning.

Commending Family and Individual Strengths

We routinely commend family and individual strengths, competencies, and resources observed during interviews. Commendations differ from compliments. A commendation is an observation of patterns of behavior that occur across time (e.g., "Your family members are very loyal to one another."), whereas a compliment is usually an observation of a one-time event (e.g., "You were very praising of your son today."). Families coping with chronic, life-threatening, or psychosocial problems commonly feel defeated, hopeless, or unsuccessful in their efforts to overcome or live with these problems. In many cases, families coping with health problems have not been commended for their strengths or made aware of them (McElheran & Harper-Jaques, 1994). We choose to emphasize strengths and resilience rather than deficits, dysfunctions, and deficiencies in family members.

Immediate and long-term positive reactions to commendations indicate that they are effective therapeutic interventions (Bohn, Wright, & Moules,

2003; Houger Limacher & Wright, 2003, 2006; McLeod & Wright, 2008; Moules, 2002; Wright & Bell, in press). Robinson (1998) offers further credence to this belief with her study that explored the processes and outcomes of nursing interventions with families suffering with chronic illness. The families in this study reported the clinical nursing team's "orientation to strengths, resources, and possibilities to be an extremely important facet of the process" (Robinson, 1998, p. 284). Perhaps surprisingly, focusing on strengths was most significant and influential for the women in these families. In addition, families who internalize commendations offered by nurses appear more receptive to other therapeutic interventions that are offered.

Another fluent and moving piece of research focused on the commendation interventions offered in practice at the Family Nursing Unit of the University of Calgary. A key uncovering both families and nurses reported and reiterated the value and power of commendations that brought forth "goodness" that helped alleviate suffering (Houger Limacher & Wright, 2003, 2006). This bringing forth of "goodness" becomes a relational phenomenon in the context of the nurse–patient and nurse–family relationship. The routine practice by nurses of commending family and individual strengths is a particular way of being in clinical practice. This notion is best exemplified in the following quote: "We become our conversations and we generate the conversations that we become" (Maturana & Varela, 1992).

In one family, an adopted son's behavioral and emotional problems had kept the family involved with health-care professionals for 10 years. The nurse commended this family by telling them that she believed they were the best family for this boy because many other families would not have been as sensitive to his needs and probably would have given up years ago. Both parents became tearful and said that this was the first positive statement made to them as parents in many years.

By commending a family's competence, resilience, and strengths and offering them a new opinion or view of themselves, a context for change is created that allows families to then discover their own solutions to problems and enhance healing. Changing the view families have of themselves frequently enables families to view the health problem differently and thus move toward solutions that are more effective. Box 4-1 suggests helpful hints for offering interventions.

Offering Information and Opinions

The offering of information and opinions from health-care professionals is one of the most significant needs for families experiencing illness, especially if the illness is complex. Families most desire information about developmental issues, health promotion, and illness management (Levac, Wright, & Leahey, 2002; Robinson, 1998). For example, helping parents to understand and help their children is a common but important intervention for families (Levac, Wright, & Leahey, 2002). Nurses can teach families about

---

Box 4-1 Helpful Hints for Offering Commendations

- Be a "family strengths" detective and look for opportunities to commend families when strengths are discovered and uncovered.
- Ensure that sufficient evidence for the commendation is present; otherwise it may sound insincere and overly ingratiating.
- Use the family's language and integrate important family beliefs to strengthen the validity of the commendation.
- Offer commendations within the first 10 minutes of meeting with a family to enhance the practitioner–family relationship and to increase family receptivity to later ideas.
- Routinely include commendations to families at the end of an interaction or meeting and before offering an opinion.

From Levac, A.M., Wright, L.M., & Leahey, M. (2002). Children and families: Models for assessment and intervention. In J. Fox (Ed.), *Primary health care of infants, children, and adolescents* (2nd ed.) (p. 13). St. Louis: Mosby, reprinted by permission.

normal physiological, emotional, and cognitive characteristics as well as identify developmental tasks or goals of children and adolescents that can be affected or altered during times of illness (Manassis & Levac, 2004). One family found it useful when the nurse explained that siblings of children experiencing life-shortening illnesses commonly develop symptoms as a result of feelings of loneliness because parents are intently focused on their ill child. Box 4-2 suggests helpful hints for offering information and opinions.

Families with a hospitalized member have indicated that obtaining information is a high priority. Many families have expressed to us their frustration at their inability to readily obtain information or opinions from health-care professionals. Nurses can offer information about the impact of chronic or life-shortening illnesses on families. They can also empower families to obtain information about resources. We have learned that this latter approach is even more useful in some circumstances. Offering educational information has been found to be an "essential intervention as it reassured family members about certain aspects of the illness and reduced their level of stress" (Duhamel & Talbot, 2004, p. 24).

One complex clinical example concerns a family of two aging parents and their 34-year-old son, who had severe multiple sclerosis. The parents were constant, devoted caregivers but had not had any respite for several months. The nurse asked the son if he would be willing to challenge his beliefs about his "helplessness." The nurse asked him to take the leadership role in exploring possible resources for caregivers so that his parents could have a vacation. Because of his search, the son discovered that he was eligible for many financial benefits of which he had previously been unaware, including benefits to hire professional caregivers. Shortly afterward,

Box 4-2 Helpful Hints for Offering Information and Opinions

- Use language that is relevant, clear, and specific.
- Provide easy-to-read literature; write out key points on a small card.
- Inform families of community support groups and resources. Determine if these resources have been helpful to families who have used them and how.
- Build on family abilities by encouraging family members to independently seek resources. Inquire about the family's reaction after seeking resources.
- Offer ideas, information, and reflections in a spirit of learning and wondering (for example, "I wonder what would happen if you tried a slightly different approach to talking with Manisha about sex and birth control. Perhaps you might...").
- Do not be invested in the outcome. If the family does not apply the teaching materials, be curious about what did not fit for them rather than becoming judgmental and angry with the family.

From Levac, A.M.C., Wright, L.M., & Leahey, M. (2002). Children and families: Models for assessment and intervention. In J. Fox (Ed.), *Primary health care of infants, children, and adolescents* (2nd ed.) (p. 13). St. Louis: Mosby, reprinted by permission.

the son arranged for 24-hour in-home nursing care when his parents took a vacation. His parents reported that they felt much less stressed and that their son was much happier. He began making efforts to walk using parallel bars, which he had not done in several months.

In this case example, the nurse offered an opinion that empowered the son to change his cognitive set. The intervention fit the cognitive domain and results took place in the affective and behavioral domains of family functioning.

INTERVENTIONS TO CHANGE THE AFFECTIVE DOMAIN OF FAMILY FUNCTIONING

Interventions aimed at the affective domain of family functioning are designed to reduce or increase intense emotions that may be blocking families' problem-solving efforts. The following interventions are examples of ways to change the affective domain of family functioning.

Validating or Normalizing Emotional Responses

Validation of intense affect can reduce or cushion feelings of isolation and loneliness and help family members to make the connection between a family member's illness and their emotional response. For example, after diagnosis of a life-shortening illness, families frequently feel out of control or frightened for a period. It is important for nurses to validate these strong emotions and to reassure and offer hope to families that in time they will adjust and learn new ways to cope. In one clinical example, the nurse normalized changes in sexuality following a couple's experience with a cardiac condition. As a result, the wife reported, "I felt that the question regarding our sexuality was well put, because [the nurse] applied it to couples in general. The fact that others are going through the same experience, well I thought it was good to know. It is a very personal and private question, and you presented it well" (Duhamel & Talbot, 2004, p. 25).

Encouraging the Telling of Illness Narratives

Too often, family members are encouraged to tell only the medical story or narrative of their illness rather than the story of their own unique experience of their illness, or *illness narrative*. However, when nurses encourage family members to tell their illness narratives, not only are stories of sickness and suffering told but also stories of strength and tenacity (Wright & Bell, in press). Through therapeutic conversations, nurses can create a trusting environment for open expression of family members' fears, anger, and sadness about their illness experience (Tapp, 2001; Wright & Bell, in press). These conversations are particularly important for complex family types involving multiple parents and siblings. Having an opportunity to express the impact of the illness on the family and the influence of the family on the illness from each family member's perspective validates their experiences. Duhamel and Talbot's (2004) study, which utilized the CFIM and this particular intervention, found that nurses agreed about the importance of encouraging family members to share their experiences of cardiac illness during and after the hospitalization period. Also, family members commented that through these types of clinical sessions, they were able to vent emotions, which provided tremendous relief from suffering, healed psychological wounds, and enabled family members to acknowledge one another's experiences.

Listening to, witnessing, and documenting illness stories can also have a profound impact on the nurse. This approach is very different from limiting or constraining family stories to symptoms, medication use, and physical treatments. By providing a context for family members to share the illness experience, nurses allow intense emotions to be legitimized.

Drawing Forth Family Support

Nurses can enhance family functioning in the affective domain by encouraging and helping family members to listen to each other's concerns and feelings. This technique can be particularly useful if a family member is embracing some constraining beliefs when a loved one is dying or has died (Moules et al, 2004, 2007; Wright & Nagy, 1993). Through fostering opportunities for family members to express feelings about this painful experience, the nurse can enable the family to draw forth their own strengths and resources to support one another. The nurse can be the catalyst that facilitates communication between family members or between the family and other health-care professionals. This type of family support can prevent families from becoming unduly burdened or defeated by an illness. Intervening in this manner is especially important in primary health-care settings.

INTERVENTIONS TO CHANGE THE BEHAVIORAL DOMAIN OF FAMILY FUNCTIONING

Interventions directed at the behavioral domain help family members to interact with and behave differently in relation to one another. This change is most often accomplished by inviting some or all family members to engage in specific behavioral tasks. Some tasks are given during a family meeting so that the nurse can observe the interaction; other tasks or homework assignments are given for family members to complete between sessions. In some cases, the nurse must review with the family the details of the particular task or experiment in order to verify that the family understands what has been suggested. The following interventions are examples of ways to change the behavioral domain of family functioning.

Encouraging Family Members to be Caregivers and Offering Caregiver Support

Family members are often timid or afraid to become involved in the care of their ill family member unless a nurse supports them. However, in our experience, we have found that family members greatly appreciate opportunities to help their hospitalized family member. They report that it makes them feel less helpless, anxious, and out of control. Of course, family caregivers are also susceptible to the well-known phenomenon of caregiver burden. Health professionals must be alert to the risks involved in family caregiving and be willing to intervene when necessary by offering caregiver support. Caregiver support can be defined as a provision of the necessary information, advocacy, and support to facilitate primary patient care by people other than health-care professionals. LeNavenec and Vonhof (1996) offer the notion of "one day at a time" as a useful coping strategy for families with a member experiencing dementia. We encourage nurses to weigh with family members the ethical balance between too much caregiving and not enough caregiving.

Encouraging Respite

Family caregivers commonly do not allow themselves adequate respite. Too frequently, family members feel guilty if they need or want to withdraw themselves from the caregiving role. Even the ill member must occasionally disengage himself or herself from the usual caregiving and reject another person's assistance. Each family's need for respite varies. Factors affecting respite include the severity of the chronic illness, availability of family members to care for the ill person, and financial resources. All of these issues must be considered before a nurse can recommend a respite schedule. Caregiving, coping, and caring for one's own health need to be balanced.

One example of a way to balance needs is to recommend that a family buy a less expensive prosthesis and use the extra money for a family vacation. Another example of encouraging respite is to recommend that a mother and father with a leukemic child have the grandparents babysit for a day while the couple spends time together. Such "time-outs" or "times away" are essential for families facing excessive caregiving demands.

Devising Rituals

Families engage in many types of rituals: daily (such as bedtime reading), yearly (such as Thanksgiving dinner at Grandma's), and cultural (such as ethnic parades). Nurses can suggest therapeutic rituals that are not or have not been observed by the family. Roberts (2003a) defines rituals as:

> ... co-evolved symbolic acts that include not only the ceremonial aspects of the actual presentation of the ritual, but the process of preparing for it as well. It may or may not include words, but does have both open and closed parts which are "held" together by a guiding metaphor. Repetition can be a part of rituals through the content, the form, or the occasion. There should be enough space in therapeutic rituals for the incorporation of multiple meanings by various family members and clinicians, as well as a variety of levels of participation. (p. 9)

Nurses are also contributing to the literature about rituals, as evidenced by a very comprehensive piece about rituals, routines, recreation, and rules by Fomby (2004). She emphasizes the use of family rituals for health promotion and claims the following benefits: cohesiveness among family members, a sense of family pride, continuity, understanding, closeness, and love.

In our clinical practice, we have observed that chronic illness and psychosocial problems frequently interrupt the usual rituals. Roberts (2003b) offers a poignant narrative of her experience with cancer and describes how rituals can "mark the path" of healing when a devastating illness emerges. Rituals are best introduced when there is an excessive level of confusion, and they can provide clarity in a family system (Imber-Black, Roberts, & Whiting, 2003). For example, parents who cannot agree on parenting practices commonly give conflicting messages to their families. This can result in chaos and confusion for their children. The introduction of an odd-day/even-day ritual (Selvini-Palazzoli, et al. 1978) can typically assist the family. The mother could experiment with being responsible for the children on Mondays, Wednesdays, and Fridays, and the father on Tuesdays, Thursdays, and Saturdays. On Sundays, they could behave spontaneously. On their "days off," parents could be asked to observe, without comment, their partner's parenting.

CLINICAL CASE EXAMPLES

The following clinical case examples illustrate the use of the CFIM. In these actual examples, interventions were chosen to facilitate change in all three domains (cognitive, affective, and behavioral) of family functioning. Remember, it is not always necessary or efficient to try to 'fit' interventions to all three domains of family functioning simultaneously. Whether this can be done successfully depends on how well the family is engaged, and it depends on prior assessment of the nature of the illness, problems, or concerns.

Clinical Case Example 1: Difficulty Putting 3-Year-Old Child to Bed

To illustrate a specific family intervention aimed at all three domains of family functioning, let us consider a parenting problem commonly presented to community health nurses (CHNs): young parents having difficulty putting their young children to bed each night. The parents' efforts are generally met with annoyance from the child, then anger, and then tears. In their efforts, the parents also become frustrated and commonly end up angry with each other as well as with their child. The family intervention offered was information and opinions. In describing this case example, we will also discuss executive skills the nurse can use to operationalize the intervention. These skills are also outlined in Chapter 5.

Parent–Child System Problem. Parents' chronic inability to get their 3-year-old to go to bed and stay there at required time.

DOMAINS OF FAMILY FUNCTIONING	INTERVENTION: OFFERING INFORMATION AND OPINIONS
Cognitive	Offer a parenting book that explains what bedtime means to children and suggests how to put children to bed.
Affective	Inform the parents that it is important to admit their frustrations to one another, especially if one spouse made an effort to put the child to bed but has not been successful. The other parent may give emotional support (e.g., "You tried real hard, dear; he's a handful").
Behavioral	Teach the parents that, when they put their son to bed, they should not respond to his efforts to gain attention (e.g., asking for a glass of water). Rather, parents should be sure that these needs have been attended to as part of his bedtime rituals. Warn parents that, before they can change their child's behavior of leaving his bed or continually calling them to his bedroom, his behavior will worsen for a few nights while he makes greater efforts to get his parents to respond. If the parents continue in a matter-of-fact way to put him back in his room and respond "no" to any further requests, his behavior should improve dramatically in a few nights.

Clinical Case Example 2: Elderly Father Complains His Children Do Not Visit Often Enough

Next, let us consider a clinical example that illustrates the intervention of encouraging family members to be caregivers and offering caregiver support. This intervention entails inviting family members to be involved in the emotional and physical care of the patient and offering support. The problem described in this case example was related to us by a nurse in a geriatric setting. Again, the accompanying executive skills to operationalize the interventions are given.

Parent–Child System Problem. An elderly father wants his adult children to visit more often; the adult children do not enjoy visiting because their father always complains that they do not visit often enough.

DOMAINS OF FAMILY FUNCTIONING	INTERVENTIONS: ENCOURAGING FAMILY MEMBERS TO BE CAREGIVERS AND OFFERING CAREGIVER SUPPORT
Cognitive	Teach the adult children that their father is having behavioral difficulty remembering their visits (short-term memory deficits), a common phenomenon of aging. Therefore, they need not remind him of when they visited last.
Affective	Empathize with the father, for example, by saying that you understand that it must be lonely at times being a resident in a geriatric care center. The adult children might appreciate knowing that their parent is lonely so that they can respond appropriately. Therefore, advise the father to avoid complaining to the children and, instead, tell them how lonely he feels sometimes and that he is happy that they come to visit.
Behavioral	Advise the adult children to stop giving excuses for why they cannot visit more often. Instead, obtain a guest book or calendar and write down each visit. Write down who visited, on what day, and perhaps any interesting news so that the aging parent may read this between visits.

We believe very strongly that, in the preceding examples, many other interventions and executive skills could have been offered. There is no one "right" intervention, only "useful" or "effective" interventions. How useful or effective an intervention is can be evaluated only after it has been implemented. The element of time must be taken into account. With some interventions, the change or outcome may be noted immediately. However, in many cases, changes (outcomes) are not noticed for a long time. Most problems do not occur overnight; therefore, their resolutions also require reasonable lengths of time. Change can be observed, as Bateson (1972) states, as "difference which occurs across time" (p. 452).

Clinical Case Example 3: Enuresis and Discipline Problems with Child

To illustrate that change is observed over time, we now offer two more actual case examples of clinical work, from beginning to end, with the emphasis on the interventions that were used. In the first case, a family was referred to one of our graduate nursing students with the complex presenting problems of enuresis and disciplinary problems at school in the eldest child, an 8-year-old boy. The family was composed of the father, age 28, self-employed; the stepmother, age 21, homemaker; and two sons, ages 8 and 6. The couple had been married for approximately 1 year. The family was seen (both as a whole family and in various subsystems) for six sessions over 13 weeks from initial contact to termination. A thorough family assessment (using the CFAM model) revealed problems in the whole family system, in the parent-child subsystem, and at the individual level.

Whole-Family System Problem. Adjustment to being a stepfamily. When the couple married, a new family was formed and all family members had to adjust to a new family structure. After being married for only a short time, the stepmother found herself thrust into a parenting role when she and her husband became responsible for his two children, ages 8 and 6. The birth mother had deserted the children after living with them for 2 years in her home. The children had to adjust to a new set of parents, new surroundings, and no contact with their biological mother.

In the first session, the graduate nursing student acknowledged that the problems the family was experiencing were a usual part of the adjustment of stepfamilies. The intervention of offering information and opinions was directed at the cognitive area of family functioning. This new information seemed to relieve the parents a great deal. In addition, the student gave advice by encouraging the parents to allow the children to have contact with their biological mother when she again sought them out. Initially, the parents were hesitant about this suggestion, but they later stated that they understood that this contact was important for the children. The eldest child's enuresis was conceptualized as a response to the adjustment to a stepfamily and the loss of his mother. This new opinion, also directed at the cognitive domain of family functioning, had a very positive effect on the family. The enuresis improved dramatically over the course of treatment.

Parent–Child Subsystem Problem. Maladaptive interactional pattern between stepmother and eldest son (Fig. 4-4). Because of the initial experience of the loss of their father (as a result of the biological parents' divorce) and then the abandonment by their biological mother, the children, particularly the eldest child, feared being abandoned again. Thus, the eldest child, hoping to be reassured that he would not be abandoned again, frequently reminded his young stepmother that she was not his real mother. Initially, the stepmother made efforts to reassure him, but she eventually withdrew

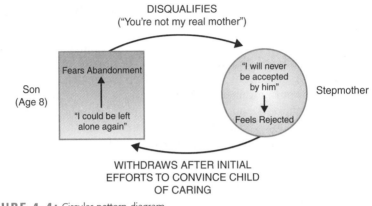

FIGURE 4-4: Circular pattern diagram.

in frustration and felt rejected. This encouraged the child to maintain the maladaptive interactional pattern because he perceived this withdrawal as further evidence that he would again be abandoned. The vicious cycle was evident.

In deciding which interventions to offer the family, the graduate nursing student was at first overwhelmed by the complexity of their situation. Then, she considered which area had the most leverage for change. She encouraged the stepmother to stop withdrawing and to offer the child continual and sustained reassurance by stating, "I know I am not your mother, but your father and I love and care for you and want to look after you. We will not leave you." This intervention of parent support and education was aimed at the behavioral, affective, and cognitive domains of family functioning. The behavioral task proved quite successful. The stepmother reported that when she offered more reassurance to the boy, he stopped rejecting her. With decreased rejection, the stepmother was able to offer even more reassurance. Thus, a virtuous cycle began. The nursing student also offered commendations of family strengths (an intervention directed at the cognitive domain of family functioning) to the stepmother for her efforts to fulfill her role, saying that she was an exceptionally warm and caring young mother. The stepmother reported that she felt more relaxed in her parenting after this intervention.

Individual Problem. Eldest child's behavioral problems at school. To further assess this behavioral problem, the graduate nursing student met with the child's teacher at school and discussed the problem twice with the teacher by telephone. The stepmother was also present during the session at school.

The main objective of the interventions was to enhance the eldest child's self-esteem by focusing on his positive behavior. The teacher agreed to implement an intervention focused at the behavioral domain of family functioning: to acknowledge the child's positive behavior in front of his classmates to give him a different status than "class clown." The graduate student also recommended that the stepmother minimize her contact with the school and allow the teacher to assume more responsibility for the boy's behavior in class. Within a few weeks, the teacher reported a positive change in the child's behavior at school. The parents expressed great satisfaction about their child's improvement.

On termination with this family, the graduate student recommended to the parents some readings on stepfamilies and informed them of a self-help group for stepfamilies. These two interventions of offering ideas and opinions in books and providing information on community resources were targeted at all three domains of family functioning: cognitive, affective, and behavioral.

It might seem that the interventions chosen by the graduate student in the above example were "simple." However, we believe that, in many cases, nurses either try to use overly complex interventions to address issues or they have difficulty collaborating with the family to determine areas with leverage for change. In both cases, we have found that nurses commonly become frustrated and immobilized by the complexity of the family situation. A thorough exploration of the presenting issue and then an offering of interventions designed to ameliorate that problem generally works best to foster change.

Clinical Case Example 4: Social Isolation and Physical Complaints of Elderly Woman

During one of our undergraduate nursing students' field placement in a community-health facility, she encountered a family whose presenting problems were social isolation and frequent physical complaints from the 78-year-old widowed mother. The widow lived in a government-subsidized, one-bedroom apartment. She had 6 adult children (5 sons, ages 51, 48, 41, 37, and 35; and 1 daughter, age 44) and 12 grandchildren. Five of the children were married, and all six lived in the same city as their mother. The family was seen as a whole and in various subsystems for eight home visits over a period of 2 months. After a thorough family assessment (using the CFAM model) and individual assessments, the following core problem was identified.

Whole-Family System Problem. The mother's lack of social contact beyond her immediate family. It became apparent that this older woman was overly dependent on her adult children and, therefore, did not make an effort to be involved with her peers or in social activities appropriate to her age-group. This resulted in frequent disagreements between the mother and the children over the frequency of visits with the mother. The problem was further exacerbated by the fact that the mother had no friends. After the death of her husband, approximately 10 years earlier, she had lived intermittently with some of her children, but for the past 4 years had been living alone in a one-bedroom apartment. At the time of intervention, the youngest son visited most often and did the mother's grocery shopping.

The nursing student's first significant intervention was to broaden the context in order to expand her view and understanding of this family's concerns. Thus, the student initially interviewed the mother alone and then interviewed her with her youngest son (the adult child who visited most frequently). Then the student took on the ambitious task of arranging an interview with the mother and her six children. This was a significant effort on the student's part to create a context for change by obtaining each family member's view of the problem. In the interview with the mother and her youngest son, the mother agreed to contact the children. However, when the student followed up with the mother, the mother said that she had not called any of her children because she expected her youngest son to do it. This was further evidence of the mother's overdependence on her children. Because the youngest son was anxious to have the meeting take place, he had taken on the task of inviting all of his siblings to an interview with his mother and the student.

At the family interview, all of the siblings were present and two of their spouses attended as well. Interestingly, the daughters-in-law were more vocal than their husbands and stated that they were very involved with their mother-in-law. In this large family interview, the mother's social isolation (apart from her family) was discussed. Through the process of circular questioning, the expectations for family contact of both the mother and children were assessed. Initially, the student encouraged the family to explore solutions to their mother's lack of social activities and peer interactions (an intervention aimed at the behavioral domain of family functioning). To this intervention, the family responded that they had no ideas beyond what they had already tried. Therefore, the student suggested more-specific interventions in an attempt to uncover solutions to the mother's social isolation.

This important interview revealed that the woman had always relied on her children for her main social interaction. She had never been a "joiner." In the past few years, she had even discontinued her attendance at church. Throughout her life, she had few close friends. The assessment also revealed that, collectively, the children had generally been supportive of their mother. Each week, she had lunch with one or more of them. They included her in all special family occasions. However, the children always had to initiate contact. They were genuinely concerned about their mother's loneliness and lack of additional social contact but had exhausted their ideas for changing her situation.

One of the first interventions the nursing student attempted was directed at both the cognitive and behavioral domains of family functioning: offering information regarding community resources that are available to older people. Specifically, the student made the family aware of the Community Services Visitor Program. The mother agreed to contact this program, and the children agreed to provide support. The mother also expressed interest in becoming involved in a choir again. The student offered to accompany her to a senior citizens' choir practice and introduce her to other participants.

The final major intervention discussed in that family session was directed at the behavioral domain. The student nurse asked the mother if she would initiate contact with one of her children during the next week. After the contact, the child would ask the mother to come for a visit as soon as possible. This intervention was important because interest of family members in an older parent's activities typically increase the parent's motivation. It is important to emphasize that the mother was involved in and receptive to these interventions.

The effects and outcomes of these interventions were as follows:

- The mother followed through on contacting the Community Services Visitor Program. The coordinator of the program then contacted the mother and arranged for a regular visitor.
- The student nurse accompanied the mother to the senior citizens' choir. The older woman enjoyed the experience and telephoned two of the other women in the choir afterward!
- The mother took the initiative to contact a couple of her children, and they, in turn, invited her for a family visit, which she accepted. The children reported that they enjoyed having their mother call them, and this new dynamic appeared to increase their own desire to have more frequent contact with her.

In subsequent interviews, the student nurse encouraged the mother to reconnect with her church. The student also solicited the support of the children in this endeavor by requesting that they take an interest in and inquire about their mother's church and choir activities when they called her.

Because this mother was accustomed to a good deal of family support, it was not appropriate to remove that support totally. However, physical instrumental support (i.e., doing things for the mother) was reduced without the mother feeling abandoned. Verbal (emotional) support for the mother's attempts at independence was most appropriate. When the mother began to increase her social contacts and activities, her nonspecific physical complaints decreased.

The student concluded treatment with this woman in a face-to-face interview. To involve the children in the termination process, the student sent a therapeutic letter (Hougher Limacher & Wright, 2006; Moules, 2002, 2003; Wright & Bell, in press) to each of them. This letter, written by the student and her faculty supervisor, is printed below verbatim. It beautifully highlights the major interventions and again solicits further assistance from the children. In addition, the student very nicely included some of the family strengths in the letter. Hopefully, the change process in this particular family will continue to evolve long after this nursing student's termination of the therapeutic relationship with them.

Dear (real names omitted to preserve confidentiality):

I wish to thank you for your help and cooperation in my family assignment. I enjoyed meeting each of you and appreciated your individual input and assessment of your family. Your willingness to work together is certainly an excellent family strength.

I visited your mother on several occasions during my time with the Outreach Program. She continued to express her desire to be more socially independent. She has been able to make some increased community contact. She attended the choir and several of the choir ladies have called her to encourage her in continued participation. She met with the gentleman from the church and spoke with his wife. The coordinator of the visitor program visited; she is arranging for a friend who will visit with your mother. Hopefully, they will develop some outside interests together. She has also been out to shop on her own on a few occasions.

I did contact Kerby Centre, as well as other seniors from Carter Place who go there, but was unable to find anyone going to the Wednesday lunch or any other suitable transportation. I have discussed this with your mother and she felt it might be something she could pursue on her own in the future.

Your mother expressed positive feelings about her attempts to be more socially active. However, she still looks to her children for her main support. At times, I found she needed more encouragement not to overly worry about her health to the point that she thinks she is unable to participate in any activities. I believe that each of you may help your mother by encouraging her in this area. I might suggest that if she says that she is unwell that she see her doctor. If there is no serious problem, gentle support for her independent activities might be helpful. This may be somewhat difficult at first, but if you are able to present a united front to your mother and support each other in a mutual approach to her being more socially active, she may be more able to accomplish this.

I am very impressed with the cohesiveness of your family and the continued concern and support you show toward your mother. Thank you very much again for letting me work with you.

Yours truly,
Leslie Henderson
Undergraduate Nursing Student
Faculty of Nursing, University of Calgary

This therapeutic letter sent by the student is an intervention in and of itself (Moules, 2002, 2003; White & Epston, 1990; Wright & Bell, in press). In addition, several interventions were outlined in the letter. These interventions were aimed at all three areas of family functioning. Specifically, the student offered commendations and opinions directed at the cognitive domain of functioning. She invited the adult children to encourage their mother, which aimed at changes in the behavioral domain. By summarizing the clinical work with the family in the form of a therapeutic letter, the student intended to effect changes in both the affective and cognitive domains of family functioning. This exemplary clinical work is a stellar example of effectively involving families in health care by the use of family assessment and intervention models with clear treatment goals by a student committed to improving family functioning and softening suffering.

CONCLUSIONS

Interventions can be straightforward and simple or as innovative and dramatic as the nurse deems necessary for the health or illness problems presented. Interventions intended to promote health and manage illness should be based on the assumption that individual health behaviors are strongly influenced by those around us, and that family general well-being can promote the physical health of its members. All interventions should be directed toward the treatment goals collaboratively generated by the nurse and the family. As nurses learn to actively engage and thoroughly assess families; clearly identify problems, concerns, and suffering; and set treatment goals, the process of conceptualizing, choosing, and offering specific interventions with each family becomes more rewarding and effective. The ultimate goal, of course, is to aid family members in discovering new solutions to help soften or alleviate emotional, physical, and/or spiritual suffering.

References

Bateson, G. (1972). *Steps to an ecology of mind: Collected essays in anthropology, psychiatry, evolution, and epistemology.* New York: Ballantine Books.

Bateson, G. (1979). *Mind and nature.* New York: E.P. Dutton.

Bohn, U., Wright, L.M., & Moules, N.J. (2003). A family systems nursing interview following a myocardial infarction: The power of commendations. *Journal of Family Nursing, 9*(2), 151–165.

Campbell, T.L. (2003). The effectiveness of family interventions for physical disorders. *Journal of Marital and Family Therapy, 29*(2), 545–583.

Deatrick, J.A. (1998). Integrative review of intervention research with children who have chronic conditions and their families. In M.E. Broome, et al. (Eds.), *Children and families in health and illness.* Thousand Oaks: Sage Publications.

Duhamel, F., & Dupuis, F. (2004). Guaranteed returns: Investing in conversations with families of cancer patients. *Clinical Journal of Oncology Nursing, 8*(1), 68–71.

Duhamel, F., & Talbot, L.R. (2004). A constructivist evaluation of family systems nursing interventions with families experiencing cardiovascular and cerebrovascular illness. *Journal of Family Nursing, 10*(1), 12–32.

Feeley, N., & Gottlieb, L.N. (2000). Nursing approaches for working with family strengths and resources. *Journal of Family Nursing, 6*(1), 9–24.

Fomby, B.W. (2004). Family routines, rituals, recreation, and rules. In P.J. Bomar (Ed.), *Promoting health in families: Applying family research and theory to nursing practice* (3rd ed.). Philadelphia: Saunders.

Holtslander, L. (2005). Clinical application of the 15-minute family interview: Addressing the needs of post-partum fathers. *Journal of Family Nursing, 11*(1), 5–18.

Houger Limacher, L., & Wright, L.M. (2003). Commendations: Listening to the silent side of a family intervention. *Journal of Family Nursing, 9*(2), 130–135.

Hougher Limacher, L., & Wright, L.M. (2006). Exploring the therapeutic family intervention of commendations: Insights from research. *Journal of Family Nursing, 12,* 307–331.

Imber-Black, E., Roberts, J., & Whiting, R.A. (Eds.). (2003). *Rituals in families and family therapy* (Revised Ed.). New York: Norton.

Leahey, M., & Harper-Jaques, S. (1996). Family-nurse relationships: Core assumptions and clinical implications. *Journal of Family Nursing, 2*(2), 133–151.

LeNavenec, C., & Vonhof, T. (1996). *One day at a time: How families manage the experience of dementia.* Westport, CT: Greenwood Publishing Group – Auburn House.

Levac, A.M.C., Wright, L.M., & Leahey, M. (2002). Children and families: Models for assessment and intervention. In J.A. Fox (Ed.), *Primary health care of infants, children, and adolescents* (2nd ed.) (pp. 10–19). St. Louis: Mosby.

Loos, F., & Bell, J.M. (1990). Circular questions: A family interviewing strategy. *Dimensions of Critical Care Nursing, 9*(1), 46–53.

Manassis, K., & Levac, A.M. (2004). *Helping your teenager beat depression: A Problem-solving approach for families.* Bethesda, MD: Woodbine House.

Maturana, H.R. & Varela, F. (1992). *The tree of knowledge: The biological roots of human understanding.* Boston: Shambhala Publications, Inc.

McElheran, N.G., & Harper-Jaques, S.R. (1994). Commendations: A resource intervention for clinical practice. *Clinical Nurse Specialist, 8*(1), 7–10.

McLeod, D.L., & Wright, L.M. (2008). Living the as-yet unanswered: Spiritual care practices in family systems nursing. *Journal of Family Nursing.14(1),* 118–141.

Moules, N.J. (2002). Nursing on paper: Therapeutic letters in nursing practice. *Nursing Inquiry, 9*(2), 104–113.

Moules, N.J. (2003). Therapy on paper: Therapeutic letters and the tone of the relationship. *Journal of Systemic Therapies, 22*(1), 33–49.

Moules, N.J., et al. (2004). Making room for grief: Walking backwards and living forward. *Nursing Inquiry,* 99–107.

Moules, N.J., et al. (2007). The soul of sorrow work: Grief and therapeutic interventions of families. *Journal of Family Nursing, 13*(1), 117–141.

Roberts, J. (2003a). Setting the frame: Definition, functions, and typology of rituals. In E. Imber-Black, J. Roberts, & R. Whiting (Eds.), *Rituals in families and family therapy.* New York: Norton.

Roberts, J. (2003b). Rituals and serious illness: Marking the path. In E. Imber-Black, J. Roberts, & R. Whiting (Eds.), *Rituals in families and family therapy.* New York: Norton.

Robinson, C.A. (1998). Women, families, chronic illness, and nursing interventions: From burden to balance. *Journal of Family Nursing, 4*(3), 271–290.

Robinson, C.A., & Wright, L.M. (1995). Family nursing interventions: What families say makes a difference. *Journal of Family Nursing, 1*(2), 327–345.

Rungreangkulkij, S., & Gilliss, C.L. (2000). Conceptual approaches to studying family caregiving for persons with severe mental illness. *Journal of Family Nursing, 6*(4), 341–366.

Schober, M., & Affara, F. (2001). *The family nurse: Frameworks for practice.* Geneva: International Council of Nurses.

Selvini-Palazzoli, M., et al. (1978). A ritualized prescription in family therapy: Odd days and even days. *Journal of Marriage and Family Counseling, 4*(3), 3–9.

Selvini-Palazzoli, M., et al. (1980). Hypothesizing circularity-neutrality: Three guidelines for the conductor of the session. *Family Process, 19*(3), 3–12.

Tapp, D.M. (2001). Conserving the vitality of suffering: Addressing family constraints to illness conversations. *Nursing Inquiry, 8*(4), 254–263.

Thorne, S., & Robinson, C.A. (1989). Guarded alliance: Health care relationships in chronic illness. *Image: The Journal of Nursing Scholarship, 21*(3), 153–157.

Tomm, K. (1984). One perspective on the Milan systemic approach: Part II. Description of session format, interviewing style and interventions. *Journal of Marital and Family Therapy, 10*(3), 253–271.

Tomm, K. (1985). Circular interviewing: A multifaceted clinical tool. In D. Campbell & R. Draper (Eds.), *Applications of systemic family therapy: The Milan approach* (pp. 33–45). London: Grune & Stratton.

Tomm, K. (1987). Interventive interviewing: Part II. Reflexive questioning as a means to enable self-healing. *Family Process, 26*(6), 167–183.

Tomm, K. (1988). Interventive interviewing: Part III. Intending to ask linear, circular, strategic, or reflexive questions? *Family Process, 27*(1), 1–15.

Watson, W.L., & Nanchoff-Glatt, M. (1990). A family systems nursing approach to premenstrual syndrome. *Clinical Nurse Specialist, 4*(1), 3–9.

White, M., & Epston, D. (1990). *Narrative means to therapeutic ends.* New York: Norton.

Wright, L.M., & Bell, J.M. (in press). *Beliefs and illness: A model for healing.* Calgary, AB: 4th Floor Press.

Wright, L. M., & Leahey, M. (1987). Families and life-threatening illness: Assumptions, assessment, and intervention. In M. Leahey & L.M. Wright (Eds.), *Families and life-threatening illness* (pp. 45–58). Springhouse, PA: Springhouse Corp.

Wright, L.M., & Leahey, M. (Producers). (2000). *How to do a 15 minute (or less) family interview.* [DVD]. Calgary, Canada: www.familynursingresources.com.

Wright, L.M., & Leahey, M. (Producers). (2001). *Calgary Family Assessment Model: How to apply in clinical practice.* [DVD]. Calgary, Canada: www.familynursingresources.com.

Wright, L.M., & Leahey, M. (Producers). (2002). *Family nursing interviewing skills: How to engage, assess, intervene, and terminate with families.* [DVD]. Calgary, Canada: www.familynursingresources.com.

Wright, L.M., & Leahey, M. (Producers) (2003). *How to intervene with families with health concerns.* [DVD]. Calgary, Canada: www.familynursingresources.com.

Wright, L.M., & Leahey, M. (Producers) (2006). *How to use questions in family interviewing.* [Videotape]. Calgary, Canada: www.FamilyNursingResources.com

Wright, L.M., & Levac, A.M. (1992). The non-existence of non-compliant families: The influence of Humberto Maturana. *Journal of Advanced Nursing, 17,* 913–917.

Wright, L.M., & Nagy, J. (1993). Death: The most troublesome family secret of all. In E. Imber-Black (Ed.), *Secrets in families and family therapy* (pp. 121–137). New York: Norton.

Chapter **5**

Family Nursing Interviews: Stages and Skills

Once nurses have a clear, conceptual framework for assessing and intervening with families, they can then begin to consider the various new competencies and skills needed for family interviews. The skills deemed necessary by various authors on family work reflect each author's particular theoretical orientation and unique preference regarding how to approach and resolve problems. Therefore, the skills delineated in this chapter are based on our postmodernist worldview. This includes, but is not limited to, the theoretical foundations of systems theory, cybernetics, communication theory, biology of cognition, and change theory that inform the Calgary Family Assessment Model (CFAM) and Calgary Family Intervention Model (CFIM).

We favor a strengths- and resiliency-based, problem- and solution-focused, time-effective approach. We emphasize that families possess the ability to solve their own problems and suffering. Our task as nurses is to help them find and facilitate their own solutions to their emotional, physical, or spiritual suffering. We do not propose that we know what is "best" for families. We embrace the notion that the world has multiple realities—in other words, that each family member and nurse sees a world that he or she brings forth through interacting with others through language. We encourage openness in ourselves, our students, and our families to the diversity of difference among us. However, to be involved in helping families change requires that nurses possess certain essential competencies and skills.

In the previous chapters, we discussed the theoretical knowledge base that is necessary to begin to competently assess and intervene with families. We also offered two practice models (the CFAM and CFIM) as frameworks to conceptualize family dynamics and offer specific family interventions. This chapter focuses on the specific beginning-level skills necessary for relational family nursing interviews.

The literature on family work that has appeared in the past 30 years indicates that myriad skills can be used when working with families (Tomm & Wright, 1979; Wright & Bell, in press).

Various professional nursing associations have made efforts to identify the necessary competencies for practice. However, the two most significant documents with regard to the specific development of family nursing skills and competencies are those published by the International Council of Nurses (ICN). The first was titled *The Family Nurse: Frameworks for Practice* developed by Madrean Schober and Fadwa Affara (2001). These ideas were further expanded when on May 12, 2002, the ICN selected the theme for the International Nurses Day to be "Nurses Always There for You: Caring for Families" and produced a document with the same title (International Council of Nurses, 2002). In the document is outlined the "nine star family nurse." We offer it below to demonstrate the vastness of the possibilities of caring for families.

The Nine-Star Family Nurse: Multi-skilled with diverse roles

Nurses working with families play multiple roles, depending on the family needs and the settings for care, which can include the home, health-care facilities, temporary refugee shelters or the streets. In an effort to capture the full range of the nurse's work with families, we will refer to the key roles in terms of the nine-star nurse. The roles of the nine-star family nurse include:

■ Health educator: Teaching families formally or informally about health and illness and acting as the main provider of health information.

■ Care provider and supervisor: Providing direct care and supervising care given by others, including family members and nursing assistants.

■ Family advocate: Working to support families and speaking up on issues such as safety and access to services.

■ Case finder and epidemiologist: Tracking disease and playing a key role in disease surveillance and control.

■ Researcher: Identifying practice problems and seeking answers and solutions through scientific investigation alone or in collaboration.

■ Manager and coordinator: Managing, collaborating and liaising with family members, health and social services and others to improve access to care.

■ Counselor: Playing a therapeutic role in helping to cope with problems and to identify resources.

■ Consultant: Serving as consultant to families and agencies to identify and facilitate access to resources.

■ Environmental modifier: Working to modify, for example, the home environment so that the disabled can improve mobility and engage in self-care.

The nine-star family nurse uses a number of these roles to identify health risks, a health problem or a need, and to address the situation working singly or in partnership with families, other health professionals and community groups. (p. 10).

A major challenge in determining core competencies for family work is to distinguish what can be called "general skills and knowledge"—which are needed by all nurses working with clients—from unique, advanced practice skills and knowledge, particularly those of family nurses. Another challenge is to delineate sufficient competencies to cover the range of practice and yet not specify so many that the practitioner is overwhelmed. In an attempt to do this, Leahey, Southern, and Harper-Jaques (2007) developed ladders for family nursing skills and integrated family nursing into mental health urgent care practice in a community health setting (Southern, et al. 2007). Using Benner's (2001) levels, they outlined skills for family nursing from the novice to expert level.

Simply stating general skills such as "the student must be able to label interactions accurately" says nothing about how that skill can be achieved. The use of specific learning objectives helps to remove the mystery from what a family nurse interviewer does. Thus, the learning objectives or skills become a tentative "map" for the interview. It is essential to highlight, however, that the correlation of skills with client outcomes has not yet been established. The skills described in this chapter emerge from our theoretical orientation and application of the CFAM and CFIM practice models. These skills become the nurse behaviors that are unique to working with families. Of course, each nurse also has his or her own unique genetic and personality makeup and history of interactions, and these personalize the application of these skills.

EVOLVING STAGES OF FAMILY NURSING INTERVIEWS

Within the context of a therapeutic conversation between a nurse and a family, four major stages of family nursing interviews can be identified:

- Engagement
- Assessment
- Intervention
- Termination.

These stages evolve throughout the interview. They tend to follow a logical sequence during both the course of a given interview and the overall course of contact. For example, a nurse engages family members and terminates with them not only at the end of each interview, but also at the beginning and end of the entire contact. Of course, there are times when a nurse may have to return to a previous stage. For example, interventions may be offered too quickly before a thorough assessment has been completed. Other times, the nurse might want to revisit the engagement stage if a new family member attends a meeting.

In the first stage, *engagement,* the nurse exercises skills that invite himself or herself and the family to establish and maintain a therapeutic relationship. Our preferred stance or posture with families is to be collaborative and consultative (Leahey & Harper-Jaques, 1996). We also encourage a posture of curiosity and interest in the family. This implies greater equality and respect for the family's resiliency and resourcefulness. As long as there is an atmosphere of curiosity, judgment and blame are kept at bay.

The nurse brings to the relationship expertise about promoting health and managing illness, and family members bring their own expertise about their understanding of health and their illness experiences. It is this synergy of combined expertise that can generate new outcomes to constraining situations. Factors that appear to inhibit engagement by the family interviewer are the lack of creating a context for change, and confrontation or interpretation too early in treatment. Additional ideas and suggestions for the engagement stage are given in Chapters 6 and 7.

Assessment, the second stage, includes the substages of problem identification and exploration plus delineation of a strengths and problems list. During this stage, the nurse enables the family to tell the story about their particular situation. The story is different for each family. It may be an illness story; a story of loss and grief; a story of uncertainty about the health of family members (e.g., a child's developmental delay or undiagnosed symptoms); a story about terror, war, and unwanted migration; or a story of a desire to promote or maintain healthy lifestyles and avoid obesity or alcoholism that has plagued a family. We stress that the conversation between the nurse and the family is in and of itself part of the therapeutic discourse (Tapp, 2001; Wright & Bell, in press). That is, if the nurse attends only to the signs and symptoms of disease, both the nurse and family will find themselves in a discourse emphasizing pathology. Alternative discourses that emphasize "right answers" rather than an understanding of the family's frustrations, sufferings, dilemmas, and yearnings would be equally unhelpful.

Beginning nurse interviewers generally lack a clear, stepwise rationale to guide the collecting and processing of data during an interview. Thus, some beginners commonly spend an inordinate amount of time collecting vast amounts of information. Frequently, this information is tangential to the presenting problem and is not usable. Alternatively, beginners sometimes rush into inappropriate treatment because they do not have a clear formulation of the presenting problem. It is better, however, for beginners to err on the side of taking longer than usual to complete the initial assessment than to prematurely rush to the intervention stage. Nurses in family work must remember that assessment is an ongoing process. Thus, the strengths and problems list may change over time as the nurse's conceptual understanding of the family becomes more systemic. Ideas for conducting a time-effective 15-minute interview are given in Chapter 8. Information on what areas to assess and how to integrate and document the data is available in Chapters 3 and 11, respectively.

The third stage, *intervention*, is really the core of clinical work with families. It involves providing a context in which the family may make small or significant changes. There are numerous ways to intervene, and treatment plans should be co-constructed and tailored by the nurse and family to match each family situation. Chapter 4 (The Calgary Family Intervention Model) offers examples of specific interventions that can be used by nurses, and Chapter 9 gives ideas of the kinds of questions that can be used in family interviewing.

Termination, the last stage, refers to the process of ending the therapeutic relationship between the nurse and the family in a manner that allows the family not only to maintain but also to continue constructive changes, new understandings, and facilitative beliefs. Therapeutic termination encourages the family's ability to solve problems in the future. Specific ideas for therapeutic termination are described in Chapter 12.

TYPES OF SKILLS

Each stage of family interviewing requires three types of skills:

- Perceptual
- Conceptual
- Executive

Cleghorn and Levin's (1973) identification and categorization of these three skill types are considered a seminal contribution. Tomm and Wright (1979) used the perceptual, conceptual, and executive skills framework as a guide for their comprehensive outline, which offered examples of therapist functions, competencies, and skills in each category over the evolution of a family interview. In our text, we have kept Wright's previous identification of particular perceptual, conceptual, and executive skills across the four stages of family interviews. However, we have adapted the perceptual, conceptual, and executive skills to be congruent with nurses who are just beginning to practice with families. Although we believe these skills are most descriptive of the work of beginning family nurse interviewers, we do not wish to imply that the skills are only used with "simple" family situations. Rather, we recognize that all nurses, from beginner undergraduates to experienced practicing nurses, deal with complex family situations on a day-to-day basis. These skills provide a framework for relational family nursing practice irrespective of the complexity of the family's presenting issue.

The skills that we have identified fit within the context of our particular practice models—namely, the CFAM and CFIM. Perceptual and conceptual skills are paired because what we perceive is so intimately interrelated with what we think; in many cases, separating the perceptual from the conceptual component is difficult. Perceptual and conceptual skills are then matched with executive skills.

Perceptual skills relate to the nurse's ability to make relevant observations. The nurse's own age, ethnicity, gender, sexual orientation, race, and class are but a few of the factors that influence his or her perceptions. The perceptual skills required in individual interviewing are much different from those required in family interviewing. This difference can be explained by the fact that, in family interviewing, the nurse is involved in observing multiple interactions and relationships simultaneously; the interaction among family members and the interaction between the nurse and the family are simultaneous.

Conceptual skills involve the ability to give meaning to the observations that the nurse made. They also involve the ability to formulate one's observations of the family as a whole, as a system. Nurses must always be cognizant that the meanings derived from observations are not "the truth" about the family; instead, they represent efforts to make sense of observations.

We believe that a student entering the nursing field has intuitive perceptual and conceptual skills that have been learned in other roles in previous life experiences. The student, however, is unaware of many of these skills. As a nurse, he or she needs to develop an overt awareness of the perceptual process. Perceptual and conceptual skills are the basis of the executive skills.

Executive skills are the observable therapeutic interventions that a nurse carries out in an interview. These skills, or therapeutic interventions, elicit responses from family members and are the basis for the nurse's further observations and conceptualizations. As can be readily seen, the interview process embedded within the therapeutic conversation is a circular phenomenon between the nurse and family. The process is highly influenced by the nurse's and family members' gender, ethnicity, class, and race. Of course, the types of therapeutic interventions offered by the nurse are highly dependent on his or her clinical expertise and experience in working with families.

DEVELOPMENT OF FAMILY NURSING INTERVIEWING SKILLS

In the education of nurses developing family nursing skills, emphasis should be placed first on the development of perceptual and conceptual skills. This can be accomplished by several methods. Lectures and readings are helpful. Role-playing, practicing reflective inquiry, and observing and analyzing video-tapes or DVDs of actual family interviews are all useful and effective ways to increase perceptual and conceptual skill accuracy. For this reason, we have developed *The "How to" Family Nursing Series*, available on DVD at the Family Nursing Resources website (www.familynursingresources.com). This DVD series currently comprises five educational programs, which present live clinical scenarios that demonstrate family nursing in actual practice, including interviews with families with young children, middle-aged families, and later-life families. The health problems and health-care settings are varied, as are the ethnic and racial groups. The emphasis is on demonstrating how to practice these skills. The DVD most related to this chapter is *Family Nursing Interviewing Skills: How to Engage, Assess, Intervene, and Terminate* (Wright & Leahey, 2002). See page 345 for a full description of each DVD and for ordering information.

Application of family nursing interview skills in family nursing labs is one of the most meaningful skill-development opportunities for both graduate and undergraduate nurses. Moules and Tapp (2003) offer some creative, innovative ideas and exercises for educators conducting family nursing labs for undergraduate students. In their research, they found that experiential and interactive, inquiry-based activities aimed at creating personal, meaningful, relational family nursing practice received positive student feedback. For example, the authors shifted from using role plays to using a questioning exercise to emphasize reciprocity between the family and the nurse interviewer. After selecting one student in the group, every other student asks questions of that student based on their knowledge and experience of that person as a classmate or friend. The power and timeliness of interventive questions quickly become evident to the students at a very personal level. The exercise continues until each student has had the opportunity to be the questioned member. Moules and Tapp (2003) also fashioned a commendations exercise aimed at offering students the opportunity to genuinely look for, find, and then offer a sincere acknowledgement to a real student. The exercise was designed in a similar fashion to the questioning exercise, with one student receiving commendations offered by other group members. Moules and Tapp reported that the experiential, personal component of these exercises enriched students' valuing of relational family nursing practice.

If a nurse is unable to perform a specific executive skill, it is useful to find out whether he or she has developed a perceptual and conceptual base for that particular skill. This is the value of matching these skills in pairs. We encourage nurses to reflect on their practice to distinguish their unique areas of strength and weakness in the conceptual, perceptual, or executive areas.

Family assessment is generally well taught at the baccalaureate level and in masters and doctoral programs specializing in community and/or family nursing in North America. However, family interventions and the accompanying skills at both the undergraduate and graduate levels still need to be greatly enhanced and improved. On the global scene, a study in Nigeria revealed that the limited focus on family nursing theory in basic and post-basic nursing curricula was deemed inadequate to develop the knowledge and skills necessary for all practicing nurses to embrace family-focused care (Irinoye, Ogunfowokan, & Olaogun, 2006). However, these researchers did find that a survey of postgraduate curricula showed that master's and doctorate-degreed nurses specializing in community health nursing have a theoretical base in family nursing theory, although they did not elaborate as to whether specific skills were taught or supervision provided. Live supervision of clinical practice with families, particularly at the graduate level, is regularly provided in very few locations worldwide (Wright & Bell, in press). Case discussion and process recording remain the predominant method of supervision in the development of family nursing skills. However, live supervision is essential to developing and achieving therapeutic competence in nursing practice with families (Chesla, Gilliss, & Leavitt, 1993; Tapp & Wright, 1996; Wright, 1994; Wright & Bell, in press). Feeling supported through supervision, having competence emphasized, and hearing about specific in-session behaviors contribute to increased self-confidence. Observing peers as a mirror of one's own development and seeing one's own internal experience as normal were reported as helpful to increasing self-confidence. Learning from peers is useful in two ways: first, when a novice asks the inexperienced clinician for suggestions, the novice is able to see that the peer can be a valuable resource; second, as the inexperienced clinician seeks out consultation from a novice, the novice is able to see himself or herself as competent with the person to whom they are offering consultation.

It is especially encouraging to note the increase in the family nursing literature of descriptions and reports of how nurse-educators both in academia and in practice settings are committed to enhancing the development of family nursing skills. Specific examples in the literature include teaching students to "think family" (Green, 1997), to offer family nursing workshops within practice settings (LeGrow & Rossen, 2005; Simpson, et al., 2006), to integrate family nursing into everyday practice in mental health urgent care (Southern, et al., 2007), and to practice family nursing skills in structured family nursing labs within undergraduate nursing programs (Moules & Tapp, 2003; Tapp, et al., 1997). These articles offer evidence for the continuing and deepening efforts to enhance and increase nursing students' and practicing nurses' competencies and skills in their care of families.

Specific skills for interviewing families are listed in logical sequence in Table 5-1. However, during the course of an actual interview, the nurse need not follow this outline rigidly. Rather, this outline serves as a "map of interviewing" that allows considerable flexibility in application. The family's cultural norms for giving and receiving information can provide a guide for the pacing of the meeting. We cannot emphasize enough the importance of the nurse and the family developing a collaborative working relationship during the interview.

Protinsky and Coward (2001) found that the main developmental theme emerging from their study of seasoned interdisciplinary family clinicians was the integration of their personal and professional selves. The participants reported a synthesis accumulated from a set of personal and professional experiences that were now part of their expertise. They no longer spoke solely from a theoretical perspective. We have found this to be true also in our own lives; our personal and professional experiences are now more integrated into our practice of relational family nursing.

Table 5-1	Family Interviewing Skills for Nurses

STAGE 1: ENGAGEMENT

PERCEPTUAL/CONCEPTUAL SKILLS	EXECUTIVE SKILLS
1. **Recognize that an individual family member is best understood in the context of the family.**	1. **Invite all family members who are concerned or involved with the problem, suffering, or illness to attend the first interview.**
That is, no individual exists in isolation.	For example, grandparents or other relatives or friends living inside or outside of the home should also be invited to attend if they are involved with the problem or illness.
2. **Appreciate that initial efforts to involve both spouses/parents enables, from the onset, a more holistic view of the family and increases engagement.**	2. **Employ all efforts to initially involve both spouses/parents in initial sessions.**
That is, fathers should definitely be involved for effective family work.	The spouses/parents have the greatest influence on the identification, understanding, and resolution of the problem, softening suffering and/or managing illness.
3. **Recognize that providing a clear structure to the interview reduces anxiety and increases engagement.**	3. **Explain to family members the purpose, length, and structure of the interview and ask if they have any questions relating to the interview.**
That is, people generally feel anxiety related to the uncertainty of being in a new setting and of not knowing how to behave in the situation. Structure is particularly important if the family is experiencing a crisis.	For example, say: "I thought we could spend about 10 minutes together discussing the issues that you are concerned about."
4. **Recognize that initially members are most comfortable talking about the structural aspects of the family.**	4. **Ask each family member to relate information with regard to name, age, work or school, years married, and so forth.**
That is, note nonverbal cues indicating level of comfort, such as taking coat off, adequate versus minimal time spent talking, and participating in versus ignoring conversation.	For example, introduce yourself directly by giving your name and either shaking hands or making some physical contact (such as touching a baby's head). After introductions, ask questions about information that is familiar to all family members because this type of conversation is familiar to the family members and is least threatening.

STAGE 2: ASSESSMENT

PERCEPTUAL/CONCEPTUAL SKILLS	EXECUTIVE SKILLS
1. **Realize the importance of having a conceptual assessment map to understand family dynamics.**	1. **Explore the components of the structural, developmental, and functional aspects of CFAM to assess strengths and problem areas.**
That is, a conceptual assessment map provides the nurse with several possible courses for focused exploration.	Not all components of CFAM need to be explored if they are not relevant to the present issues, problems, or illness.
2. **Realize the importance of beginning a family assessment by obtaining a detailed description and history of the presenting problem, concern, or illness.**	2. **Ask each family member, including the children, to share his or her knowledge and understanding of the presenting concern.**

Continued

Table 5-1	Family Interviewing Skills for Nurses—*cont'd*

STAGE 2: ASSESSMENT

PERCEPTUAL/CONCEPTUAL SKILLS	EXECUTIVE SKILLS
That is, the presenting problem usually serves as an entry point for the family to seek help. Focusing on addressing the problem is time-effective.	For example, ask the father: "How do you see the problem?" or ask the whole family, "What is the main problem or issue that each of you would like to see changed?"
3. **Realize that the presenting problem is commonly related to other concerns in the family.**	3. **Explore with the family if there are other problems or concerns connected to the presenting problem.**
That is, a child's temper outbursts may be related to family conflict (e.g., the child may be triangulated into a family conflict over caring for the grandmother).	For example, say: "We have been talking for some time about the problem of Theo's refusal to take his meds in the mornings. I am wondering if there are any other problems the family is presently concerned about."
4. **Realize that eliciting differences generates more specific information for family assessment.**	4. **Inquire about differences between individuals, between relationships, and between various points in time.**
That is:	For example:
(a) Clarification of differences between individuals is a significant source of information about family functioning.	(a) To explore differences between individuals, ask the child: "What is expected of you before you go to bed at night?" and then ask, "Who is the best, mother or father, at getting you to do those things in the evening?"
(b) Clarification of differences between relationships is a significant source of information about family structure and alliances.	(b) To explore differences between relationships, ask: "Do your father and Ingo argue more or less than your father and Hannah about how to care for your younger sister?"
(c) Clarification of differences in family members or in relationships at various points in time is a significant source of information about family development.	(c) To explore differences before or after important points in time, ask: "Do you worry more, less, or the same about your husband's health since his heart attack?"
5. **Use the information obtained from the family assessment to begin formulating hypotheses in the form of a strengths and problems list.**	5. **Obtain verification of the nurse's understanding of strengths and problems by listing them to the family for their agreement and eventually recording them.**
Offering conclusions or a summary of the nurse's assessment ideas enhances engagement and collaboration and allows for self-correction. That is, structural, developmental, and functional strengths and problems may be present at various systems levels. For example, whole family system issues:	For example, say: "We have identified that being a new single parent and also having to cope with your child (who has a developmental delay) leaving home are your two major concerns. We have also discussed that your family is very well respected in the Latino community. Have I understood things correctly?"
(a) Structural: Adjusting to new family form of single-parent household. (b) Developmental: Family in life cycle stage of children leaving home. (c) Functional: Family belief that "Father would be displeased with us for still crying about his death."	

Table 5-1	Family Interviewing Skills for Nurses—*cont'd*

STAGE 2: ASSESSMENT

PERCEPTUAL/CONCEPTUAL SKILLS	EXECUTIVE SKILLS
6. **Assess whether any of the identified problems are beyond the scope of the nurse's competence.**	6. **Tell the family whether you will continue to work with them on problems. (If a decision is made to refer them to another professional, proceed to Stage 4A: Termination.)**
That is, it is appropriate to consider referral when medical symptoms have not been fully assessed or long-standing emotional or behavioral problems exist.	For example, tell the family: "Now that I have a more complete understanding of your concerns, I think it is necessary to have your son's headaches checked out medically. I would like to refer you to a pediatrician."
7. **Recognize that a more extensive inquiry into the most pressing problems is necessary before intervention plans can be implemented.**	7. **Seek the family's opinion of which issue they perceive as most important and/or where there is the greatest suffering, and explore it in depth. If the family cannot agree, then discuss the lack of consensus.**
That is, initially families are usually most concerned with the presenting problem or the area of greatest suffering.	For example, ask: "About which of the problems we have discussed today are you most concerned?"
8. **Recognize that the assessment is complete when sufficient information has been obtained to formulate a treatment plan.**	8. **State your integrated understanding of problems to the family and obtain their commitment to work on a specific problem.**
That is, nurses sometimes rush into inappropriate treatment because they are without a clear understanding of the presenting problem or other significant related problems.	For example, say: "Because everyone agrees that Soon's bulimia is connected to the other addictions in the family, I would like to suggest that we focus on this problem for three interviews. Would you be willing?"

STAGE 3: INTERVENTION

PERCEPTUAL/CONCEPTUAL SKILLS	EXECUTIVE SKILLS
1. **Recognize that families possess problem-solving abilities.**	1. **Encourage family members to explore possible solutions to problems and to soften suffering.**
That is, recognizing that families not only possess the capability to change but also can identify and implement solutions for how to change helps the nurse avoid becoming over-controlling or over-responsible.	For example, say: "Sanjeshna, you have mentioned that your mother is too blaming of herself. Do you have any ideas of what she could do to blame herself less about experiencing a chronic illness?"
2. **Recognize that interventions are focused on the cognitive, affective, and behavioral domains or areas of functioning in families, as described in the CFIM.**	2. **Plan interventions to influence any one or all three of the domains of functioning described in the CFIM.**
That is, it is not always necessary or efficient to design interventions for all three domains of functioning simultaneously.	For example: (a) Cognitive: Invite the family to think differently. (b) Affective: Encourage different affective expression. (c) Behavioral: Ask the family to perform new tasks either within or outside of the interview.

Continued

Table 5-1	Family Interviewing Skills for Nurses—*cont'd*

STAGE 3: INTERVENTION

PERCEPTUAL/CONCEPTUAL SKILLS	EXECUTIVE SKILLS
3. **Recognize that lack of information of an educational nature can inhibit the family's problem-solving abilities.**	3. **Provide information to family members that will enhance their knowledge and facilitate further problem solving.**
That is, when given additional information, many families can provide their own creative and unique solutions to problems.	For example, the nurse can ask family members if they would like to hear about some typical reactions of a 3-year-old to a new baby or about the aging process of an older adult with Alzheimer's disease. This type of intervention targets the family's cognitive domain of functioning.
4. **Recognize that persistent and intense emotions can often block the family's problem-solving abilities.**	4. **Validate family members' emotional responses, when appropriate.**
That is, families who predominantly experience emotions such as sadness or anger are often unable to deal with problems until the emotional constraint is removed.	For example, family members suppressing grief over the loss of another family member may only need confirmation of the normal grieving process to work through their bereavement. This type of intervention targets the family's affective domain of functioning.
5. **Recognize that suggesting specific tasks or assignments can often provide a new way for family members to behave in relation to one another that will improve problem-solving abilities.**	5. **Assign tasks or assignments aimed at improving family functioning.**
That is, some tasks can facilitate changes in the structure of the family or family rules or rituals.	For example, suggest that the father and son spend one evening a week together in a common activity; suggest to the mother and father that one parent put the children to bed on odd days and the other on even days. This type of intervention influences the family's behavioral domain of functioning.

STAGE 4: TERMINATION

A. IF CONSULTATION OR REFERRAL IS NECESSARY:

1. **Recognize that families appreciate additional professional resources when problems are quite complex.**	1. **Refer individual family members or the family for consultation or ongoing treatment.**
That is, nurses cannot be expected to have expertise in all areas.	For example, say: "I feel that your family needs professional input beyond what I can offer for Tracey's learning disability. Therefore, I would like to refer you to the learning center in the city. They have more expertise in dealing with these types of problems."

B. IF FAMILY INTERVIEWING WITH NURSE CONTINUES:

1. **Recognize the importance of evaluating the family interviews or meetings at regular intervals.**	1. **Obtain feedback from family members about the present status of their problems or level of suffering and initiate termination when the contracted problems have been resolved or sufficient progress has been made.**

Table 5-1	Family Interviewing Skills for Nurses—*cont'd*
B. IF FAMILY INTERVIEWING WITH NURSE CONTINUES:	
That is, evaluating the progress of family interviews leads to more focused and purposeful time spent with the family.	Families normally do not lead problem- or suffering-free lives. Rather, what is important is their feeling of confidence to cope with life's challenges and stresses.
2. Recognize when dependency on the nurse inadvertently may have been encouraged.	**2. Mobilize other supports for the family if necessary, and begin to initiate termination by decreasing the frequency of sessions.**
That is, many interviews over a prolonged period can foster excessive dependency.	For example, nurses can inadvertently provide "paid friendship," with mothers in particular, unless they mobilize other supports such as husbands, friends, or relatives.
3. Recognize family members' constructive efforts to solve problems or soften suffering.	**3. Summarize positive efforts of family members to resolve problems and lessen suffering whether or not significant improvement has occurred.**
That is, the family's perception of progress is more significant than the nurse's perception.	For example, comment: "Your family has made tremendous efforts to find ways to care for your elderly father at home while still attending to your children's needs."
4. Recognize that backup support by professional resources is appreciated by individuals and families in times of stress.	**4. End the family interviews with a face-to-face discussion when possible. If appropriate, extend an invitation for additional family meetings should problems recur or if the family desires consultation.**

CONCLUSIONS

The family interviewing skills (perceptual, conceptual, executive) discussed in this chapter function as a guide or a map for nurses working with families. Thus, through the implementation of these skills, beginning family nurse interviewers can progress through the four stages of the interview by engaging families; assessing strengths and problems; deciding whether to intervene or to refer families; and terminating with the family. These stages of a family interview, with their accompanying skills, are another useful blueprint for nurses working with families. We strongly encourage nurses to tailor the use of these skills to each family's unique context and their relationship with the family. The nurse and family converse and collaborate together and bring forth old and new stories of suffering, problems, resiliencies, strengths, competence, and problem resolution. The ethnicity, culture, class, sexual orientation, and race of the nurse and family members will, of course, influence their collaboration.

References

Benner, P. (2001). *From novice to expert: Excellence and power in clinical nursing practice.* New Jersey: Prentice-Hall.

Chesla, C.A., Gilliss, C.L., & Leavitt, M.B. (1993). Preparing specialists in family nursing: The benefits of live supervision. In S.L. Feetham, et al. (Eds.), *The nursing of families: Theory, research, education, and practice* (pp. 163–76). Newbury Park, CA: Sage Publications.

Cleghorn, J.M., & Levin, S. (1973). Training family therapists by setting learning objectives. *American Journal of Orthopsychiatry, 43*(3), 439–446.

Green, C.P. (1997). Teaching students how to "think family." *Journal of Family Nursing, 3*(3), 230–246.

International Council of Nurses (2002). *Nurses always there for you: Caring for families.* Geneva, Switzerland: Author.

Irinoye, O., Ogunfowokan, A., & Olaogun, A. (2006). Family nursing education and family nursing practice in Nigeria. *Journal of Family Nursing, 12*(11), 442–447.

Leahey, M., & Harper-Jaques, S. (1996). Family-nurse relationships: Core assumptions and clinical implications. *Journal of Family Nursing, 2*(2), 133–151.

Leahey, M., Southern, L., & Harper-Jaques, S. (2007). *Integrating family nursing into mental health: Ladders for learning.* Presented at the 8th International Family Nursing Conference, Bangkok, Thailand.

LeGrow, K., & Rossen, B.E. (2005). Development of professional practice based on a family systems nursing framework: Nurses and families' experiences. *Journal of Family Nursing, 11*(2), 38–58.

Moules, N.J., & Tapp, D.M. (2003). Family nursing labs: Shifts, changes, and innovations. *Journal of Family Nursing, 9*(1), 101–117.

Protinsky, H., & Coward, L. (2001). Developmental lessons of seasoned marital and family therapists: A qualitative investigation. *Journal of Marital and Family Therapy, 27*(3), 375–384.

Schober, M., & Affara, F. (2001). *The Family Nurse: Frameworks for Practice.* Geneva, Switzerland: International Council of Nurses.

Simpson, P., et al. (2006) Family Systems Nursing: A Guide to Mental Health Care in Hong Kong. *Journal of Family Nursing, 12*(8), 276–291.

Southern, L., et al. (2007). Integrating mental health into urgent care in a community health centre. *Canadian Nurse, 1,* 29–34.

Tapp, D.M. (2001). Conserving the vitality of suffering: Addressing family constraints to illness conversations. *Nursing Inquiry, 8*(4), 254–263.

Tapp, D.M., & Wright, L.M. (1996). Live supervision and family systems nursing: Postmodern influences and dilemmas. *Journal of Psychiatric and Mental Health Nursing, 3,* 225–233.

Tapp, D.M., et al. (1997). Family skills labs: Facilitating the development of family nursing skills in the undergraduate curriculum. *Journal of Family Nursing, 3*(3), 247–266.

Tomm, K.M., & Wright, L.M. (1979). Training in family therapy: Perceptual, conceptual, and executive skills. *Family Process, 18*(3), 227–250.

Wright, L.M. (1994). Live supervision: Developing therapeutic competence in family systems nursing. *Journal of Nursing Education, 33*(7), 325–327.

Wright, L.M., & Bell, J.M. (in press). *Beliefs about illness: A model for healing.* Calgary, AB: 4th Floor Press.

Wright, L.M., & Leahey, M. (Producers). (2002). *Family nursing interviewing skills: How to engage, assess, intervene, and terminate with families.* [DVD]. Calgary, AB: www.familynursingresources.com

Chapter 6

How to Prepare for Family Interviews

Nurses who work in various types of settings often ask, "How do I prepare for a family interview?" For many nurses, family meetings happen by chance, such as when family members are visiting their loved one in the hospital. For others, family presence in emergency departments or intensive care units is an accepted practice, and nurses are expected to interact with family members. However, only 5% of nurses work in units with a written family presence protocol (Duran, et al, 2007). For some nurses, interviews are a planned event and may be initiated by either the family or the nurse. Some nurses must overcome the belief that they would be intruding on the family visit if they were present in the patient's room. For many nurses, tension caused by the time required to set up an interview, develop a relationship with the family, and intervene effectively is a major challenge to overcome. Time tension is something that health-care professionals need to learn to manage; otherwise, they can become immobilized by it. We suggest that nurses cannot afford *not to* attend to families!

For both the nurse and the family, the first interview or family meeting is often filled with anxiety. We believe that the less anxious the nurse is, the more he or she invites confidence in family members, thereby reducing their anxiety. The purpose of this chapter is to help reduce the nurse's anxiety by discussing how to plan for the first and subsequent interviews. How to develop hypotheses related to the purpose of the interview is also addressed. Concrete issues are then presented, such as deciding on the interview setting, deciding who will be present, and contacting the family by telephone. Ideas are also offered for the nurse to reflect on the type of relationship that is most desirable to be co-constructed with a family.

HYPOTHESIZING

Before meeting the family for the first time, the nurse should develop an idea of the purpose of the interview and an understanding of the family's context.

For example, a nurse in primary care who is conducting an interview to understand how the family is coping with a chronic or life-threatening illness will conduct it differently than a nurse who is trying to assess family violence, abuse, or some other specified problem. In the latter example, either the family or some other agency may have already identified the problem. Also, if a family were in crisis, for example, having just received news of an untimely death of a family member, the context for the interview would be different than if the family were not experiencing a crisis. Another purpose for an interview could be for the nurse to discover parents' desires about whether or not they want to remain at their child's side during complex invasive procedures and resuscitation. Offering family members a choice was a practice Dingeman, et al (2007) found parents preferred. Indeed, many family members felt it was their right to see what was being done for their loved ones, but parents need not feel obligated to be present. Inquiring how family members would like to be involved in the patient's home care or hospitalization could be another reason for a family meeting. Depending on the purpose of the interview, the types of questions asked and the flow of the therapeutic conversation may be quite different. See Chapters 4, 7, 8, 9, and 10 for clinical examples of interviews.

We are heartened by the work of Burke, et al (2001), who studied the effects of stress-point intervention with families of repeatedly hospitalized children. They hypothesized that each additional hospitalization has unique challenges and could be more stressful than previous ones. A family-focused supportive intervention called Stress-Point Intervention by Nurses (SPIN) was designed to reduce family problems. The findings from a three-site clinical trial with random assignment of nurses and families to experimental (SPIN) and control (usual care) groups indicate that parents who received SPIN were more satisfied with family functioning and had better parental coping after hospitalization than parents who received usual care. The intervention was based partly on CFAM and CFIM and involved " a) identifying the family's own particular stressful issues surrounding the expected or anticipated hospitalization, b) developing a plan with the parents to handle these specific issues and c) following up to praise strengths and successes, modify, and evaluate the success of the intervention" (Burke, et al, 2001, p. 138). It is the follow-through on these types of hypotheses that we find encouraging for the further development of relational family nursing practice.

In our clinical supervision with nurses, we have encouraged them to generate hypotheses related to the purpose of the meeting before the interview. Several authors have defined the term *hypothesis*. In one of their earliest works, Selvini-Palazzoli, et al (1980) refer to a hypothesis as a formulation based on information that the clinician processes regarding the family to be interviewed. They believe that a hypothesis establishes a starting point for tracking relational patterns. Fleuridas, Nelson, and Rosenthal (1986) define hypotheses as "suppositions, hunches, maps, explanations, or alternative explanations about the family and the 'problem' in its relational context" (p. 115). For them, the purpose of a hypothesis is to connect family behaviors with meaning and guide the interviewer's use of questions. A hypothesis provides order for the interviewing process. It introduces a systemic view of the family and generates new views of relationships, beliefs, and behaviors. Tomm (1987) considers a hypothesis to be a "conceptual posture." He advocates for the interviewer to adopt a posture or stance of hypothesizing to deliberately focus his or her cognitive resources in order to generate explanations. Preferably, the hypothesis should be circular rather than linear to maximize the therapeutic potential.

The essence of all these definitions is similar: A hypothesis is a tentative proposition or hunch that provides a basis for further exploration. For example, we know from stress theories and from our own personal and professional experiences that the time of diagnosis of an illness is generally stressful and, in many cases, symptoms temporarily become worse.

Using this as a hypothesis, the nurse can arrange a family interview to discuss the impact of the diagnosis on the family, the family's response to the illness, and the family's expectations of the nurse. In this way, the nurse can explore family patterns of adjusting to the diagnosis and also the family members' ideas of the types of relationships they would like to have with health-care providers. The hypothesis provides general direction for the nurse interviewer in exploring with this particular family their unique adjustment to a diagnosis.

The value of curiosity and naïveté for the nurse working with families, especially in immigrant and marginalized populations, cannot be overestimated. Cultural naïveté and respectful curiosity can be as significant as or more significant than knowledge and skill. Cathryn Ladoux, whose son suffered with Duchenne's muscular dystrophy, reminded us of the importance of cultural context to hypothesizing (Patterson, 1997). She states:

> When a child in our tribe acquires a disability or a chronic illness, we believe that this child is here to remind us that something is out of balance with the universe. We must pay attention to all this child will teach us, for in this way, we will be guided to discover what we need to know to move toward balance. (p. 237)

It is important for us to point out how our thinking about hypotheses has changed as we work toward operating within a postmodernist paradigm and shift from a modernist point of view. Our attention has shifted from what *we* think about what patients and families are telling us, to trying to grasp what *they* think about what they are telling us. Weingarten (1998) offers a useful exercise that she and Roth developed to help clinicians notice this postmodernist shift to what she calls "radical listening" and attending to the other. For example, a family is describing a clinical or personal situation. One nurse listens and notices what the family is saying. This nurse asks herself: What am I thinking about what the family is saying? What hypotheses do I have about this family in their situation? How am I organizing the information I am taking in? Do I see patterns here? What are they? Another nurse listens to the family describing a personal situation. This nurse asks herself: What is the family saying? What do I think *they* think about what *they* are saying? Weingarten (1998) states that the second interviewer generates hypotheses having to do with what the family might be thinking, feeling, or meaning. The first nurse listens more to her own thinking and follows a modernist tradition. The second nurse is more attuned to the family, and her thinking is more consistent with a collaborative, respectful appreciation of the family's worldview. Her hypothesis includes a consideration of the influence of the family's spirituality, ethnicity, class, race, gender, and other such diverse factors on the conversation.

We are quite drawn to this idea: "How is it possible to make cultural distinctions about work done in the culture where the nurse was born and raised?" We encourage clinicians to listen to the family's talk of suffering, make space for their words and voices, and enter into the family's meaning to work with them to soften their suffering. This is a very important skill in relational practice.

How to Generate Hypotheses

Hypotheses can be formulated from many bases. For example, they can be based on information the family provided or ideas about the family gathered during hospital admission, during visiting hours, or from the other staff. The information may consist of opinions, observations of behavior or interactive patterns, and other data. In considering this information, we encourage nurses to ask themselves what they think the other staff thinks about what they are saying. We believe the most relevant hypotheses are generally based on information already provided by the family. Hypotheses can also be based on the nurse's previous experience and knowledge. This experience and knowledge can involve families whom the nurse believes to have similar ethnic, racial, or religious or spiritual backgrounds. The nurse may recall similar problems, symptoms, or situations and similar interactive patterns noticed with previous patients and families. He or she may generate a hypothesis based on knowledge about family development and life cycle stages, research literature, or another conceptual framework that he or she finds most relevant. We encourage nurses to include in their hypotheses ideas about a family's strong spirit, generosity of heart, devotion to one another, deep caring, and commitment. These are enduring qualities that families can draw upon in times of stress.

In addition to formulating hypotheses based on information from or about the family or previous experience and knowledge, nurses may develop hypotheses based on whatever is salient or relevant to them about the health problem or risk that is encountered at this particular time. For example, if a recent tragedy has occurred in the immediate community, the nurse may find such information relevant in generating a hypothesis about what might be most meaningful for this particular family at this point.

We believe that it is important for nurses to state (to themselves) their hypotheses explicitly and consciously before the interview. We do not concur with those who state that hypotheses are unnecessary. Our belief is that a nurse cannot *not* hypothesize or think about a family before the meeting. It is important for nurses to explicate their hunches so that these thoughts may be refined and made transparent as nurse and family engage in the interview process. Presession hypothesizing is viewed as a way to start focusing on the family, churning up the grey matter, making connections, and generating questions. It should not involve preparing an agenda for the session that is imposed on the family regardless of what the family members desire and despite changes that may have occurred since the last session (see Chapter 10 for ideas of how to avoid these kind of mistakes).

The guidelines for designing hypotheses (Box 6-1) have been adapted from the work of Fleuridas, Nelson, and Rosenthal (1986). We encourage nurses to generate hypotheses that are useful. We do not believe that there is one "correct" or "right" hypothesis. Rather, the goal is to generate useful explanations that lead to desired outcomes. We believe that stories are authored through conversations. The story that is co-constructed between the nurse and the family is uniquely personal. We cannot know which hypotheses will fit for a particular family or where people's stories will go. We can only attune ourselves one piece at a time to the story as it unfolds.

We encourage nurses to design hypotheses that are circular rather than linear. That is, a hypothesis that includes all the components of the system (e.g., the family *and* the nurse) is most likely to be more circular than one that includes *either* the nurse *or* the family. (See Chapters 2 and 3 for a more in-depth discussion regarding circularity.) The hypothesis should be related to the family's concerns. This is important because, as previously stated, a

---

Box 6-1 Guidelines for Generating Hypotheses

- Choose hypotheses that are useful.
- Generate the most helpful explanations of the family's behaviors for this particular time.
- Understand that there are no "right" or "true" explanations.
- Include all participants in the "problem-organizing system" to make the hypothesis as systemic as possible.
- Relate the hypothesis to the family's presenting concerns so the interview can proceed along the lines most relevant to the family (versus those relevant to the nurse).
- Make the hypothesis different from the family's hypothesis to introduce new information into the system and avoid being entrapped with the family in solutions that are not working.
- Be as quick to discard unhelpful hypotheses as you are to generate new ones.

hypothesis guides the interview. For example, if the nurse develops a hypothesis that is unrelated to the family's concerns, he or she will ask questions that do not relate to the family's reason for coming to the interview or health-care facility.

The nurse who is attuned to the family's concerns will listen for openings, through questions and reflective discussion, of problem-saturated stories and unique outcomes (see Chapter 7). These outcomes, or "sparkling events," would not have been predicted in light of the problem-saturated story. We remind ourselves that it is clinicians' certainty that can oppress and constrain opportunities to hear the patient's and family's story as they experience it.

We also encourage nurses to design a hypothesis that is different from the family's explanation or hypothesis. For example, a family may have the explanation that Puichun is a "bad daughter" who is shirking her responsibility by not caring for her elderly mother in her own home. The nurse, on the other hand, may develop an alternate hypothesis that fits the same data. The nurse's hypothesis might be that Puichun is overwhelmed by having to take care of her two preschool children while maintaining a full-time job. Thus, she is stretched to the limit in also trying to take responsibility for her elderly parent. Furthermore, Puichun's elderly mother may be sensitive to her stress and thus may be reluctant to live with her.

Once hypotheses have been designed, the nurse can use them to guide the interview. The nurse can ask questions of each member and note the responses to questions, thus confirming, altering, or rejecting a hypothesis. In conversation with families, the nurse should be sure to pay attention to the small and the ordinary. We agree somewhat with the notion that the starting point for hypotheses is arbitrary and intuitive but that hypotheses are either validated or invalidated by evidence (i.e., they may be confirmed, rejected, or modified). We remain acutely aware that our notion of validation and evidence is just from our "observer perspective."

Hypothesizing and interviewing constitute a reciprocal cycle and are interdependent. The nurse develops a hypothesis, asks questions, converses with the family about the "problem" and its influence on their lives, and gathers evidence that either confirms or refutes the nurse's hypothesis. Box 6-2 illustrates questions, adapted from the work of Watson (1992), that invite hypothesizing about the system and the problem. As new information is generated, the nurse modifies the previous hypothesis and evolves a more useful one. The goal of the interview is to bring forth the family's resources to deal with the presenting issue. More information about how to conduct family interviews is provided in Chapters 7 to 10.

| **Box 6-2** | Questions That Invite Hypothesizing About the System and the Problem |

Who

Who is in the system? Who are the key players?

Who first noticed the problem?

Who is concerned about the problem?

Who is affected by the problem? (most, least)

Who is interested in keeping things the same? (most, least)

Who referred the system?

What

What is the problem at this time?

What is the meaning that the problem has for the system and for different members of the system?

What solutions have been attempted?

What question(s) do I feel obliged to ask?

What beliefs perpetuate the problem?

What beliefs might be identified as core beliefs?

What beliefs are perpetuated by the problem?

What problems and solutions perpetuate the beliefs?

Why

Why is the system presenting at this time?

Where

Where has the information about this problem come from?

Where does the system see the problem originating?

Where does the system see the problem and the system going if there is no change or if there is change?

When

When did the problem begin?

When did the problem begin in relation to another phenomenon of the system?

When does the problem occur?

When does the problem not occur?

How

How might a change in the problem affect other parts of the system (key players, relationships, beliefs)?

How does a change in one part of the system affect another part of the system or the problem?

How will I know when my work with this system is over?

How might my work with this system constrain the system from finding its solution?

Leahey and Wright (1987) provide an example of how alternative hypotheses can be generated before the first family meeting:

> A nurse working in an extended-care facility noted that the family, especially the 9- and 10-year-old children, avoided visiting their 41-year-old mother who had Huntington's disease, and that the patient's symptoms worsened around visiting days. The children seemed depressed and withdrawn every time they came to the nursing unit on their monthly visits. During case conferences, the staff wondered whether there might be a connection between the family's avoidance and the patient's flailing and head banging. They generated several hypotheses to explain why the family might be avoiding the patient and why the patient's symptoms seem to exacerbate around the time of the family visits.
>
> One hypothesis pertained to the children's belief that head banging and flailing were controllable. Perhaps the children felt that their mother was not trying to control herself so she would not have to return home to care for them. This made them angry and they avoided her. An alternate hypothesis concerned the children's conflicting loyalties toward their mother and the aunt who took care of them. Perhaps they felt that if they visited too often, their aunt might think they did not appreciate her care. Thus they spaced out their visits and seemed depressed and withdrawn. They demonstrated both loyalty to their aunt and affection for their mother.
>
> Yet a third hypothesis involved the children's fears of developing Huntington's disease themselves. They avoided visiting and showed sadness because of their own expectations of contracting the disease. (p. 60)

Having generated several hypotheses about the family and the problem in its relational context, the nurse arranged a meeting with the family. The purpose of the interview was to clarify how the family members wanted to be involved with the patient and how the staff could be most helpful to them. The nurse's hypotheses were relevant to the purpose of the interview. She did not know if the frequency of the family visits was a "problem" for either the children or the patient. Rather, the staff had identified the problem. Thus, the nurse chose to frame the purpose of the meeting as one in which the staff wanted to know how they could be most helpful to both the family and the patient during the patient's hospitalization. The patient and family were partners in care with the staff rather than the family being the object of care.

INTERVIEW SETTINGS

A family interview or meeting can take place anywhere: in the home (e.g., kitchen, living room, patient's bedroom); in an institution (e.g,. bedside, urgent care center, nurse's clinic or office, used treatment room); or in the community (e.g., interviewing room, school, office, health clinic, on the street where a homeless family "resides"). Depending on the purpose of the clinical interview, some settings are more conducive to therapeutic conversation than others. Nurses and families, therefore, need to consider the advantages and disadvantages of various settings. They should be flexible in choosing a setting that is appropriate for the specific purpose of the interview. We believe families should be offered a choice of setting whenever possible.

Home Setting

Many nurses interview families in their home setting. There are some concrete advantages to interviewing in the home. Infants, children of all ages, and very old seniors are able to be present more easily. Chances are increased for meeting significant but perhaps elusive family members, such as boarders, adolescents, or grandparents. Firsthand acquaintance with the physical environment is also possible. For example, the presence of staircases and the display of family photographs can be observed. The nurse can also experience the family's social environment; for example, rituals of eating, challenges with mobility, or who answers the doorbell can be noted.

In addition to the concrete advantages to interviewing in the home, there are also other advantages. These are particularly important if the nurse is from a different social class or ethnic background than the family. Articulate middle-class parents may report only the most exemplary family interactions in the office or school. The nurse may thus have difficulty understanding how the apparent competence of the parents and the banality of the reported parent–child incidents are in such sharp contrast to the degree of behavioral upset manifested by the child. Lower-class families sometimes have difficulty bridging the gap and explaining their situation to middle-class nurses who are unfamiliar with their home milieu. For example, a nurse suggests that an older woman prepare her husband several small meals a day rather than one very large meal, which he is unable to consume. The nurse did not know (and the family members were too embarrassed to mention) that the family shared cooking facilities with other people in their apartment building. A home interview can thus give the nurse a clearer direction for therapeutic suggestions and can enhance the relationship between the family and nurse.

Disadvantages of using the home setting for family interviews include the increased administrative and personal cost involved in traveling. In addition, the meeting may suffer from more disruptions and may require the nurse to structure the interview flexibly. Nurses should also be aware that a family's home is their sanctuary. If family members are asked in their own home to share intense and deep emotions, they are often left without a retreat. For example, if abuse is an issue, the nurse should anticipate that the family's affective disclosure would be quite intense. Perhaps they will need more physical and psychological space to deal with the issues than their home permits. On the other hand, if the purpose of the interview is to facilitate shared grieving over the loss of a family member, the home setting might be ideal.

Snyder and McCollum (1999) reported that their interns who did in-home therapy experienced both positive and negative challenges. They liked and cared about the clients a great deal and felt humbled by their warm reception into their clients' homes. Ideas about therapeutic boundaries and hierarchy, confidentiality, and the timing and pacing of interventions were challenged. The interns reported doubts and confusion about the usefulness of intervention after they had experienced first-hand the economic deprivation of their clients. These interns also reported that they developed strategies for addressing their anxiety, such as giving themselves "permission" to work with the family in a unique, nonclinical way. They learned to manage time in the meetings, keep a focus, and remind clients of the overarching, jointly constructed goals for the meetings. Thomas, McCollum, and Snyder (1999) noted that the interns' experiences in clients' homes had significant effects on their in-clinic work. One intern reported, "Getting stuck with clients worries me less than before. Experiencing Head Start families in their homes has taught me there are small opportunities even when their world seems to go under. That makes me more confident and comfortable to hold clients' hopelessness and helplessness and be with them to develop strategies to get unstuck, rather than trying to rescue them" (p. 186).

The nurse can tell the family that he or she would like to have an interview in the home "to get a better feel for their situation." Explain that, in your experience, there are frequently interruptions to an interview in the home (e.g., telephone calls, cell phones, neighbors dropping in, children wanting to put on the television or do computer games). Ask, "How should we handle this if it comes up?" In this way, you have already set the stage for work, rather than for visiting, and for a specific purpose to the interview. One way to handle social offerings, such as coffee or a cold drink, is to say, "Thanks, but maybe we could work first and then have coffee afterward." The work and social boundaries are thus clearly identified. Keep in mind that although this boundary might be useful for some nurses working with certain ethnic groups, such a boundary might be offensive to families from other ethnic groups or from rural areas.

Office, Hospital, or Other Work Setting

The greatest advantage of using the work setting for the interview is that the setting is the nurse's base. Therefore, the nurse can capitalize on the opportunity and adapt the setting to the needs of the interview. Fewer telephone calls, mobile phones, and visitor interruptions are also possible. Furthermore, the nurse has a greater opportunity to obtain consultation from colleagues when interviewing the family in the work setting.

Disadvantages of interviewing in the work setting concern issues of context. A family might be intimidated by the professional trappings (e.g., large institution, plush furniture, complicated equipment) and therefore display anxiety or reluctance to talk. Frank (1991), a sociology professor who experienced cancer, described the reluctance he and his wife had about sharing information in the hospital setting because of the lack of privacy:

> One incident can stand for all the deals I made during treatment. During my chemotherapy I had to spend three-day periods as an inpatient, receiving continuous drugs. In the three weeks or so between treatments I was examined weekly in the day-care part of the cancer center. Day care is a large room filled with easy chairs where patients sit while they are given briefer intravenous chemotherapy than mine. There are also beds, closely spaced with curtains between. Everyone can see everyone else and hear most of what is being said. Hospitals, however, depend on a myth of privacy. As soon as a curtain is pulled, that space is defined as private, and the patient is expected to answer all questions, no matter how intimate. The first time we went to day care, a young nurse interviewed Cathie (my wife) and me to assess our "psychosocial" needs. In the middle of this medical bus station she began asking some reasonable questions. Were we experiencing difficulties at work because of my illness? Were we having any problems with our families? Were we getting support from them? These questions were precisely what a caregiver should ask. The problem was *where* they were being asked.
>
> Our response to most of these questions was to lie. Without even looking at each other, we both understood that whatever problems we were having, we were not going to talk about them there. Why? To figure out our best deal, we had to assess the kind of support we thought we could get in that setting from that nurse. Nothing she did convinced us that what she could offer was equal to what we would risk by telling her the truth. (p. 68)

Suggestions for how beginning interviewers can maximize privacy in hospital settings are given later in this chapter.

Another disadvantage of using the institution for interviewing can be the inadvertent fostering of the belief that pathology resides in the individual—for example, "Mom's the sick one. We're only coming to help Mom get over her depression." This attitude is particularly evident if the mother has been hospitalized on a psychiatric unit. This disadvantage can be handled by using the family's willingness to "help Mom." The interviewer can reframe or discuss the mother's hospitalization in a positive light, for example, by saying, "Perhaps your mother's hospitalization has provided the family with an opportunity to all work together in a new way."

How to Use the Work Setting

Some places have elaborate interviewing rooms, but most nurses must make do with the usual hospital or clinic setting. Therefore, they may have to negotiate with coworkers for space and privacy. We recommend that you choose a private place where you will not be interrupted. For example, an unused patient room or an office is often more quiet than a four-bed room with curtains, a visitor's lounge, or a waiting area. Remove any important or intimidating equipment (such as machines and monitors). The discussion area should ideally be sparsely furnished with movable chairs and no big desks, couches, or examining tables. This allows family members to control their own space, move closer or further away from someone, and not worry about children touching hospital equipment. A few quiet toys, such as rubber or cloth hand puppets or paper and crayons, are useful to have readily available in the room. Books and magazines should not be available during the interview because they give a mixed message to the family, especially to adolescents. The participants should expect to discuss issues; they should not expect to read during the interview.

Acquaint yourself with the physical layout of the room before the session. This is likely to increase your feelings of comfort when first meeting the family. At the beginning of the interview, if children are present, you can say to the parents, "I'd like you to handle the children in whatever way you usually do. That will give me a better idea of how things go at home." If the baby starts to cry, observe who comforts the baby. If the noise level gets beyond your tolerance, notice what tolerance level the family has. Unless absolutely necessary, try to avoid giving behavioral directives (e.g., "Watch out for that plant," or "Don't touch Dad's chest tube") during the first interview unless they are required for safety. Valuable information can be lost by imposing your standards of behavior. At the same time, be sure to structure the interview to avoid chaos.

At the end of the session, assess the influence of the work setting. Ask family members if they behaved differently than they usually do: for example, "Did the children behave better or worse today than they usually do?" or "Were family members more or less talkative than usual?"

WHO WILL BE PRESENT

Deciding who will be present for the first and subsequent interviews is important. This decision is generally determined mutually by family members and the nurse. In our early days of working with families, we thought it imperative that *all* family members be present for family interviewing. However, we have signifcantly changed in our thinking about who should come to the meetings. We now believe that a nurse can develop hypotheses, assess, and intervene with a family regardless of who is in the interviewing room. The number of people in the room does not reflect the unit of treatment. Rather, what is more important is how the nurse conceptualizes human suffering, problems and solutions.

We find the idea of "problem-determined systems" very helpful in our clinical practice. The appropriate description for the system of treatment is the problem-determined system rather than the individual, the couple, the family, or the larger system. People are under the influence of problems; *they* are not the problem. This notion allows us to avoid becoming mired in the concept of "dysfunctional" family, work group, and so forth. We do not find it useful to use the term "dysfunctional family." People in active communication regarding a problem are the problem-determined system. We do not believe that problem-determined systems are fixed. Rather, they are fluid—always changing, never stable. As the problem definition changes, so does the membership of people involved in describing a problem. The goal of interviewing is the dissolving of the problem or the softening of suffering.

The role of the nurse is simply to engage in conversation with those who are relevant to the problem resolution in such a way that there is a co-evolved, new reality or language system, and therefore a dissipation of the problem or shared belief that a problem exists. Through therapeutic conversations, the nurse creates a context wherein the participants in a problem-determined system no longer distinguish what they are thinking and talking about as a "problem." The nurse knows that change has occurred when the concerned membership of a problem-determined system can think and talk of their shared problems differently.

Although we believe in problem-determined systems, we also believe that nurses who are beginning to interview families will generally find it easiest to invite everyone living in the household to be present for the first interview. In this way, the nurse can more easily elicit information from members who most likely have a description of the problem. To begin family work by interviewing one person is to begin with a handicap, but it is still possible to inquire about family functioning even if seeing only one family member. If the problem concerns a couple, we usually try to have both spouses together for the first meeting. Similarly, if the issue is parenting related and it is a heterosexual couple, then the father, mother, and child should all be invited to the meeting.

The more people present, the more information it is possible to gather and the more viewpoints and descriptions of the influence of the problem can be considered. Family members at the first interview might include the young children, the grandparent "who never has much to say," and the nephew "who just moved in for the weekend." Sometimes the most significant thing that the nurse is able to accomplish in a family interview is just to bring the whole family together in one spot at one time to discuss an important issue. We believe it is very useful, when deciding who to invite to the first meeting, to consider the network of professional resources involved with the family as well as the family members themselves. We believe that relational family nursing is best practiced in context.

Nurses frequently question whether they should include psychotic family members, those who are mentally or cognitively handicapped, or elderly family members who are experiencing dementia or Alzheimer's disease in the first interview. Generally, the answer is yes. Including these members provides the nurse with an opportunity to talk with the family about the impact of the psychosis, mental handicap, or dementia on the family. In addition, it shows the nurse how the family and individual interact to deal with the presenting problem. A clinical example may help to illustrate this point. A family requested help for their 6-year-old daughter, who was "regressing, having imaginary friends, and refusing to play with peers or go to school." During the initial interview, the little girl walked over to the door and turned the doorknob. The nurse asked her not to leave the room. In response, the family members said that she was not leaving but rather "was letting the cat out the door." The nurse looked a bit startled because there was no cat in the room. The nurse then asked the other children how they knew that this was what the little girl was doing and proceeded to inquire if this was how they usually responded to the child's behavior. Had the "psychotic child" not been present, the nurse would have been unaware of the siblings' contribution to perpetuating the presenting problem.

Deciding who should be present for the first meeting is an important indicator of the collaborative nurse–family relationship. A conversational partnership is encouraged. It is important for the nurse to be aware of who is in relevant conversation with whom about the problem outside the interview room. Given the ever-increasing use of telecommunication devices such as e-mail, chat rooms, Skype, Facebook, and text messaging, it is useful for nurses to inquire not just about the family contacts in the immediate vicinity but also those online. We must respect family members' ideas about *what* is germane to the conversation and *who* should be involved in it. We recommend that all decisions about who should be involved in meetings, when, and what is talked about are determined collaboratively, conversation by conversation.

FIRST CONTACT WITH THE FAMILY

The way in which the nurse makes the first contact with the family conveys an important message to the parents and the children. We believe that the quality of the nurse's relationship with the family in addition to manners and etiquette are important ingredients for accountable therapeutic engagement. Although manners and etiquette may seem like superficial concepts, they can help manage deep currents of tension and ease potentially awkward situations. Manners such as respect, tact, and humility can go a long way in establishing the nurse–family relationship. Madsen (2007, p. 98) suggests that "there is a long history of tension between professionals and poor and working-class people that is often invisible to professionals but painfully apparent to the poor and working classes."(See Chapter 8 for more ideas about using manners in relational practice.) By inviting each person in the household to the family meeting, the nurse implicitly states that each is a significant family member and each has a role to play in understanding, describing, and dealing with the problem.

The rationale for involving as many family members as possible can be explained in several ways. If a baby is in the intensive care nursery, the nurse might use the following explanation: "When a baby is in the intensive care nursery, we frequently find that family members are concerned and often anxious as well. Bringing family members together results in more information for the whole family on how best to help the baby." Another idea is for the nurse to say: "Years ago fathers and family members were kept out of the delivery room and out of the hospital units. We've learned, though, how important it is to have family members present for special events such as the birth of a baby. Now we recognize that it is even more important for family members to be present and involved in health care when there is some type of illness. Family members know and care about each other. In many cases, they have a lot to offer each other."

With families experiencing a crisis, such as the diagnosis of a stage 4 glioblastoma brain tumor in a previously healthy 62-year-old father, nurses may want to focus on providing physical information relating to the patient. Nurses can also see if the family is interested in hearing about services for families coping with the sudden onset of a life-threatening illness. They may state that in times of crisis families often find comfort in meeting with health professionals so that they can gain accurate, up-to-date patient information. Nurses are aware from their knowledge of crisis theory that the time frame for intervention is limited because crises are self-limiting. Assertiveness and a calm demeanor are generally useful postures for nurses to take when a family is overwhelmed by a crisis.

Spouses sometimes agree to come for an interview but object to either having the children present or taking the children out of school. One way to handle the latter problem is to have meetings before school, during the lunch hour, after school, or in the evening. If this is not possible because of the nurse's work schedule, the nurse may say, "I understand your concern about the children missing school. In my experience, however, children have a tremendous amount to contribute to a family interview. They generally feel quite relieved when they see that the family is dealing with an issue about which they may have been worrying. Schools also are usually quite agreeable to children missing an hour."

How to Set Up an Appointment

The purpose of the initial telephone contact with the family is to set up an appointment for an interview, explain the rationale for involving family members, and determine with the family who will be present at the interview. Naturally, both nurse and family gather much useful information about each other over the telephone. Telephone contact is therefore part of the development of a collaborative working relationship, and the nurse should treat it as such.

Generally, the first telephone contact sets the stage for subsequent interviews. Our advice is to pay careful attention to this contact, whether you call the family to set up an appointment or a family member calls you. The following is a sample first telephone contact:

Mother: Hello.

Nurse: Mrs. Rodriquez, this is Amrita Virk. I'm the community health nurse in your neighborhood.

Mother: Yes.

Nurse: I understand that you have a new baby. It's our practice to come out and visit all families with new babies.

Mother: Oh, I didn't know that.

Nurse: Yes, we usually do a physical examination of the baby and discuss feeding or other concerns.

Mother: Oh, that seems like a good idea. The doctor didn't tell me much about feeding.

Nurse: Sure, we can get into that during our visit. I was just calling to set up a time that would be convenient for your family and for me. I would like to see the whole family because usually, when a new baby arrives, the child has a great impact, not just on the mother but on the father and other children as well.

Mother: You can say that again! My 2-year-old usually seems to like his baby sister, but last night I saw him pinch her.

Nurse: Yes, these are the kind of things that we can discuss when the whole family and I get together. The meeting will probably take about an hour. I have some time available on Tuesday at 10 or on Thursday at 3. Which would be best for you, the baby's father, and the children?

Mother: Tuesday isn't good because my son is going to the doctor that day. Thursday would be better since my husband works shifts and gets off at 2:30. But I should tell you that my husband didn't like the last nurse because she made some negative comments about his tattoos and piercings.

Nurse: Let me reassure you, I'm fine with people expressing themselves in body art. Would a 3:00 appointment give him enough time to get home, or should we make the appointment at 3:15?

Mother: Yes, 3:15 would be better.

Nurse: I look forward to seeing you and the whole family then.

Mother: Yes, me too.

Nurse: Goodbye.

Mother: 'Bye.

In the previous selection, the nurse was clear, confident, focused, and accommodating. The nurse set forth the purpose of the interview and who she thought should be involved. She invited the family to a "meeting" by stating that this is the agency's usual practice. She responded directly to Mrs. Rodriquez' concern about tattoos and piercings. Whether the nurse refers to her collaborative time with a family as a "meeting" or an "interview" is arbitrary; it's most important that the nurse use the most palatable language with families based on the context in which she encounters families. The nurse took charge by identifying and introducing herself without apologies and offered specific appointment times. Furthermore, the nurse received much information that can be useful in the family meeting:

"The doctor didn't tell me much about feeding."

"I saw [the 2-year-old] pinch her."

"My son is going to the doctor..."

"...my husband works shifts..."

It is not possible to provide written guidelines to cover all the various situations that nurses will encounter in trying to set up a family interview. Davis Kirsch and Brandt (2002) offer some suggestions for involving fathers based on their telephone research:

- Emphasize the value and importance of fathers' perceptions and observations.

- Demonstrate respect for the father's time by asking if the telephone call was made at a convenient time.

- Use positive verbal cues (e.g., common courtesies, personal titles, a cheerful and interested tone of voice, positive phrases, carefully timed pauses and probes, and affirming remarks) in order to maintain rapport.

Each family presents different challenges for the nurse, and vice versa. Therefore, each interview must be approached with flexibility. A unique approach is always the rule in clinical practice. Each telephone contact demands a slightly different plan of action to invite family members to an interview or to elicit the family's permission for a home visit. We strongly encourage nurses, especially community health nurses, to plan their telephone calls and appointments to maximize efficiency and the possibility of developing a collaborative partnership with the family. We generally do not recommend that appointments be set up by email, as there can be issues of confidentiality and ambiguity about how promptly the email will be responded to and by whom. However, we do recognize that, in some rural or very remote areas, setting up and even offering family meetings may be done online via Skype, email, or iChat. Online family meetings may prove to be very useful if a face to face meeting is not possible.

RESISTANCE AND NONCOMPLIANCE

Often in our clinical supervision with nurses, we have been asked how to deal with resistant or noncompliant families. When nurses ask this, they are generally referring to families whom they perceive to be "in denial," oppositional, or noncompliant with ideas and advice that could promote, maintain, or restore health. The family is designated as noncompliant when they do not respond to particular nursing interventions; nurses often interpret this behavior as unwillingness or a lack of readiness to change (Wright & Levac, 1992).

We do not use the terms *resistance* and *noncompliance* anymore, because we have not found them clinically useful in relational family nursing practice. Resistance was initially used to describe a client's reluctance to uncover or recover from some anxiety-filled experience. The clinician's job was often to uncover this material, but when this area of the client's life was touched on, the client was seen to resist the interviewer's effort. Resistance is still generally viewed as "located" in the client and is often described as something the client "does." This is a linear view that implies that problems with adherence to treatment regimens reside within individuals and families, not in the interactions or relationships between individuals. We disagree with this view because we see the idea of resistance as a *product* of client–interviewer interaction. We believe that resistance and noncompliance are not terms describing a unilateral phenomenon but rather an interactional phenomenon.

Rather than using the terms resistance and noncompliance, we have found the multidirectional terms *cooperation* and *collaboration* to be very useful clinically. When nurses think of how they work collaboratively with families, they are less likely to impose their will on the family. They tend to open space for the family and to be more tentative and receptive to the family's point of view.

The theory behind the "death of resistance" (de Shazer, 1984) has emerged since the first edition of *Nurses and Families*. The result has been a dramatic increase in a solution-focused, strengths-based, and resiliency orientation to family interviewing (de Shazer, 1991; Hougher Limacher & Wright, 2006; Lipchik & de Shazer, 1986; Madsen, 2007; Walsh, 2003). With emphasis on a solution comes an increasing emphasis on change, cooperation, and collaboration. We are especially partial to the work of Miller and Duncan (2000), who advocate client-directed, outcome-informed clinical work as compared to a model-driven focus. The "common factors" (Hubble, Duncan, & Miller, 1999) associated with positive outcomes include:

■ Extratherapeutic factors, including clients' beliefs about change, strengths, resiliencies, and chance-occurring positive events in clients' lives (40%)

- The client–therapist relationship experienced as empathic, collaborative, and affirmative in focusing on goals, method, and pace of treatment (30%)
- Hope and expectancy about the possibility of change (15%)
- Structure and focus of a model or approach organizing the treatment (15%).

Another orientation that we have embraced is the narrative approach initially developed by White and Epston (1990). This approach provides far more positive direction for our work than the negative labels of resistance and noncompliance, which previously left us stymied in our clinical practice. They open us to reflect on conversation, language, and possibilities rather than pathologizing labels. We agree with Madsen (2007) that relational practice can be seen as a cross-cultural negotiation in which the two parties interact in a mutually influencing relationship, a two-way street.

How to Deal With a Hesitant Family Member

A spouse may be hesitant to attend the family session for several possible reasons. Each requires a different approach on the part of the nurse. The following are a few common situations that interviewers encounter:

1. "My husband would never come to a family interview. He thinks that my mother's stroke and how to handle it are my responsibility."
   Ask what the wife thinks about her husband attending the interview. If she believes her mother's chronic illness is *her* responsibility and has very little to do with her husband, she will not be interested in inviting her husband to a family interview. You would need to engage in conversation with the wife to see if she wants to alter *her* cognitive set *before* you start talking to her about her husband.

2. "My husband wouldn't want to come to a family interview. Besides, I wouldn't know how to get him there."
   If the wife would like her husband to attend but does not know how to invite him, you can explore with her why she feels her husband might be hesitant. There could be several reasons:

   - He may view the problem as his wife's, not his own.
   - The timing of the interview might be inconvenient.
   - The thought of going to a hospital might be repugnant ("seeing all those sick people").
   - He may be afraid of being blamed for not taking a more active role in his mother-in-law's care.

   You can ask the wife if she thinks any of these feelings or thoughts might be stopping her husband from becoming involved. After she has speculated on the reasons for her husband's hesitance and her own desire for him to be present, you can discuss with her some alternate ways to engage him:

■ She can discuss with her husband how *she needs his help* to deal with her mother's illness.

■ She can find out convenient times for her husband to come to a half-hour meeting.

■ She can tell him exactly where the interview will be held (e.g., not in the patient's room but in an office).

■ She can tell him that *the nurse is most hesitant* to see only parts of the family for a meeting.

That is, if you saw only the wife with her mother, there could be a danger that the husband would feel left out and perhaps blamed. If he were present, however, this could not happen. He could help you to understand more fully the relationship between his wife and her mother. The wife can let him know that he has a unique view of the family—a view that only he can provide. Most husbands do not like to be left out of the original planning and decision making. Once they have a fuller understanding of the purpose of a family interview, they are often quite agreeable to attending.

Although it may involve a little persuasion, when nurse-interviewers ask that the husband attend and state that they need him to be there, they are likely to have few problems with absent husbands. Conversely, nurses are likely to have difficulties in this area if they are timid or inconsistent in requesting the husband's presence.

Piercy (2003) offers an interesting description of a not unfamiliar couple interaction pattern frequently encountered in engaging the "less articulate, less emotionally available partner [who is] generally (but not always) the husband" (p. 61):

> Often the woman wants more emotional intimacy, and the man isn't sure what to say or do. (That wasn't part of throwing a football.) If anything, the more the woman demands intimacy, the more the man tharns. (Tharning is wonderful word from the book *Watership Down*. In the book, rabbits tharn. That is, they freeze in one spot when they are frightened.) Men often tharn when their partners beg for more intimacy. And, of course, the more the man tharns, the more frustrated the woman becomes. Because of her frustration she presses for more intimacy. This frightens and immobilizes the man more, he tharns again, and the painful repetitive cycle is in full gear. (p. 62)

Ideas for interrupting such a negative circular pattern might include suggesting to the woman that she *stop pursuing* the husband to attend the family meeting. Rather, the wife could write down some questions and invite him to discuss them with her for 10 minutes at the kitchen table the next evening. (This gives him a heads up regarding the questions, specifies the time frame, and identifies a place. These strategies can all help to reduce tharning.) Sample questions include:

- Let's talk about any times in our relationship that we pulled together as a team. How was that for each of us?
- What can we do now to show each other we're uniting as a team to, for example, stand up to the impact of depression on Erica and our family?

We believe it is important for nurses to recognize that husbands and wives may be at different stages in their desire to seek help. Some of this may be attributable to gender differences, with females generally more likely than males to utilize social support networks. Women are more than twice as likely as men to speak to someone about their problems. It seems likely, then, that wives would lead the discussion regarding assistance and help their husbands along the process.

Another idea for inviting an anxious or a threatened family member to an interview is to suggest that the person be asked to be present as an observer, just to see what is happening. Also, the person can come whenever he or she is "in the mood" as a historian, an accuracy checker, or a consultant. If these suggestions are followed, it is important to ask the "observer" or "historian" to react at the *end* of the interview to what the family has discussed in the session. Gradually, as the family member continues to observe sessions, he or she often becomes more comfortable and is willing to participate *during* the interview. This may be a particularly useful way of engaging some adolescents. Telling the member not to talk places no direct pressure on that member to participate. Silent members are often closely attuned to the process and, when a sensitive area is broached, they forget their defensive stance and join in the process. Other times, they may remain silent but hear the information.

How to Deal With Family Nonengagement and Referral Sources

If you have difficulty engaging the family on the telephone, you may need to contact the referral source. That is, physicians frequently tell a patient on discharge, "The nurse will be out to check up on you and see how you are doing." When you contact the patient, the patient may have forgotten what the physician said, may be confused about the purpose of the visit, or simply may not be interested in being "checked up on." Sometimes in situations of suspected child abuse, the physician may contact the nurse and ask him or her to "drop in on the family just to see if there is any abuse." You may then find yourself in an awkward situation, trying to explain the purpose of your visit to a family who may be reluctant to have you come. One way to approach this is to say: "Doctor Fishkin asked me to set up a visit with your family to discuss issues about raising children. Dr. Fishkin feels that most families who have infants and preschoolers as close together as yours sometimes find it helpful to talk to a nurse." In approaching the situation this way, you have clearly indicated that it is on Dr. Fishkin's request that you are calling, and you have attempted to normalize the purpose of the interview. If, however, the family is still reluctant to have you visit, initiate contact with the physician and have the physician set the stage for future work with the family. You should not consider this inability to engage a family your fault or the fault of the family's resistance, but rather as a problem of inadequate preparation by the referral source.

Several other ideas have emerged over the past few years about dealing with referral sources. We find it best for interviewers to avoid focusing prematurely on family dynamics if the request for the interview comes from another agency or if the interview is compulsory. Treatment failure often ensues because of powerful conflict between the family and the referral source. In such situations, we recommend that the nurse engage the family and conceptualize their work together as collaboration to deal not with family issues per se, but with dynamics between the family and the agency. In this way, the interviewer can join with the family around a problem such as, "That school is always making trouble for us." Thus, the focus of the nurse's work would not be on family dynamics but on work with the family to "get the school off their case."

Selvini (1985) also has talked about the problem of the sibling as the referring person. She advocates that special attention be paid to the influence of this person (generally a "most competent and prestigious family member") on the nurse–family contract. We believe that the interviewer must identify and grapple with the expectations of the person referring the "problem family" for assessment. Some useful questions to ask include:

- Why is this referral being made to me at this time?
- What is the relationship between the referral source and my agency?
- Who is paying? For whom? For what?
- What are the expectations of the hierarchy within which I work?
- If the referral source is unhappy with the assessment, who will hear about it?
- If I am unhappy about the assessment process, who will hear about it?

In any situation in which nonengagement occurs, the nurse must realize that the reluctance provides important information about the dynamics between the interviewer and the family. The hypothesized reason that a person is not present should be explored at the first interview. For example, we were once asked to consult with the family members of a 59-year-old woman who was terminally ill with cancer. The hospital staff nurse arranged the interview for a time convenient for the husband and adult daughter. However, only the daughter and the mother showed up for the interview. In exploring the reasons that the husband did not attend, we discovered that he was 73 years old and in poor health himself, a fact unknown to the hospital staff. By asking the adult daughter about the impact of her mother's illness, we also discovered information about the father's absence. The daughter wept openly about her mother's impending death. She then stated, "If you think I'm a basket case, you should see my father. He's in worse shape than I am." Thus, in this situation, the husband's absence from the interview provided important information about the family's emotional state. It is important for nurses to understand reluctance as a systems phenomenon rather than an individual issue. In this case, we hypothesized not only that the father was reluctant to attend but that the adult daughter was trying to protect him.

IDEAS ABOUT THE NURSE–FAMILY RELATIONSHIP

Since the first edition of this book, there has been a steady increase in the attention paid to the "therapeutic conversation," meaning the therapist acting with, rather than on, patients. Madsen (2007) has advocated self-reflection in relation to dominant societal ideas and practices, intimate relationships past and present, the client–therapist relationship, gender, sexual thoughts, and strong feelings. We believe that nurses cannot avoid their influence on families. Nurses and families inevitably influence each other, but not always with predictable results. We are concerned not about influencing or not influencing, but about understanding the quality and nature of the relationship.

We believe that families and nurses each have their own health-care system. Families provide diagnosis, advice, remedies, and support to their members in both sickness and health. They have constraining and facilitating beliefs about the illness (Wright & Bell, in press). Nurses also have their own constraining and facilitating beliefs, theories, opinions, recommendations, and remedies about managing problems or illness that they share with families. Leahey and Harper-Jaques (1996) have outlined five assumptions relating to the family–nurse relationship and the clinical implications of each assumption. Emphasis is on both the nurse's *and* the family's contribution to establishing and maintaining the relationship. We believe that it is useful for a nurse to reflect on his or her potential contribution to the relationship *before* meeting with a family. It is also helpful for the nurse to reflect with the family about their working relationship at the end of their contract. More ideas on this topic are provided in Chapter 12.

The five assumptions related to the family–nurse relationship are as follows:

Assumption 1: The Family–Nurse Relationship is Characterized by Reciprocity. The family and nurse are connected in a pattern that is quite distinct from the positivist-based idea of two separate components, either family or nurse. It is the "fit" between the family and the nurse that is important to foster a collaborative partnership. Trust is a process that evolves over time. If the nurse wishes to foster a reciprocal relationship, he or she can reflect on the sample questions in Box 6-3.

Assumption 2: The Family–Nurse Relationship is Nonhierarchical. Each person's contribution is sought, acknowledged, and valued. Conversation is

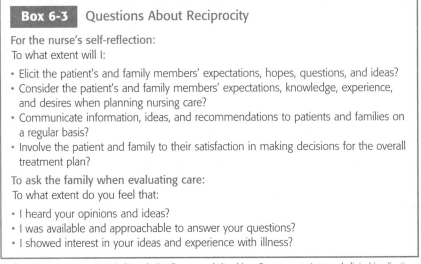

Leahey, M., & Harper-Jaques, S. (1996). Family-nurse relationships: Core assumptions and clinical implications. *Journal of Family Nursing, 2*(2), 133–151. Copyright 1996 by M. Leahey and S. Harper-Jaques. Reprinted by permission of Sage Publications, Inc.

a co-construction of ideas and mutual discoveries. Both the nurse and the family remain aware, however, that they are bound by moral, legal, and ethical norms. Tapp's research (2000) identifies useful practices to counterbalance hierarchy and expert professional views: "offering commendations, coevolving a description using the family's language, exploring the illness story and the medical story, asking questions that invite reflection, and initiating conversations about family members' preferences" (p. 69). Madsen (2007) suggests that the clinician examine the stance that clients hold toward problems. Do the clients believe they have some influence over the problem and want to do something about it? Or, perhaps the clients don't see themselves as having a problem? Or, this is a problem, but I have no control over it? Connecting with clients' intentions, hopes, and preferred view of self is a way for the nurse to demonstrate respect and collaboration. (More ideas on this topic are given in Chapter 7).

Box 6-4 contains some sample questions that nurses can ask themselves and the family about hierarchy.

Assumption 3: Nurses and Families Each Have Specialized Expertise in Maintaining Health and Managing Health Problems. Families who live with chronic conditions develop expertise in managing symptoms, adapting their environments, and adjusting their lifestyles. They live "near illness," "along side of illness," and "with illness" (Fergus, 2000). When they meet with nurses, they bring a wealth of information and personal expertise to the encounter. Nurses, through their education and experience, also bring expertise to the relationship with the family. Out of this mutually respectful encounter, the family members' confidence in self-management of a disease can be enhanced.

Box 6-4   Questions About Hierarchy

For the nurse's self-reflection:
- To what extent am I imposing my beliefs on the family? Allowing the family to impose their beliefs on me?
- How well do the expectations between the family and I match?
- When there is a mismatch, whose opinion usually predominates?
- How frequently are decisions about the patient's health care made mutually by the patient, family, and me?

To ask the family when evaluating care:
- Overall, what percentage of time were decisions about your health care made in a mutual way between you and me?
- To what extent did I help you feel more in control of your health?

Leahey, M., & Harper-Jaques, S. (1996). Family-nurse relationships: Core assumptions and clinical implications. *Journal of Family Nursing, 2*(2), 133–151. Copyright 1996 by M. Leahey and S. Harper-Jaques. Reprinted by permission of Sage Publications, Inc.

Diabetes management, for example, depends largely on self-regulation. We believe that more traditional compliance models relying on pressure to follow recommendations need to be replaced by patient-empowerment models. Nurses risk starting to believe they really know what the best answers are for a family or a particular problem. We agree with Tapp (2000) that "these beliefs can become oppressive when the expert has the expectation that their advice must be obeyed" (p. 81). Nurses can think about their own expertise and the family's expertise as they prepare to meet with a family to discuss managing a particular health problem. Developing and nurturing a kernel of appreciation and respect for the client is foundational to a therapeutic alliance. Box 6-5 provides sample questions that the nurse can consider.

Box 6-5   Questions About Expertise

For the nurse's self-reflection:
- What do I know about the family's ideas and plans for care during this course of treatment?
- What can I learn from this family about their experiences in living with this health problem?
- What knowledge and expertise do I have to offer this family?
- How does this family demonstrate its trust in my expertise?
- Who in the family has the most expertise in getting grandpa to take his medications?

To ask the family:
- What are the things that you or other family members do to help you to relieve the pain?
- What ways have you found most useful to invite your father to take care of his own personal needs?

Leahey, M., & Harper-Jaques, S. (1996). Family-nurse relationships: Core assumptions and clinical implications. *Journal of Family Nursing, 2*(2), 133–151. Copyright 1996 by M. Leahey and S. Harper-Jaques. Reprinted by permission of Sage Publications, Inc.

Assumption 4: Nurses and Families Each Bring Strengths and Resources to the Family–Nurse Relationship. Nurses who use a resource-identification lens strive to draw forth the family's cultural, ethnic, spiritual, and other beliefs that have been helpful in dealing with the health problem. Nurses also bring to the relationship their own life experience, clinical intuition, and cultural, ethnic, spiritual/religious, and educational background. Box 6-6 offers sample questions that nurses can ask themselves about how they would like the relationship with the family to be focused on strengths.

Assumption 5: Feedback Processes Can Occur Simultaneously at Several Different Relationship Levels. Nurses have often focused on family dynamics and interactional patterns within family systems. More recently, however, they have begun to address family–nurse relationships and reflect on their own patterns with families. Rarely do nurses address the interactive patterns that can simultaneously occur at different relational levels. Box 6-7 offers sample questions that the nurse can consider about the family–nurse relationship.

Box 6-6 **Questions About Strengths**

For the nurse's self-reflection:
• Will my actions and comments acknowledge the strengths and abilities of this family?
• What interventions can I use to further enhance this family's strengths?
• How am I inviting this family to trust my knowledge and skill in helping them with this health problem?
• What are the strengths that I bring to this relationship?

Leahey, M., & Harper-Jaques, S. (1996). Family-nurse relationships: Core assumptions and clinical implications. *Journal of Family Nursing*, 2(2), 133–151. Copyright 1996 by M. Leahey and S. Harper-Jaques. Reprinted by permission of Sage Publications, Inc.

Box 6-7 **Questions About The Family–Nurse Relationship**

For the nurse's self-reflection:
To what extent did my relationship with the patient and family help to:

• Increase their knowledge? Insight? Coping?
• Increase *my* knowledge? Insight?
• Improve or enhance their emotional well-being? My emotional well-being?
• Improve the patient's physical health?
• Build stronger relationships between the patient and family members?

To ask the family when evaluating care:
To what extent did our meetings together:

• Meet your needs?
• Contribute to your having an increased sense of confidence in living with your illness?

Leahey, M. & Harper-Jaques, S. (1996). Family-nurse relationships: Core assumptions and clinical implications. *Journal of Family Nursing*, 2(2), 133–151. Copyright 1996 by M. Leahey and S. Harper-Jaques. Reprinted by permission of Sage Publications, Inc.

CONCLUSIONS

In preparing for family interviews, it is important for nurses first to remind themselves of the purpose of the meeting and then to generate hypotheses related to this purpose. Box 6-8 outlines areas for nurses to consider in preparing for family interviews. Decisions about the interview setting and who will be present flow from ideas about who has a description of the problem and who is a customer for change. These ideas are the result of a collaborative relationship between the nurse and the family.

Box 6-8 Helpful Hints for Planning a Family Meeting

Before Initiating a Family Meeting, the Nurse Needs To:
• Ascertain the purpose and benefit of a family meeting from the family's perspective.
• Explain why a family meeting may be beneficial to the family.
• Determine who in the family agrees that a problem exists, and who might be willing to come to a family meeting.
• Mutually determine with the family when and where a meeting could take place (home, office, school).
• Read literature about working with families experiencing similar health problems to better understand the issues, concerns and lived experiences of that specific population.
• Begin to formulate hypotheses (explanations about the family's behaviors that connect the family system and the particular problem).
• Prepare linear and circular questions that will elicit relevant data about family structure, development, and function. (See the discussions of CFAM in Chapter 3 and CFIM in Chapter 4 for examples of questions.)

Levac, A.M.C., Wright, L.M., & Leahey, M. (2002). Children and families: Models for assessment and intervention. In J.A. Fox (Ed.), *Primary health care of infants, children, and adolescents* (2nd ed.) (pp. 10–19). St. Louis: Mosby. Copyright 2002. Adapted with permission from A.M.C. Levac, L.M. Wright, & M. Leahey.

References

Burke, S.O., et al. (2001). Effects of stress-point intervention with families of repeatedly hospitalized children. *Journal of Family Nursing, 7*(2), 128–158.

de Shazer, S. (1984). The death of resistance. *Family Process, 23*(1), 11–21.

de Shazer, S. (1991). *Putting difference to work.* New York: Norton.

Davis Kirsch, S.E., & Brandt, P.A. (2002). Telephone interviewing: A method to reach fathers in family research. *Journal of Family Nursing, 8*(1), 73–84.

Dingeman, R.S., et al. (2007). Parent presence during complex invasive procedures and cardiopulmonary resuscitation: A systematic review of the literature. *Pediatrics, 120* (4), 842–854.

Duran, C.R., et al. (2007). Attitudes toward and beliefs about family presence: A survey of healthcare providers, patients' families, and patients. *American Journal of Critical Care, 16*(3), 270–279.

Fergus, K.D. (2000). When illness intrudes. *Journal of Couples Therapy, 9*(3/4), 113–124.

Fleuridas, C., Nelson, T., & Rosenthal, D. (1986). The evolution of circular questions: Training family therapists. *Journal of Marital and Family Therapy, 12*(2), 113–127.

Frank, A.W. (1991). *At the will of the body: Reflections on illness.* Boston: Houghton Mifflin.

Hougher Limacher, L., & Wright, L.M. (2006). Exploring the therapeutic intervention of commendations: Insights from research. *Journal of Family Nursing, 12(3),* 307–331.

Hubble, M.A., Duncan, B.L., & Miller, S.D. (1999). Introduction. In M.A. Hubble, B.L. Duncan, & S.D. Miller (Eds.), *The heart & soul of change: What works in therapy* (pp. 1–19).Washington, DC: American Psychological Association.

Leahey, M., & Harper-Jaques, S. (1996). Family-nurse relationships: Core assumptions and clinical implications. *Journal of Family Nursing, 2(2),* 133–151.

Leahey, M., & Wright, L.M. (1987). Families and chronic illness: Assumptions, assessment, and intervention. In L.M. Wright & M. Leahey (Eds.), *Families and chronic illness* (pp. 55–76). Springhouse, PA: Springhouse.

Levac, A.M.C., Wright, L.M., & Leahey, M. (2002). Children and families: Models for assessment and intervention. In J.A. Fox (Ed.), *Primary health care of infants, children, and adolescents* (2nd ed.) (pp. 10–19). St. Louis: Mosby.

Lipchik, E., & de Shazer, S. (1986). The purposeful interview. *Journal of Strategic and Systemic Therapies, 5(1),* 88–99.

Madsen, W.C. (2007). *Collaborative therapy with multi-stressed families.* New York: The Guilford Press.

Miller, S.D., & Duncan, B.L. (2000). Paradigm lost: From model-driven to client-directed, outcome-informed clinical work. *Journal of Systemic Therapies, 19(1),* 20–33.

Patterson, J.M. (1997). Meeting the needs of Native American families and their children with chronic health conditions. *Families, Systems and Health, 15(3),* 237–241.

Piercy, F.P. (2003). Communication questions for couples: A structure to engage the less articulate, less emotionally available partner. *Journal of Couple and Relationship Therapy, 2(1),* 61–65.

Selvini, M. (1985). The problem of the sibling as the referring person. *Journal of Marital and Family Therapy, 11(1),* 21–34.

Selvini-Palazzoli, M., et al. (1980). Hypothesizing circularity-neutrality: Three guidelines for the conductor of the session. *Family Process, 19(3),* 3–12.

Snyder, W., & McCollum, E.E. (1999). Their home is their castle: Learning to do in-home family therapy. *Family Process, 38(2),* 229–242.

Tapp, D.M. (2000). The ethics of relational stance in family nursing: Resisting the view of "nurse as expert". *Journal of Family Nursing, 6(1),* 69–91.

Thomas, V., McCollum, E.E., & Snyder, W. (1999). Beyond the clinic: In-home therapy with Head Start families. *Journal of Marital and Family Therapy, 25(2),* 177–189.

Tomm, K. (1987). Interventive interviewing: Part I. Strategizing as a fourth guideline for the therapist. *Family Process, 26(1),* 3–13.

Walsh, F. (Ed.) (2003). *Normal family processes : Growing diversity and complexity* (3rd ed.). New York: Guilford Press.

Watson, W.L. (1992). Family therapy. In G.M. Bulechek & J.C. McCloskey (Eds.), *Nursing interventions: Essential nursing treatments* (2nd ed.) (pp. 379–391). Philadelphia: W.B. Saunders.

Weingarten, K. (1998). The small and the ordinary: The daily practice of a postmodern narrative therapy. *Family Process, 37(1),* 3–16.

White, M., & Epston, D. (1990). *Narrative means to therapeutic ends.* New York: Norton.

Wright, L.M., & Bell, J.M. (in press). *Belief and illness: A model to invite healing,* Calgary, AB: 4th Floor Press.

Wright, L.M., & Levac, A.M. (1992). The non-existence of non-compliant families: The influence of Humberto Maturana. *Journal of Advanced Nursing, 17,* 913–917.

Chapter

How to Conduct Family Interviews

Once a nurse and a family have decided to meet together, the nurse can begin to consider how to conduct the meeting. Just as there are stages in the whole interviewing process, there are also stages in initial family interviews. An awareness of these stages provides the nurse with a general interview structure and can help to allay the nurse's anxiety.

In this chapter, we present guidelines for each stage of an initial family interview. After this, we address the stages involved in the entire interviewing process.

GUIDELINES FOR FAMILY INTERVIEWS

The following stages generally occur in initial interviews:

1. *Engagement stage,* in which the family is greeted and made comfortable.

2. *Assessment stage:*

   a. **Problem identification,** in which the nurse explores the family's presenting concerns and/or suffering

   b. **Relationship between family interactions and health problem,** in which the nurse explores the family's typical responses to the health problem and how the health problem is affecting their family life and relationships

   c. **Attempted solutions,** in which the family and nurse talk about the solutions the family has tried and their effects on the presenting issues

   d. **Goal exploration,** in which the nurse draws together the information and the family specifies what goals, changes, or outcomes they are seeking (note: if family members are suffering from the impact of an illness, it is also important to clarify if they desire an alleviation or softening in their suffering in the emotional, physical, and/or spiritual domains)

3. *Intervention stage,* in which the nurse and family collaborate on areas for change
4. *Termination stage,* in which the nurse and family end the interview

Engagement Stage

During the engagement, or first stage of the interview, the nurse and family begin to establish a therapeutic relationship. Engagement has several purposes (Box 7-1). The goal in this stage is for family members and the nurse to develop a mutual alliance. In the beginning, the nurse is often perceived as a stranger, unknown and potentially helpful or unhelpful. Because family members do not know what to expect from the nurse, he or she must establish a relationship with the members by demonstrating understanding, competence, and caring. Family nursing is relational nursing practice, acknowledging the expertise and knowledge of families (Tapp, 2000).

We encourage nurses to consider the type of relationship that they would like to establish with families over the course of time. Thorne and Robinson (1989) have described various stages of the evolution of relationships between families experiencing chronic illness and their health-care professionals: naïve trust, disenchantment, and guarded alliance. They propose that naïve trust among the chronically ill, their families, and health-care providers is inevitably shattered in the face of unmet expectations and conflicting perspectives. Anxiety, frustration, and confusion often result in disenchantment. Trust can then be reconstructed on a more guarded basis so that the chronically ill patient, the family, and the nurse can continue to engage in health-care activities. Thorne and Robinson (1989) state that this reconstructed trust is highly selective and is based on revised expectations of the roles of both patient and provider. They suggest that there are four relationship types in guarded alliance: hero worship, resignation, consumerism, and team playing. In hero worship and team playing, the trust dimension is high, whereas in resignation and consumerism, it is low. Both team playing and consumerism place a high value on competence,

---

| **Box 7-1** | Purpose of Engagement |

- To promote a positive nurse–family relationship by developing an atmosphere of comfort, mutual trust, and cooperation between the practitioner and the family
- To recognize that the family members bring strengths and resources to this relationship that may have previously gone unnoticed by health-care professionals
- To prevent potential practitioner–family misunderstandings or problems later on in the therapeutic relationship

Levac, A.M.C., Wright, L.M., & Leahey, M. (2002). Children and families: Models for assessment and intervention. In J.A. Fox (Ed.), *Primary health care of infants, children, and adolescents* (2nd ed.) (p. 11). St. Louis: Mosby. Copyright 2002. Adapted with permission.

whereas hero worship and resignation put a low value on competence. Important ABCs for the engagement of families with children are provided in Box 7-2.

Reciprocal trust is a critical dimension to consider during the engagement phase of family interviewing. The nurse helps the patient and family to feel more confident in their own competence in managing illness. To develop a high degree of trust in the nurse, the patient and family are encouraged to explicitly state their expectations for health care. The nurse provides the opportunity for family members to express their desires. If the patient and family are to have a high degree of trust in their own competence, family members and health-care providers must acknowledge the family's resources. We agree with Griffith (1995) that there is no completely open conversational space. We have found her ideas helpful in continuing to move from a stance of certainty to wonder. She outlines four "certainties" that constrain opportunities to hear the family's story as they experience it. Although she applies these to religion, we have used them in our teaching and continually try to apply them when talking with families experiencing chronic or life-threatening illness.

Box 7-2 The ABCs of Engaging Families		
A	B	C
Assume an active, confident approach.	Begin by providing structure to the meeting (time frame, orientation to the context).	Create a context of mutual trust.
Ask purposeful questions that draw forth family assessment data.	Behave in a curious manner, and take an equal interest in all family members, whether present or not.	Clarify expectations about your role with the family.
Address all who are present, including small children.	Build on family strengths by offering commendations to the family.	Collaborate in decision making, health promotion, and health management.
Adjust the conversation to children's developmental stages.	Bring relevant resources to the meeting (list of agencies, phone numbers, pamphlets).	Cultivate a context of racial and ethnic sensitivity. Commend family members.

Levac, A.M.C., Wright, L.M., & Leahey, M. (2002). Children and families: Models for assessment and intervention. In J.A. Fox (Ed.), *Primary health care of infants, children, and adolescents* (2nd ed.) (p. 11). St. Louis: Mosby. Copyright 2002. Adapted with permission.

Constraint #1: I know what your illness is like for you because I have the same or a similar illness.
Constraint #2: I know what your illness is like for you because I know what you mean when you talk about suffering.
Constraint #3: I know why your illness has happened to you—because you have not lived a healthy life.
Constraint #4: I know how you should manage your illness and you could too if you follow what I say!

One way of reminding ourselves not to fall into the trap of certainty and expertness on the family's situation has been to develop a strong sense of curiosity. When initiating engagement, we assume a position of neutrality or curiosity. Cecchin (1987) draws connections between neutrality or curiosity and hypothesizing. He maintains that curiosity is a delight in the invention and discovery of multiple patterns. "Curiosity helps us to continue looking for different descriptions and explanations, even when we cannot immediately imagine the possibility of another one...hypothesizing is connected to curiosity. Hypothesizing has more to do with technique. Curiosity is a stance, whereas hypothesizing is what we do to try to maintain this stance" (p. 411). We believe that curiosity nurtures circularity and is useful in the development of hypotheses. We have found hypothesizing, circularity, and curiosity to be extremely important components of our clinical work. We agree with Cecchin (1987), who states, "circular questioning can be understood as a method by which a clinician creates curiosity within the family system and therapy system" (p. 412). See Chapters 2 and 3 for more information about circularity, and see Chapter 6 for additional ideas about hypothesizing. We have found that, by using hypothesizing, circularity, and curiosity, we have become more open to families and they, in turn, have developed more reciprocal trust in us. The family perceives the nurse as curious when he or she does not take sides with any one member or subgroup. Nurses who are curious are seen as aligned with everyone and no one in particular at the same time. They are seen as nonjudgmental and accepting of everyone.

Increased societal, professional, and personal experiences with fear and suffering have caused us to engage clients in more personal, open ways than ever before, especially since September 11, 2001. The societal experiences of large-scale death and both foreign and domestic terrorism (e.g., the Oklahoma bombing, the Virginia Tech massacre, Hurricane Katrina) have made our relationships with families more human and less clinical, and thus more transparent. Our own personal sufferings and losses of family members and friends enhance this transparency. Our therapeutic relationships in recent years have felt different, less formal, and more connected as we experience similar fears and suffering when crisis events erupt or illness or loss occurs.

Wright and Bell (in press) pose a reflective question when they ask, "Are clinicians to remain neutral and non-hierarchical when confronted with illegal or dangerous behaviors?" They answer this important question by stating that each family functions in the way that members desire and in a way that they determine most effective. However, being part of a larger system, clinicians are bound by moral, ethical, legal, cultural, and societal norms that require them to act in accordance with those norms in regard to illegal or dangerous behavior. Cecchin (1987) assented that, in these situations, "clinicians may need to take a different position—one which is distinct from a non-hierarchical, collaborative stance. Confronted by illegal behavior, a clinician may have to abandon a curious, therapeutic manner and become a social controller" (p. 409) in order to conform to the moral or legal rules and their consequences.

To enhance engagement, the nurse must provide structure, be active and empathic, and involve all members of the family. To provide structure, the nurse might say something such as, "We'll meet now for about 10 minutes so that I can get a better sense of your expectations and any concerns you have about hospitalization. We can then talk about what I might be able to help you with. How does that sound to you?" By stating the structure at the beginning of the meeting, the nurse reduces the family's anxiety about how long they will meet and also gives some direction for the conversation.

One way in which the nurse can be active during the engagement phase of the interview is to find out who is present. Many times, we have found that "extra" family members attend interviews in the hospital. Leahey, Stout, and Myrah (1991) found an attendance rate of 94% of families invited to meetings on an inpatient mental health unit in a Canadian community hospital. Extra family members attending interviews held constant over a 7-year period. In many cases, family members of whom the nurse was unaware showed up for the family meeting. For example, extended family members or ex-spouses might have been invited by the patient or other family members who believed it was important for them to be present.

Some nurses have found it useful to start an interview by working with the family in constructing a genogram or ecomap (see Chapter 3). Duhamel and Campagna's genograph (2000) is a particularly helpful educational tool that can assist nurses in drawing genogram and determining what questions to ask. Families generally find that constructing a genogram is an easy way to involve themselves in giving the nurse relevant information. The genogram can be obtained reliably and accurately in a brief interview. Furthermore, genograms obtained by a health-care provider are likely to have more influence on care and health outcomes than those completed by the patient or health assistant and placed on file.

At the start of the interview, the nurse should ask questions of each member. This is particularly important for nurses working with families with adolescents. Engaging adolescents by asking what their favorite computer games or school subjects are and why, whether they play any sports, what musical groups they like, and whether they have any special talents and hobbies can sometimes be useful. The purpose of these questions is to start establishing a shared habit (between the nurse and the young person) of discussion and bantering about the young person's opinions about personal aspects of their lives. However, we do not recommend that this type of conversation go on for longer than 5 minutes because it seems easier for families to engage around the presenting problem than to make small talk of a general nature.

Nurses should initially attempt to spend an equal amount of time with each family member. We suggest that the nurse ask the same question or a similar one of each member to gather each person's ideas about a particular topic. We believe that when families answer questions, they are not retrieving particular experiences. Rather, in the conversation with the clinician, family members put forth their own unique storytelling of their experiences, suggest beginnings and endings for these experiences, and highlight portions of experience while diminishing or excluding others.

Examples of questions used to foster a collaborative working relationship and engagement have been offered by Levac, Wright, and Leahey (2002). These provide an implicit message to family members that the practitioner cares about them. They also open space for the family to exert more power in the conversation, voice concerns, and clarify the working arrangement. Some examples are:

- What was most useful and least useful in your past working relationships with health professionals like me?
- If you become frustrated with our work, would you be open to having a conversation with me about your concerns?
- On a scale of 1 to 10 (with 1 being very low and 10 being very high), how well do you think I understand your situation?
- In what ways was our discussion useful to each of you?

Both students and practicing nurses have often asked us for tips on how to deal with verbose clients. Some ideas we have found helpful include:

- Letting the person tell his illness story or particular concern
- Setting the timeframe at the beginning such as "we have 20 minutes to meet; what are the most important things that we need to discuss?"
- Saying, "I know we only have time to skim the surface today in talking about your experiences, so what shall we focus on?"
- Explaining, "I'm not connecting what you're telling me with the reason you've come in today. Could you help me out on this, please?"
- Taking a break to pull your thoughts together or to seek a consult.
- Stopping the discussion and setting limits such as, "We can spend 10 minutes talking about the poor addictions services in this city and 10 minutes on what you said your goals were and how you're addressing them. How does that sound as a plan for today?"

■ Using humor and interrupting by saying something such as, "Seems like we could talk all day about this issue, but I'm mindful of the time."

■ Determining who is most interested in the client being seen if the client has been referred by another health professional. "The note from your physician indicated she wants you to have.... Is this your understanding of why you are here today? Did you have another goal for our meeting?"

If the engagement between the nurse and family does not proceed well or if a fit cannot be established, we recommend that the nurse take a metaposition and reflect on the relationship. We have found the following ideas about relationships with families helpful to keep in mind in our clinical practice.

1. Both the health-care provider and patient are experts. The patient is expert in the illness story and, usually but not always, the health-care provider is expert in the physiology of the disease process, illness management, and softening suffering.

2. The health-care provider will try to facilitate change, but the ultimate agent of change is the patient.

3. To construct a workable management plan, the patient's and the health-care provider's interpretation of the symptoms must both be acknowledged.

The engagement stage may also be thought of as the phase of the interview in which a context for change is created that constitutes the central and enduring foundations of the therapeutic process (Wright & Bell, in press). Wright and Bell suggest that all obstacles for change need to be removed during this stage so that a full and meaningful nurse–family engagement may be made. Examples of obstacles to change include a family member who does not want to be present or attends the meeting under duress, previous negative experiences with health-care professionals, and unrealistic or unknown expectations of the referring person about treatment. Most central to this stage, however, is that the family should feel that the nurse is willing to listen and witness their voice, to "do hope," as Weingarten (2000) calls it. However, hope does not reside within one individual; it is not solitary or alone. Hope is something we do with others. "It is the responsibility of those who love you to *do hope* with you" (Weingarten, 2000, p. 402). Especially during the engagement phase, nurses should follow the clients' lead, listening for and adopting their language, worldview, goals, ideas about the problem, and experiences with the change process. We encourage nurses to get to know their clients outside of the influence of the problem and connect with them in their lives. For example, a nurse could appreciate their experience as skilled immigrants who have made tremendous sacrifices to stand up to oppressive regimes, learn a new language, and make a significant move to a new country. She could wonder how this stamina might now serve the family as they stand together against chronic pain.

We have found Madsen's ideas (2007) about the importance of relational stance helpful when engaging with multistressed families. He describes several relationship difficulties:

- Loss of connection with the family can occur when clinicians' reactions to clients run the gamut of emotions, including judgment, fear, despair, resignation, and avoidance.

- Loss of competence can occur when the clinician feels overwhelmed by the nature of the problems confronting multistressed families, the inadequate patchwork of available services, and the apparent lack of progress in change.

- Loss of direction can occur when clinicians feel overwhelmed by the multitude of problems, not knowing where even to begin work, and by personal emotional reactions to the family's plight.

- Loss of hope can occur if the clinician gets caught in the cycle of despair and resignation.

- Loss of balance can occur if clinicians romanticize the strengths and resiliencies of families while ignoring or minimizing the limitations and pain that exisit in their lives.

Madsen's suggestions (2007) for engaging and intervening in these situations include the clinician's adopting an attitude of humility, becoming an appreciative ally, striving for cultural curiosity and honoring family expertise, believing in the possibility of change and building on family and community resourcefulness, working in partnership and fitting services to families, engaging in empowering processes, and making our work more accountable to clients.

If the engagement relationship is not going well, we encourage nurses to acknowedge this difficulty. For example, the nurse could tune into potential difficulties such as the client's repetitions or interruptions. The nurse could acknowledge the difficulties to the patient and say, "I'm having trouble understanding how you'd like me to help." Or, "It doesn't seem that this visit is going the way you had hoped." "I would like to work with you even though we see some things differently."

Assessment Stage

During the assessment stage, the nurse and family explore four areas: problem identification, relationships between family interaction and the health problem, attempted solutions, and goals.

Problem Identification: Exploration and Definition

During this phase of the family interview, the nurse asks family members about their main concerns, complaints, or problems. The nurse could ask, for example, "What is the problem that each family member would most like to see addressed or changed?" After exploration of each family member's perception of the most pressing concern, preferably at the end of the interview (once adequate engagement has occurred), we have found it useful to ask the "why now?" question: "What made you decide to come in today?" We assume the family probably consulted others prior to meeting with the nurse and are curious about why, at this point in time, the client chose to seek help.

Another useful question is the "one question question" suggested by Wright (1989)—that is, "If you could have only one question answered during our work together, what would that one question be?" This is a particularly effective way to elicit at the end of the clinical meeting the family's deepest concern or greatest area of suffering (Duhamel, Dupuis & Wright, in press). It provides a focus for the conversation and generates sharing of new information among family members and between the nurse and the family. For example, the husband of a 44-year-old woman with newly diagnosed multiple myeloma asked, "How can I support my wife and children better during this time?" The teenage daughter asked, "How can I learn more about my mother's illness?" The patient asked, "How long do I have to live?" The young adult son asked, "Should I avoid having my friends come over to the house so that the house can be quieter for my mother when she returns home?" These four very different questions made it clear that each family member had different concerns and issues, expectations for the interview, and expectations for the relationship with the nurse. We are drawn to Madsen's phrase, "Honor before helping," in which he reminds us how important it is not to attempt to help a family without its authorization to do so (2007).

It is important to emphasize that an effective interview does not depend on the use of any one type of question but on the knowledge of when, how, and to what purpose questions are used with particular family members at particular points in time. (For more information on various types of questions, see Chapters 4 and 9.)

Leahey and Wright (1987) give examples of how to elicit the family's concerns by asking circular questions that focus on the present, past, and future:

Present. The nurse should ask each family member, including the children, to share their knowledge and understanding of the present situation. For example, the community health nurse working with a family with teens could ask such questions as:

- What is the family's main concern now about Mobina's cyber-bullying?
- How is this concern a problem for the family now as compared with before?
- Who agrees with you that this is a problem? Is this a problem that Mobina believes she has control over?
- What is your explanation for this?

Past. In exploring the past, the nurse can again ask questions pertaining to:

- *Differences:* How was Mobina's behavior before her cyber-bullying was noticed?
- *Agreement or disagreement:* Who agrees with Dad that this was the main concern when the family lived in Uganda?
- *Explanation or meaning:* What do you think was the significance of Mobina's decision to stop using the family computer for her messaging?

Future. During the initial interview with a new family, the nurse must learn about the family's own hypotheses or beliefs about the problems. In asking the family to explain the present situation, the nurse should attempt to identify previously unrecognized connections. This might be done by asking such questions as:

- If Rahim suddenly developed renal disease, how would things be different from the way they are now?
- Does Rahim agree with you?
- If this were to happen, how would you explain the change in Mobina's relationship with Mom?

If children or adolescents are reluctant to identify concerns in the family, the nurse may need to ask the children alternative questions. Children may hesitate to disagree with their parents' description of the situation. A nurse can ask a child what he or she would like to see different in the family or how he or she would know if the problems went away. For example, one 8-year-old repeatedly stated that there were no difficulties surrounding his brother's diabetes and his mother's intense involvement with the sick child. However, when the nurse asked a future-oriented question about what differences he would notice in the family if his brother did not have diabetes, the 8-year-old said that he and his mother could go to basketball games after school. At the time of the interview, the mother had stated she was hesitant to leave the house after the boys returned from school for fear that her oldest son, Raja, would have an insulin reaction.

Other ideas for involving children in interviews have also been presented. For example, having paper, markers, and crayons in the office and using strategies such as:

- Art techniques (e.g., drawing a family picture)
- Verbal techniques (e.g., the "Columbo" strategy of taking a position of not knowing)
- Role playing or make believe
- Storytelling techniques to allow families to personify, reframe, and externalize problems
- Puppet and doll techniques to ask the family about interactions
- Experiential techniques (e.g., family sculpture or "a can of worms in action")

Relationship differences can be explored by providing props, such as scarves, hats, and glasses, to the children. This role-playing technique using props enables children and adults to display their perceptions. Another idea is to give the child an ordered array of pictures ranging from a frowning face to a smiling face and then ask, "Which one of these is most like how you and your brothers got along this week?" Engaging children through video games offers many other possibilities. Whatever strategy is used to engage young people in conversation, we are mindful of the importance of inviting active thinking by children and adolescents versus the expectation of compliance with adult thinking. This is foundational to relational practice.

In exploring the presenting concern, the nurse should obtain a clear and specific definition of the situation. We recommend that the nurse pay attention only to the problem as defined by the family, setting aside his or her own definition of the problem. We believe it is helpful to coevolve a problem description using the family's language and to initiate conversations about family members' preferences. Box 7-3 lists some factors for the nurse to consider when defining the problem.

Mauksch, Hillenburg, and Robins' (2001) have offered eight techniques (microskills and cognitive cues) that we have adapted for establishing problem focus in an initial interview:

1. Microskill: Make a list; ask "anything else" until the patient or family indicates completion.

2. Cognitive cue: Remind yourself that you need not address all problems in one visit.

| **Box 7-3** | Factors to Consider in Defining the Problem |

1. Presenting Problem
   • Specify
2. Problem Identification
   • Who in the family was the first to identify the problem? And then who?
   • When was the problem identified?
   • What were the concurrent life events or stressors at the time of identification of the problem?
   • Who else (family members, friends) agrees that it is a problem? Who disagrees?
   • How does the family understand that this problem developed (beliefs)?
3. Problem Evolution
   • What behaviors became problematic?
   • Pattern of development
   • Frequency of problem emergence
   • Time intervals of quiescence
   • Factors aggravating
   • Factors alleviating
   • Who in the family is most and least concerned?

Adapted from Family Nursing Unit records, Faculty of Nursing, University of Calgary.

3. Microskill: Place the relationship above the need to establish focus. Some patients in crisis may need to tell their story before attempting to organize their health concerns into manageable bites.

4. Microskill: Avoid premature diving. Postpone asking questions that elicit in-depth stories until the presenting problems and concerns have emerged.

5. Microskill: Ask the family to prioritize the list.

6. Cognitive cue: Ask yourself if you can address all the problems; if not, suggest follow-up.

7. Microskill: Express concerns about particular issues (such as abuse) when your rank order differs from the family's. Negotiate in a collaborative way that does not undermine the patient's autonomy.

8. Microskill: Seek confirmation and commitment. (pp. 149–50)

It is interesting to note that, despite eliciting more problems, the physicians who used these eight strategies did not use more of their scheduled time than did the control group, and they were as satisfied with their patient encounters as were physicians in the control group. We believe these findings would also hold true for nurses.

We try to remember, in our conversations with families, that each family expresses its pain and suffering in a unique way. Al-Krenawi (1998) points out that Bedouin-Arab patients routinely express their personal or family problems in proverbs. For example, a co-wife of a husband engaged in polygamy described how her husband's multiple marriages affected her deeply by saying, "My eye is blind and my hand is short." She meant that she felt unable to do anything (p. 73). Another example of how a presenting problem can be described is offered by Fraser (1998), who cites African-American couples' frequent use of metaphors to describe issues. For example, a couple experiencing major disagreement and conflict used the metaphor, "a glass wall between us, we can see each other, but we never seem to touch" (p. 142). The nurse can identify conflict among family members about the problem definition if it arises. When differences exist, the nurse should clarify the issues further to help define the problem for which the family is seeking change.

The nurse can also ask questions of each member about his or her own explanation for the current situation. It is important for nurses to attend to *how* clients talk about the concerns that prompted them to show up for a meeting. To bring a family focus to the situation when interviewing an individual, the nurse could ask the following family-oriented questions:

1. Has anyone else in the family had this problem? (This addresses family history.)

2. What do other family members believe caused the problem or could treat the problem? (This explores the individual's explanatory model and health beliefs.)

3. Who in the family is most concerned about the problem? (This helps to understand the relational context of the concern.)

4. Along with your illness and symptoms, have there been any other recent changes in your family? (This addresses family stress and change.)

5. How can your family be helpful to you in dealing with this problem? (This focuses on family support.)

Wright and Bell (in press) believe that exploring family beliefs in the first meeting and at times of crisis is particularly important. The family members are joining with the nurse and entrusting the nurse with their well-being. If they feel that their beliefs or explanations about the illness are not acknowledged, they may quickly feel marginalized. The nurse can ask, for example, their explanation or theory as to why this problem exists at this point in time. We believe it is also important to ask if the client and family have any control over the problem. The simplest way to do this is to ask direct, explanation-seeking questions such as, "What do you think is the reason for your son's violence toward his peers? Do you think Salahuddin has any control over the problem?"

Another idea is to ask clients to use their imagination to discuss an explanation. The interviewer can also offer a variety of alternative explanations or "gossip in the presence" by asking triadic questions such as, "Yael, What do you think is Zack's explanation for your mother's depression?" In exploring the family's preexisting explanations, it is essential for the interviewer to be curious and to avoid agreeing or disagreeing with the explanation.

There are several advantages to exploring the family's causal explanations, including improving cooperation between the interviewer and the family, developing systemic empathy with all family members versus selective empathy with one or two, detaching oneself from explanations provided by other professionals, recognizing and avoiding coalitions, loosening firmly held explanations, diluting negative explanations, and developing an ability to speculate with the clients about the effects of believing in one explanation or the other. Roffman (2003) calls this process of interaction "unpacking." The clinician and the family "collaborate to generate more possibilities by identifying, opening up, breaking up, and making distinctions within existing constraints" (p. 64).

Morgan (2000) offers other intriguing ideas for a thorough exploration and personification of the problem by externalizing the problem. To shift the problem from inside the person to outside of them, Morgan suggests exposing and finding out as much as possible about:

- the problem's tricks
- the problem's tactics
- the problem's way of operating
- the problem's ways of speaking: its voice, tone, the content of what it says

- the problem's intentions
- the problem's beliefs and ideas
- the problem's plans
- the problem's likes and dislikes
- the problem's rules
- the problem's purposes, desires, motives
- the problem's techniques, dreams, deceits, or lies
- the problem's allies: who stands with it or beside it, who supports it, what forces are in league with it. (p. 25)

The problem-defining process, or "co-evolving the definition," is a critical aspect of family work. Cecchin (1987) warns clinicians to accept neither their own nor the client's definition too quickly, and Maturana and Varela (1992) caution clinicians to adopt an attitude of permanent vigilance against the temptation of certainty. By remaining curious, a clinician has a greater chance of escaping the "sin of certainty," or the sin of being too invested in one's own opinion. As clinicians, nurses need to avoid becoming intoxicated with their own brightness or ideas. Rather, each nurse should ask, "What does the client want from me? What are the client's thoughts, hunches, and theories about the problem? About the extent of their control over the problem? Their solutions?" We try to always "keep the problem on the table" as we engage with families.

Relationship Between Family Interaction and the Health Problem

Once the main problems have been identified, the nurse asks questions about the relationship of family interaction to the health problem. Box 7-4 lists some factors to consider in exploring family interaction related to the presenting problem. The nurse conceptualizes the information that he or she has already gathered from the family in light of the meaning it has for the family and the hypotheses generated before the interview. For example,

---

Box 7-4	Factors to Consider in Exploring Family Interaction Related to the Problem

- Current manifestations of the problem.
- Typical responses of family members and others to the problem.
- Other current associated problems, challenges, or concerns.
- How the problem influences family functioning.
- What family members appreciate about how they have coped with this challenging situation.
- How family members understand that they have not been successful in conquering this problem (beliefs).

Adapted from Family Nursing Unit records, Faculty of Nursing, University of Calgary.

a home care nurse talking with parents caring for a technology-dependent child at home might be mindful of the parents' new role as care specialists, the transformation of family space and privacy with the introduction of multiple health-care professionals, and the financial drain on their resources.

The nurse then begins to develop additional questions that focus on interactional behaviors dealing with the three time frames of present, past, and future. Within each time frame, the nurse once again explores differences, agreements and disagreements, and explanations or meanings. It is important to emphasize that the purpose of asking these questions is not merely to gather data. Rather, the nurse and the family are coauthoring a new story to replace a problem-saturated description. That is, by asking circular questions, the nurse generates new ideas and explanations for himself or herself and the family to consider.

Present. In exploring the present situation, the nurse could ask, "Who does what, when? Then what happens? Who is the first to notice that something has been done?" The nurse should steer away from asking about traits that are supposedly intrinsic to a person, for example, being "shy." Rather, the nurse might ask, "When does Ari *act* shy?" or "To whom does he *show* shyness?" Then, "What does Jennifer do when Ari shows shyness?" The nurse can inquire about differences between individuals: "Who is better at getting grandmother to make her meals, Shanghi or Puichun?" The nurse can also inquire about differences between relationships: "Do your ex-husband and Manuel José fight more or less than your ex-husband and Nadiya?" In working with families with chronic or life-threatening illness, the nurse should explore differences before or after important events or milestones. For example, the nurse could inquire: "Do you worry more, less, or the same about your wife's health since her emergency surgery?"

In addition to exploring areas of difference, the nurse can inquire about areas of agreement or disagreement: "Who agrees with you that Brandon is most likely to forget to give your mother her eyedrops three times per day? Who disagrees with you?" The nurse should explore the family's explanation for the sequence of interaction: "How do you understand Brandon's tendency to be most forgetful about the eyedrops? Are there times when he does remember? What seems to be different about the times when he remembers?"

Past. In exploring the past, the nurse should use similar types of questions to explore:
Differences: "How was Brandon's caregiving different before he had high-speed internet? How does that differ from now?"
Agreement or disagreement: "Who agrees with Murdock that Dad was more involved in Genevieve's exercise program?"
Explanation or meaning: "What does it mean to you that, after all this time, things between your wife and her mother have not changed?"

In addition to exploring how the family saw the problem in the past, we have found it extremely useful to explore how they have seen changes in the problem. Change in the problem situation frequently occurs before the first meeting with the interviewer. If prompted, families can often recall and describe such changes. It is important to note that, in many cases, the family must be prompted to emerge from their problem-saturated view of the situation. For example, a man may tell the nurse at the community mental health center that his male partner drinks very heavily and has done this "until recently." If the nurse is attuned to inquiring about pretreatment changes, he or she will ask questions about the differences that the man has noticed recently. For example, the nurse might inquire, "Is his recent behavior the kind of change you would like to continue to have happen?" The idea of noticing exceptions to problems is one that we have used frequently in our clinical work, and we are indebted to de Shazer (1982, 1991) and White (1991) for emphasizing it.

Future. By focusing on the future and how the family would like things to be, the nurse instills hope for more adaptive interaction regarding the presenting concern. He or she also co-constructs a reality between family members and herself for a system in which the problem has dissolved. The nurse can ask questions pertaining to:

Differences: "How would it be different if your grandfather did not side with your mother against your father in managing Paola's Crohn's disease?"
Agreement or disagreement: "Do you think your mother would agree that, if your grandfather stayed out of the discussions, things would be better?"
Explanation or meaning: "Dad, if your wife stopped phoning her father for advice about Paola's Crohn's disease, what would that mean to you?"

We believe it is especially important to ask future-oriented questions when working with families dealing with hereditary disorders such as Huntington's disease. For at-risk individuals, the possibility of detecting the disease-provoking gene exists, but no treatment is available. It is not so much the test result itself that may be disrupting to family life transitions but instead the changed expectations and possibilities for the future.

There is also the stigma. Katharine Moser, in a poignant interview, discusses how she was left to confirm for herself through library books and a CD-ROM encyclopedia that she and her brothers, her mother, her aunts, an uncle, and cousins could all face the same fate as her grandfather of having the lethal Huntington's gene. Choosing to have testing at age 23 and facing her genetic heritage helped her decide how to live her life (Harmon, 2007). A study by Gallo, et al. (2005) found that parents shared genetic information based on their assessment of the child's developmental readiness and interest. Information sharing for these parents was an unfolding process that continued throughout the childhood. Because any family member may require help eventually, nurses can provide preemptive care for families experiencing these types of hereditary diseases to assist their transition through the family life cycle.

During this part of the interview, the nurse attempts to gain a systemic view of the situation and a description of the cycle of repeated interactions. These interactions may be between family members or between family members and the nurse. We stress that it is not important for the nurse to understand or agree with the problem but instead to be curious about the family's description of its positive and negative impact. We are drawn to the ideas presented by Strong (2002), who suggests using appreciative inquiry, a line of questioning that elicits and builds on appreciated practices and engages family members in discussion with each other about what works for them.

Such questions invite members to distinguish, understand, and amplify the appreciated life-sustaining forces within their family. In this way, families can take a "both/and" position. For example, they can relate the challenges of trying to raise a child with Down syndrome and discuss how raising this child has brought the family closer together and helped them pool their collective strengths and be a stronger family unit. Striking examples of how families have pooled their strengths to cope with a dying family member's illness have been recounted on numerous blogs and Facebook.

During this phase of the interview, the nurse should be able to describe the sequence of the development of the problem over time, the current contextual problem interaction, whether the family believes it has some control over the problem, the times when the problem does not show itself, and what the family members appreciate about their personal and cooperative efforts to work together.

All of the scenarios described above relate to clients that believe there indeed is a problem, believe they have some control over it, and want to see it changed. But, what of those clients who don't see themselves as having a problem and yet are referred to the nurse? They may be mandated for treatment or present under duress. For example, a 16-year-old young person verbally abused an elderly woman in his high school and then pushed her off the elevator. When asked by the principal, what happened, he said "Oh, it's nothing. We got into an argument because I didn't let her get away with that 'age stuff' and let her on the elevator first. It's no big deal." His grandmother whom he lived with stood by helplessly as the principal talked.

In situations where clients and helpers have different agendas for a meeting and different definitions of the problem, we believe it's important for the nurse not to rigidify the interaction inadvertently. That is, by insisting too early on that it *is definitely* a problem, the nurse can invite a rigid no-problem response from the client. We do not use the word "denial," as this generally just fosters an antagonistic relationship over the question of who is "right." Although we sometimes find ourselves tempted to give advice and confront the situation head-on, we have found this typically invites defensiveness and promotes shame. (Additional ideas on how not to give advice prematurely are given in Chapter 10.)

We agree with Madsen's ideas (2007) to connect with clients by eliciting their intentions, hopes, and preferred view of self. For example, the nurse could connect with the 16 year old about his willingness not to run away but instead to talk about the incident with his grandmother and the principal present. The nurse could ask if he's typically this courageous, and how has he shown couarge in the past. The nurse could openly wonder if his actions toward the older woman were in keeping with his preferred view of himself as courageous; how his friends treat his grandmother; and what his actions might have been if his grandmother had been accompanying the other woman whom he pushed.

Once the nurse has a deep appreciation of the client's intentions, hopes and preferred view of self, then the nurse can raise questions about the gap between these and the impact of the client's behavior on others. The nurse should pay extra close attention to glimmers of concern the client shows about the problem of abuse, and notice exceptions to the no-problem stance. In the context of therapeutic conversation, the client and nurse can start to build a shared proactive focus for change.

Madsen (2007, p. 113) suggests the following guidelines for engaging clients who hold a stance of "This is not a problem":

- ■ Anticipate and attempt to avoid an overresponsible/underresponsible sequence
- ■ Connect with clients' intentions, hopes and preferred view of self
- ■ Examine the gap between preferred intentions and actual effects
- ■ Build on exceptions to a no-problem stance
- ■ Build on a shared proactive focus for change

Attempted Solutions to Solving Problems

During this next phase of the assessment, the nurse explores the family's attempted solutions to the problem. Box 7-5 lists some factors to consider when exploring the family's attempted solutions. The process can begin with general questions related to the problem. For example, "What improvements have you noticed since you first contacted our clinic?" This type of question conveys the idea to families that they have the strengths and resources to change, and it assumes that changes have already occurred, which can help set in motion a positive self-fulfilling prophecy for them. Another example might be, "How have you tried to obtain information from physicians and nurses about Mandeep's condition in previous hospitalizations?"

More specific questions should then be used to identify the least and most effective solutions for achieving what the family desires. The nurse can ask when these solutions were used. For example, "What was least helpful in trying to get information from the nurses about Surjit's resuscitation? What was most effective?" The nurse can ask if any successful elements in

---

Box 7-5 Factors to Consider in Exploring the Family's Attempted Solution

- How has the family tried to resolve the problem?
- Who tried?
- With whom?
- What were the results?
- What were the events precipitating the search for professional help?
- Who is most in favor of agency help? Most opposed?
- What are the client's thoughts about the nurse's role in the change process?
- What was the sequence of events resulting in actual contact with the agency?

Adapted from Family Nursing Unit records, Faculty of Nursing, University of Calgary.

the solutions are still being used, and if not, why not. Similar types of sequences of interaction questions that focus on difference, agreement or disagreement, and explanation or meaning can be used to explore the family's attempted solutions to the presenting concerns.

White (1991) discusses the idea of attempted solutions as *unique outcomes*. These are experiences that contradict the client's dominant or problem-saturated story. Unique outcomes provide a window to what might be considered to be the alternative territories of a person's life. "For an event to comprise a unique outcome, it must be qualified as such by the persons to whose life the event relates" (p. 30). It must be judged important and significant and represent a preferred outcome and an appealing development to which people are attracted as a new possibility. White (1991) recommends "re-authoring," in which the interviewer can ask a variety of questions to facilitate the process of preferring unique outcomes. For example, he suggests the following questions:

■ How did you get yourself ready to take this step?

■ What preparations led up to it?

■ Just before taking this step, did you nearly turn back?

■ If so, how did you stop yourself from doing so?

■ Looking back from this vantage point, what did you notice yourself doing that might have contributed to this achievement?

■ What developments have occurred in other areas of your life that may relate to this?

■ How do you think these developments prepare the way for you to take these steps? (p. 30)

Morgan (2000) suggests, and we agree, that a unique outcome can be anything that the problem would not like, anything that does not "fit" with the dominant story. It "may be a plan, action, feeling, statement, quality, desire, dream, thought, belief, ability or commitment" (p. 52). For example, during a meeting with three siblings, a nurse heard a client describe a fresh unique outcome: "the other day, just after returning from my appointment with the pulmonologist, when I was tempted to smoke a cigarette, I reached instead for the cell phone to talk with my sister, Ogniana." The nurse then chose to invite the siblings to reflect on the meaning of the events they described.

White (1991) also discusses the value of what he calls "experience of experience questions." Such questions "invite persons to reach back into their stock of lived experience and to express certain aspects that have been forgotten or neglected with the passage of time" (p. 32). They "recruit the imagination of persons in ways that are constitutive of alternative experiences of themselves" (p. 32). Examples include:

> "If I had been a spectator to your life when you were a younger person, what do you think I might have witnessed you doing then that might help me to understand how you were able to achieve what you have recently achieved?"
>
> "What do you think this tells me about what you have wanted for your life, and about what you have been trying for in your life?"
>
> "How do you think that knowing this has affected my view of you as a person?"
>
> "Exactly what actions would you be committing yourself to if you were to more fully embrace this knowledge of who you are?"
>
> "If you were to side more strongly with this other view of who you are, and of what your life has been about, what difference would this make to your life on a day to day basis?" (p. 32)

In our work with families, we have frequently been told that no solutions have been attempted or that "nothing has worked." In these circumstances, we sometimes ask, "How come things aren't worse? What are you doing to keep this situation from getting worse?" Then we amplify these problem-solving strategies by asking about their frequency, effectiveness, and so forth. We also try to expand our view of typical solutions to include complementary and alternative medical and health approaches.

We also find it useful to draw on the concept of resilience in these situations. In talking with families about their resilience, we use such terms as *endurance, withstanding, adaptation, coping,* and *survival* and try to draw forth other qualities surfacing in the face of hardship or adversity. We talk about the ability to "bounce back" or make up for losses. We believe resilience is forged *through* adversity not *despite* it. Bouncing back is not the same as "breezing through" a crisis. Resilience involves multiple recursive processes over time. It is this layering and recursiveness that we inquire about when we ask families about their coping and attempted solutions.

In working with families dealing with life-threatening or chronic illness, the nurse should be aware of additional "helping agencies" involved in health-care delivery. We have found it important to ask questions such as, "Have any other agencies attempted to help you with this problem? What has been the most useful advice that you have received? Did you follow this advice? What has been the least helpful advice?" It is useful to explore the differing ideas espoused by the helping systems. If there is unclear leadership or a confused hierarchy within the helping systems, the family can be placed in a conflictual situation that is similar to that of a child whose parents continually disagree. Confusion among helping agencies can exacerbate the family's concerns. In this way, the attempted solution (assistance by helping agencies) can become an entirely new problem for both the family and other agencies. It is important for the nurse to be aware of whether this situation exists before attempting to intervene.

Having consolidated a shared view of the problem and elicited some relevant solutions, the nurse can simply state to the family that she or he would like to work with them to achieve their goals. This small but profound acknowledgement is an opportunity for the nurse to show compassion to the client and enter into a deeper relationship and collaboration.

Goal Exploration

At some point during the interview, the nurse and family establish what goals or outcomes the family expects as a result of change. Box 7-6 lists some factors for nurses to consider when exploring goals. Families are pragmatic: They are seeking practical results when they come to a health-care provider; they are "in pain" or "suffering," and their desire is to get rid of a problem. The problem may be between themselves as family members or between the family and the nurse (for example, the family desires practical information about the acceptable level of physical activity after a myocardial infarction [MI], and the nurse has not provided such concrete information). Family members may expect a large change (e.g., "My brother Sheldon will be able to walk without the aid of a cane") or a small but significant change (e.g., "We will be able to leave our handicapped daughter, Kayla, with a babysitter for 1 hour a week").

In many cases, a small change is sufficient. We believe that a small change in a person's behavior can have profound and far-reaching effects on the behavior of all persons involved. Experienced nurses are aware that small changes lead to further progress.

Goals describe what will be present or what will be happening when the complaint or concern is absent. We believe that unidimensional behavioral

---

| **Box 7-6** | Factors to Consider When Exploring Goals |

• What general changes does the family believe would improve the problem?
• What specific changes?
• What are the expectations of how the agency may facilitate change in the problem?

Adapted from Family Nursing Unit records, Faculty of Nursing, University of Calgary.

goal statements such as "I will be eating less" are not as desirable as multi-dimensional, interactional, and situational goal statements that describe the "who, what, when, where, and how" of the solution. Such a multidimensional goal statement might be, "I will be eating a small, balanced meal in the evening at the dinner table with my partner and our children; the television and computer will be off, and we will be talking to each other."

There are many ways in which the nurse can clarify the family's goals with future or hypothetical questions such as, "What would your parents do differently if they did not stay at home every evening with Snanna?" The nurse can explore future or hypothetical areas of difference ("How would your parents' relationship be different if your dad allowed your uncle to take care of Snanna one evening a week?"); areas of agreement or disagreement ("Do you think your Dad would agree that your parents would probably have little to talk about if they went out one evening a week?"); and explanation or meaning ("Tell me more about why you believe your parents would have a lot to talk about when they went out that one evening a week. What would that mean to you?").

We find it useful sometimes to combine past and future questions. For example, "If you were to tell me next week (or month or year) that you had done X, what could I find in your past history that would have allowed me to predict that you would have done X?" The questions capitalize on the "possibility to probability" phenomena at the same time as inviting a richer account of the history of the new/old story.

We have found it particularly useful in our clinical work to ask the "miracle question" (de Shazer, 1988) to elicit the family's goals. de Shazer (1991) describes the question in this way:

> Suppose that one night there is a miracle and while you are sleeping the problem …is solved: How would you know? What would be different?
>
> What will you notice different the next morning that will tell you there has been a miracle? What will your spouse notice? (p. 113)

The miracle question elicits interactional information. The person is asked to imagine someone else's ideas as well as his or her own. The framework of the miracle question (and others of this type) allows family members to bypass their causal explanations. They do not have to imagine how they will get rid of the problem but instead can focus on results. Thus, the goals developed from the miracle question are not limited to just getting rid of the problem or complaint. Clients often are able to construct answers to this "miracle question" quite concretely and specifically. For example, "Easy, I'll be able to say 'no' to cocaine," or "She'll see me smile more and come home from work with less tension."

McConkey (2002) suggests strategies for solution-focused meetings that we believe are particularly useful if a family is angry and the nurse is feeling defensive. The nurse can shift the meeting from the problem picture to the future solution picture by engaging in conversation such as this:

> Obviously, you want things to be better for your child and so do I. (Validating the parent)
> In order to make the most of this meeting, I'm going to ask you an unusual question. (Bridging statement)
> How will you know by the time you leave here today, that this meeting has been helpful? (Shifting to the future)
> When things are better, what will your son be doing? What will I be doing? What will you be doing? (Including all the stakeholders in the solution picture) (p. 192)

Nurses working with families of a patient who has a chronic or life-threatening illness commonly find family members quite vague about the changes they expect. For example, "We would like Attila to feel good about himself even though he has a colostomy." Experienced clinical nurses know that "feeling good about oneself" is very difficult to describe or measure. In this example, we recommend that the nurse ask the family to describe the smallest concrete change that Attila could make to show that he "feels good about himself." By asking for this degree of specificity about desired change early in the nurse–family relationship, we believe it is more likely that the family and nurse can accomplish the desired change.

GUIDELINES FOR THE REMAINING INTERVIEWING PROCESS

Once the nurse has completed the initial interviews or assessment, he or she can consider the entire interviewing process. The stages of the interviewing process generally include:

1. Engagement
2. Assessment
3. Intervention
4. Termination

Planning and Dealing With Complexity

After an initial assessment is completed, a beginning nurse interviewer frequently worries about whether to intervene with a family. The following questions often arise: Am I the appropriate person to offer intervention? Is the situation too complex? Do I have sufficient skills or should another professional, such as a social worker, psychologist, or family therapist, be called in?

Does every family that is assessed need further intervention? This is not to say that interventions begin only at the intervention stage. Rather, they are part of the total interview process from engagement to closure. For example, just by asking the family to come together for an interview, the nurse has intervened. Each time the nurse asks a circular question, he or she influences the family, generates new information, and intervenes.

For nurses, the decision to offer interventions, refer the family to others, or discharge them is a complex one. Several factors need to be examined before making the choice: the level of the family's functioning, the level of the nurse's competence, and the work context.

Level of the Family's Functioning

The nurse should recognize the complexity of the family situation. Some clinicians have advocated that treatment begin if the referring problem has been detected early and clearly defined procedures for management have been published. Most nurses would agree with this position but would find it very idealistic. Community health nurses and mental health nurses, in particular, often work with families who are not referred early. Some of these families present with a number of complex physical and emotional problems and are frequently involved in one crisis after another. These families offer specific challenges to the clinician.

Our recommendation is that nurses carefully assess the family's level of functioning and its desire to work on specific issues, such as management of hemiplegia after a stroke, impact of cystic fibrosis on the family, negotiation of services for elderly family members, or caring for a child with special needs. If the family is at all amenable to working on such an issue, it is incumbent on the nurse either to offer intervention or to help them get appropriate assistance by referring them to others. Guidelines for the referral process are provided in Chapter 12.

The nurse must consider ethical issues in deciding who should be treated. With the popularization of counseling, a surface inspection would seem to indicate that everyone is in need of psychotherapy in one form or another. The childless couple, the family with young infants, the family with adolescents, the single-parent family, and the aging family can all be considered candidates for psychotherapeutic aid. Many people lead psychologically constricted and difficult lives, but should they be "treated"? This is a troublesome question for helping professionals.

Our recommendation is that nurses ethically weigh two opposing positions when they make the decision to intervene with, refer, or discharge a family. One position states that if a person is potentially dangerous to self or others, that person must receive intervention. On an individual level, a suicidal or homicidal patient is such an example. On a larger system level, a family in which there is physical, sexual, or emotional abuse or violence is an example. On a community level, a person who is threatening to the community and unstable mentally might be an example.

Single-parent adoptive families as well as lesbian, gay, or bisexual couples are entitled to be considered various family forms versus alternatives to "normal" families. It is our hope that nurses will ethically and wisely consider the family's level of functioning and their own legal responsibilities. This is a necessary step before deciding to offer further treatment. This weighing of alternatives can be particularly challenging for nurses when dealing with client confidentiality, crisis situations, and nonemancipated minors. For example, a 16-year-old young woman overdosed with 30 tablets of Naproxen and was brought to the emergency room by her boyfriend. She refused to talk about what had happened and repeatedly said she did not want to talk with her parents who were in the waiting room; she text messaged her girlfriend, however, from her bed in the emergency room to say that she had overdosed. The nurse read the text message and had to weigh several options in deciding how to proceed with care. In Chapter 12, we present some ideas that we have used when we have decided not to offer additional treatment to families.

Another ethical consideration for a nurse to weigh is the balance between his or her own beliefs about a client and his or her respect for the client's situation. This is especially important with regard to issues such as sexual orientation, culture, religion, and ethnic self-determination. For example, we believe that nurses in discussing decision making at the end of life, should recognize and honor that people who are dying are still living and have the right to be in control of their lives. A real (unflinching) and ethical relationship between the patient, the staff, and the family should be maintained and valued as end-of-life issues are decided. This is particularly salient when the nurse may be unfamiliar with the views of Native American groups such as the Navajo, who hold strong beliefs about spirituality, healing, rituals concerning the end of life, and death practices. The contrasts between the beliefs of the dominant health-care system and the views of various religious groups, such as those who practice the Islamic and Hindu religions, need to be explored. With regard to homosexuality, Green (2003) has persuasively argued the firm value of respecting a client's choices and not trying to "make them" into who they are not. We believe that nurses should be able to support a client along whatever sexual orientation path he or she ultimately takes. Respect for the client's and family's sense of integrity and interpersonal relationships is the most central goal.

To avoid ethnocentrism and paternalism, some nurses have embraced certain politically correct ideas with enthusiasm. We advocate that nurses engage in critical thinking about responsible practice, safeguard human dignity, and not blindly follow injunctions to be politically correct. Nurses are responsible for their own choices in exercising independent professional judgment and moral agency. We have found it useful in our clinical work with families to be collaborative, open, and direct with them in discussing ethical dilemmas involving them.

The Nurse's Level of Competence

Nurses should consider their personal and professional capacity when choosing to work with a family. If the nurse has experienced a recent death of a family member, he or she may not be able to facilitate grieving in family members. Likewise, a nurse with strong views that people who are on disability are shirkers would be best advised not to attempt work with such families. We do not subscribe to the view that a nurse has to have personally dealt with a situation (for example, raising teenagers) to help a family. Most noteworthy in a nurse is clinical competence. We do believe, however, that the nurse should attempt to be well informed and not just offer advice that might or might not be helpful. We believe that nurses should consider scope of practice as the care for which they are competent, educated, and authorized to provide. On a professional level, the nurse needs to evaluate his or her competence by asking self-reflective questions such as: "Am I at the beginning or the advanced level of family interviewing skill?" and "Can I obtain supervision to aid in dealing with families who present with complex issues?" Each nurse should examine these questions and their answers before making a decision about intervening with a given family.

The genetic revolution is an explosive area of knowledge for nurses. Situations resulting from the application of the abundant knowledge gained from the Human Genome Project (HGP) require decisions for which there most likely will be limited precedent. Nurses and families alike struggle with uncertainty and ambiguity as new discoveries are made in the HGP. Now is an exciting and meaningful time for nurses to work alongside families dealing with new information about risk, risk expression, and treatment options.

Work Context

Considerable controversy is sometimes raised about the issue of who is competent to treat clients. This controversy involves issues of definition and professionalism. How a "family problem" and a "medical problem" are defined in a particular work setting can fuel the controversy. If a nurse who is, for example, working with a patient who has had a stroke invites the relatives to come for a class, is the nurse treating a family or a medical problem? We take the approach that the definition of the problem is less important than the solution. That is, if the whole family is involved, the definition of the problem is a question of semantics.

The issue of professional territoriality is a very thorny one with no pat answers. Sometimes the patient sees the psychologist for psychodiagnostic testing and the social worker to deal with the family and outside agencies. The role of the nurse with the family in this situation can become controversial. If the nurse does a family assessment and decides to intervene with the family, is the nurse usurping the social worker's position? Or, perhaps, is the nurse usurping the physician's position by making the decision to intervene?

One way around these dilemmas is for the nurse to consider assuming various roles in his or her work with families. For example, the nurse can serve as mediator, patient and family advocate, capacity builder for family health, empowerer, alliance builder, guide, navigator, and so forth.

There are no simple answers to complex professional and territorial issues. We urge nurses to work cooperatively to ensure the best family care possible. In general, we believe the best person to intervene in a situation is the one with the most ready access to the system level in which the problems manifest themselves. However, we believe that, in the past, nurses have been too quick to turn over family care to other professionals. Nurses are now reclaiming their important role in providing relational, family-centered care.

Changes in health-care reimbursement have required all nurses and health-care providers to examine and adapt their practices to account for the provision of timely, efficient, and cost-effective services. Managed care in its many varieties, health insurance reform, increased focus on primary care, and other complex issues have changed the face of nursing practice. The coming together of the consumer movement, health economics, and technology has huge implications for practice. Nurses have to do more than just heal their patients. Day after day, they must also attend to the socio-economic and political context of health care as well as to the survival of their careers. We believe that it is vital for nurses to find ways to thrive professionally and for families to receive optimal care. Strategies to address bureaucratic disentitlement of cultural, ethnic, racial, and other minority groups must be put forth. Models for access to health care for economically disadvantaged families need further refinement and implementation.

Accountability structures and practices need to recognize the centrality of structured power differences in our society. We believe that, as nurses work with diverse families and are increasingly transparent in this work, they will find ways to positively influence their employment contexts.

Intervention Stage

Once the nurse has decided to intervene with the family, we recommend that he or she review the CFIM (see Chapter 4). This model, which stimulates ideas about change, can help the nurse design interventions to work with the family to address the particular domain of family functioning affected: cognitive, affective, or behavioral. Helpful hints about intervention are offered in Box 7-7.

In choosing interventions, we encourage nurses to attend to several factors to enhance the likelihood that the interventions will focus on change in the desired domain of family functioning. Interventions, offered within a collaborative relationship, are not a demand but rather an invitation to change. Some factors to consider when devising interventions are outlined in Box 7-8. First, the intervention should be related to the problem that the nurse and the family have contracted to change. Second, the intervention should be derived from the nurse's hypothesis about the problem, what the family says the problem means to them, and their beliefs about the problem (Wright & Bell, in press). Third, the intervention should match the family's style of relating. (We have found in our own clinical work that we

---

Box 7-7 Helpful Hints About Interventions

• Interventions are the core of clinical work with families.
• They should be devised with sensitivity to the family's ethnic and religious background.
• They can only be *offered to* families. The nurse cannot direct change but can create a context for change to occur.
• They are offered in the context of collaborative conversations as the nurse and family together devise solutions to find the most useful fit.
• When the nurse's ideas are not a good fit for the family, the practitioner should be open to offering other ideas rather than becoming blameful of self or the family because the intervention was not chosen

---

Levac, A.M.C., Wright, L.M., & Leahey, M. (2002). Children and families: Models for assessment and intervention. In J.A. Fox (Ed.), *Primary health care of infants, children, and adolescents* (2nd ed.) (p. 18). St. Louis: Mosby. Copyright 2002. Adapted with permission.

Box 7-8 Factors to Consider When Devising Interventions

• What is the agreed-on problem to change?
• At what domain of family functioning is the intervention aimed?
• How does the intervention match the family's style of relating?
• How is the intervention linked to the family's strengths and previous useful solution strategies?
• How is the intervention consistent with the family's ethnic and religious beliefs?
• How is the intervention new or different for the family?

---

are sometimes biased toward one particular domain of family functioning, such as cognitive or affective, and that we have thus erred in devising interventions that we are most comfortable with rather than ones that the family may find most useful.) Fourth, the interventions should be linked to the family's strengths. We believe that families have inherent resources and that the nurse's responsibility is to encourage families to use these resources in new ways to tackle the problem. Fifth, the interventions should take into consideration the family's beliefs influenced by ethnicity, spirituality, race, class, gender, and sexual orientation. Sixth, the nurse should devise a few interventions so that nurse and family can consider their relative merits— for example, are these ideas new to the family or are they more of the same types of solutions that the family has already tried?

We do not believe that there is one "right" intervention. Rather, there are only "useful" or "effective" interventions. In our experience, we have found that a nurse sometimes reaches an impasse, with a family not changing, when the nurse persists in either using the same intervention repeatedly or switching interventions too rapidly. Sometimes we find that clients fail to notice responses containing possible solutions. The same can be said of nurses. Interventions are successful when constraints are lifted and important aspects of life change are noticed. The result is a clearer image of how things can be different in the future.

We have also found that sometimes the nurse is too constrained and fails to consider alternate system levels for intervention. For example, if a family does not want to hear or discuss the possibility of older adults having sexual activity at a residential care center, then the nurse may design an intervention not with the family but rather with the care center. Such an intervention with a residential care center could be to plan an in-service around the topic of HIV and older adults. The outcome is that condoms are available in the center and clients have the information they need to keep themselves safe.

With the availability of computers, PDAs, instant messaging, and telecommunication devices, we believe that nurses have become increasingly creative in finding electronic means to facilitate intervention. For example, telephone-based skill building can help dementia caregivers' sense of social support, reduce their depressive symptoms, and improve their life satisfaction in the midst of caregiving. We believe that, just as the use of computers, email, chat rooms, list serves, blogs, and cell phones for business and education has had dramatic effects on family interaction, so too has their use in health care profoundly affected nurse–family interaction.

Once the nurse has devised an intervention, he or she must attend to the executive skills (see Chapter 5) required to deliver the intervention. Part of the success of any intervention is the manner in which the intervention is offered. The family must feel confident that the intervention will promote change. The nurse also needs to show that *he or she* has confidence in the intervention or task requested and believes that it will benefit the family.

However, interventions need to be tailored to each family; therefore, the preamble or preface to the actual intervention will vary. For example, if family members are feeling very hopeless and frustrated with a particular problem, the nurse might say, "I know this might seem like a hard thing that I'm going to ask you to do, but I know your family is capable of ..." On the other hand, if the nurse is making a request of family members who tend to be quite formal with one another, then the nurse might preface it with, "What I'm going to ask you to do may make you feel a little foolish or silly at first, but you'll notice that, as you do it a few times, you will become more comfortable."

A good example of a generic intervention is the "What are you prepared to do?" question. The term "prepared" is an important word suggesting a voluntary decision to participate in the change process.

When giving a particular assignment for a family to do between sessions, the nurse should try to include all family members. It is necessary for the nurse to review with family members what the particular assignment is in order to check their understanding of what is being requested. Reviewing the assignment is a good idea, whether it is carried out within the interview or between interviews. If assignments or experiments are given between sessions, the nurse should always ask for a report at the next interview. If the family has not completed or only partially completed the assignment, the reason should be explored.

We do not subscribe to the view that families are noncompliant or resistant if they do not follow our requests. Rather, we become curious about their decision to choose an alternate course and try to learn from their response. We believe that family interviewing is a circular process. The nurse intervenes, and the family responds in its unique way. The nurse then responds to this response and the process continues. See Chapter 2 for more ideas about circularity.

During the intervention stage, the nurse must be aware of the element of time. How useful or effective an intervention is can be evaluated only after the intervention has been implemented. With some interventions, change may be noted immediately. However, more commonly, changes will not be noticed for a lengthy period. Just as most problems occur over time, problems also need an appropriate length of time to be resolved. It is impossible to state how long one should wait to ascertain if a particular intervention has been effective, but changes within family systems need to filter through the various system levels. Families themselves offer useful observations and feedback about what interventions are most useful. Robinson and Wright (1995), in discussing a study conducted by Robinson, cite that families identified interventions within two stages of the therapeutic change process that they thought were critical to healing: creating the circumstances for change and moving beyond and overcoming problems. (For further elaboration on these stages, see Chapter 1.)

More information about devising interventions is provided in Chapters 4, 8, 9, 10, and 12.

Termination Stage

The last stage of the interviewing process is known as termination or closure. It is critically important for the nurse to conceptualize how to end treatment with the family to enhance the likelihood that changes will be maintained. In Chapter 5, we outlined the conceptual, perceptual, and executive skills useful for the termination stage. In Chapter 12 we address in depth the process of termination and focus on how to evaluate outcomes.

CLINICAL CASE EXAMPLE

The following is an example of how a nurse conducted family interviews using the guidelines we have given in Chapters 6 and 7. An example of a 15-minute interview is given in Chapter 8.

Pre-Interview

Developing Hypotheses

A home health agency received a referral on the Auerswald family for home nursing services, physiotherapy, nutrition counseling, and mental health counseling. Heinz Auerswald, 51, was a paraplegic and in a wheelchair because of a multiple trauma suffered in an industrial accident. He was unemployed. Eva Auerswald, 49, a homemaker, was the primary caregiver. She was reported to be depressed. The home care nurse hypothesized that Mrs. Auerswald's depression could be related to feeling overresponsible for caring for her husband. The nurse wondered if the husband's role and beliefs might be perpetuating this. She was also curious to know what other social and professional support systems were involved and what their beliefs were about the family's health problems. During the course of the family interview, the nurse gained much evidence from both the husband and wife to confirm the usefulness of her initial hypothesis. She used this hypothesis to provide a framework for her conversation with the couple.

Relation to CFAM. The nurse generated her hypothesis based on knowledge of and clinical experience with other families in similar situations and with similar ethnic backgrounds. The nurse also based it on the structural category of CFAM (internal and external family structure, ethnicity, gender), the developmental category (middle-aged families), and the functional category (roles, power or influence, circular communication, beliefs).

Arranging the Interview
The wife stated that she did not want to discuss her depression with the nurse while her husband was awake. For the first home visit, the nurse requested that the husband and wife be interviewed together. The couple agreed to this.

Relation to CFAM. The nurse thought about family roles and gender. She speculated that Eva may be protecting her husband from her problem. In terms of the CFAM category verbal communication, the nurse speculated that clear and direct communication between Heinz and Eva might be absent or infrequent.

Interview
Engagement
The genogram data revealed that:

- The husband and wife are alone in the city; extended families and children live in other cities and visit infrequently.
- Eva had been married previously and had stayed with her first husband for 18 years, although he physically abused her. She thought it was her responsibility to protect her children.
- This was the husband's first marriage.

Relation to CFAM. The above information added some support for the nurse's initial hypothesis in terms of Eva's beliefs about responsibility and an isolated family structure.

Assessment

Problem Definition. Eva described the problem as, "Heinz has had such a hard tragedy, but now I'm the one who is depressed. It doesn't make sense." Mr. Auerswald described the problem as Eva is "worrying too much."

Relationship Between Family Interaction and Health Problem. By asking circular questions, the nurse elicited the fact that Eva had not allowed herself a break from caregiving for 2 years. Heinz encouraged her to "go out and meet people," but she stated that she was fearful he might be too lonely if she met other people. Mr. Auerswald stated that this would not be a problem for him. They both reported that Eva had recently become depressed. She cried frequently and had difficulty sleeping.

Mrs. Auerswald takes excellent physical care of Heinz and bathes him daily. He is appreciative of all her nursing care. She feels guilty about asking for help from his parents.

Attempted Solutions. Eva had recently visited her family doctor, who prescribed antidepressant medication for her. She had requested home care services once before, but she said that because "their schedule is unreliable [and she] never know[s] when they are coming," she had discontinued treatment with the nurses. On the advice of her physician, Mrs. Auerswald agreed to try home care again.

Relation to CFAM. The nurse noted that the Auerswald's problem-solving approaches were directed toward either self-sufficiency or professional resources outside the family. They sought help from the family doctor and from the home care agency only infrequently, and they were reluctant to call on extended family for assistance.

Goals. Eva's desire was to "not feel depressed, [to] feel good about myself." The smallest significant change that she was able to describe was to be able to "go out one afternoon a week without feeling guilty." Heinz was in agreement with his wife's goals.

Intervention

Consideration of CFIM. Having developed a collaborative relationship with the couple and a workable hypothesis that fit the data from the family assessment, the nurse began to consider interventions with Mr. and Mrs. Auerswald in the cognitive, affective, and behavioral domains of family functioning. The focus of intervention was Eva's depression.

Interventions and Outcome. Knowing that Mrs. Auerswald had stayed in a physically abusive first marriage for 18 years to protect her children, the nurse asked questions about beliefs and feelings of responsibility. The nurse encouraged change in Eva's beliefs by asking both husband and wife behavioral effect, triadic, and hypothetical questions about responsibility. She asked the couple to engage in behavioral experiments to try new ways of being self-responsible. Both Mr. and Mrs. Auerswald challenged their own beliefs about depression being a solely biological problem and began to take more responsibility for their own lives. Heinz stated that he wanted a bath only three times per week. Eva requested caregiving help from her mother-in-law and was able to leave her husband alone for 2 hours, three times per week while she played cards with friends. The couple reported significant improvement in her depression. The home care agency continued to provide nursing and physical therapy services for the family. The nurse and home health aide focused on supporting the couple's new beliefs about responsibility.

CONCLUSIONS

Guidelines of particular stages of family interviews for nurses to consider during an initial interview and during the whole process of interviewing have been delineated. We recommend that nurses use these guidelines as ideas and suggestions for how to maximize the effectiveness of their time with families. It is not uncommon to move back and forth between the stages of a family interview to obtain further clarity or additional assessment about the concerns. Sometimes it is even necessary to return to the engagement guidelines to strengthen the therapeutic relationship before intervention ideas are offered. Thus, there should be fluidity between these stages so that they remain truly guidelines rather than a rigid prescription for how to conduct a family interview. We also caution nurses to remember the uniqueness of every family situation and encourage them to use these guidelines with sensitivity to each clinical situation, being mindful of the family's cultural, religious, spiritual, and ethnic heritage.

References

Al-Krenawi, A. (1998). Family therapy with a multiparental/multispousal family. *Family Process, 37*(1), 65–81.

Cecchin, G. (1987). Hypothesizing, circularity, and neutrality revisited: An invitation to curiosity. *Family Process, 26*(4), 405–413.

de Shazer, S. (1982). *Patterns of brief family therapy: An ecosystemic approach.* New York: Guilford Press.

de Shazer, S. (1988). *Clues: Investigating solutions in brief therapy.* New York: Norton.

De Shazer, S. (1991). *Putting difference to work.* New York: Norton.

Duhamel, F., & Campagna, L. (2000). Family genograph. Montreal: Universite de Montreal, Faculty of Nursing. Available from *www.familynursingresources.com.*

Duhamel, F., Dupuis, F. & Wright, L.M. (in press). Families and nurses answers to the 'One Question Question': Helpful directions for clinical practice, education, and research in family nursing. *Journal of Family Nursing.*

Gallo, A.M., et al. (2005). Parents sharing information with their children about genetic conditions. *Journal of Pediatric Health Care, 19*(5), 267–275.

Green, R.J. (2003). When therapists do not want their clients to be homosexual: A response to Rosik's article. *Journal of Marital and Family Therapy, 29*(1), 29–38.

Griffith, M.E. (1995). Opening therapy to conversations with a personal God. *Journal of Feminist Family Therapy, 7*(1/2), 123–139.

Harmon, A. (March 18, 2007). Confronting life with a lethal gene: A young woman's DNA test points to an invitably grim fate. *The New York Times, CLVI*, pp. 1, 20–21.

Leahey, M., Stout, L., & Myrah, I. (1991). Family systems nursing: How do you practice it in an active community hospital? *Canadian Nurse, 87*(2), 31–33.

Leahey, M., & Wright, L. M. (1987). Families and chronic illness: Assumptions, assessment and intervention. In L.M. Wright & M. Leahey (Eds.), *Families and chronic illness* (pp. 55–76). Springhouse, PA: Springhouse Corp.

Levac, A.M.C., Wright, L.M., & Leahey, M. (2002). Children and families: Models for assessment and intervention. In J.A. Fox (Ed.), *Primary health care of infants, children, and adolescents* (2nd ed.) (pp. 10–19). St. Louis: Mosby.

Madsen, W.C. (2007*). Collaborative therapy with multi-stressed families.* New York: The Guilford Press. Second edition.

Maturana, H.R., & Varela, F. (1992). *The tree of knowledge: The biological roots of human understanding.* Boston: Shambhala Publications, Inc.

Mauksch, L.B., Hillenburg, L., & Robins, L. (2001). The establishing focus protocol: Training for collaborative agenda setting and time management in the medical interview. *Families, Systems, & Health, 19*(2), 147–157.

McConkey, N. (2002). *Solving school problems: Solution focused strategies for principals, teachers, and counsellors.* Alberta, Canada: Solution Talk.

Morgan, A. (2000). *What is narrative therapy?: An easy-to-read introduction.* Adelaide, South Australia: Dulwich Centre Publications.

Robinson, C.A. & Wright, L.M. (1995). Family nursing interventions: What families say makes a difference. *Journal of Family Nursing, 1*(3), 327–345.

Roffman, A.E. (2003). Unpacking and keeping it packed: Two forms of therapist responsivity. *Journal of Systemic Therapies, 22*(1), 64–79.

Strong, T. (2002). Constructive curiosities. *Journal of Systemic Therapies, 21*(1), 77–90.

Tapp, D.M. (2000). The ethics of relational stance in family nursing: Resisting the view of "nurse as expert". *Journal of Family Nursing, 6*(1), 69–91.

Thorne, S.E., & Robinson, C.A. (1989). Guarded alliance: Health care relationships in chronic illness. *Image: The Journal of Nursing Scholarship, 21*(3), 153–157.

Weingarten, K. (2000). Witnessing, wonder, and hope. *Family Process, 39*(4), 389–402.

White, M. (1991). Deconstruction and therapy. *Dulwich Centre Newsletter, 3*, 21–40.

Wright, L.M. (1989). When clients ask questions: Enriching the therapeutic conversation. *Family Therapy Networker, 13*(6), 15–16.

Wright, L.M., & Bell, J.M. (in press). *Beliefs and illness: A model to invite healing.* Calgary, AB: 4th Floor Press.

Chapter **8**

How to Do a 15-Minute (or Shorter) Family Interview

We added this chapter to the 3rd edition (Wright & Leahey, 2000) of our text because our professional and personal experiences made us aware that family nursing could be effectively and meaningfully practiced in just 15 minutes or less. We have been gratified by the enthusiastic and warm response of nursing students and practicing nurses to the ideas and suggestions offered in this chapter. We have listened to many commendable and inspiring stories from nurses of how these ideas have been implemented into their practice and thus how their practice with patients and families has changed in satisfying and rewarding ways. Our goal in developing these ideas was to address head-on the perception among nurses that they lack the time to involve families in their practice, and this effort seemed to resonate with many nurses. Consequently, nurses have graciously opened space to challenging one of the constraining beliefs about their practice. To further assist nurse educators and nursing students with implementing these ideas in practice, we wrote and produced an educational DVD titled *How to Do a 15-Minute (or Less) Family Interview* (see *www.familynursingresources.com* to view video clips of actual family interviews; Wright and Leahey, 2000).

"I don't have time to do family interviews" is the most common reason nurses offer for not routinely involving families in their practice. In numerous undergraduate and graduate nursing courses, professional workshops, and presentations, we have encountered this statement as the resounding reason for the exclusion of family members from health care. With major changes in the delivery of health-care services through managed care, emphasis on providing more care in the community, budgetary constraints, increased acuity, and staff cutbacks, time is of the essence in nursing practice. It is our belief, however, that families need not be banned or marginalized from health care. To involve families, nurses need to possess sound knowledge of family assessment and intervention models, interviewing skills, and questions. We believe that family nursing knowledge can be applied effectively even in very brief family meetings. We also claim that a 15-minute, or even shorter, family interview can be purposeful, effective, informative, and even healing. Any involvement of family members, regardless of the length of time, is better than no involvement.

But what is time? And what exactly can be accomplished in 15 minutes or less with a family? We have noticed that much of nursing practice time is socially and culturally coordinated, highly ritualized, and therefore honored. Nurses clearly articulate the start and ending of their shifts, their schedules, and so forth. We propose that ritualizing and coordinating meeting time with families, even if it is only 15 minutes, can also become an honored part of nursing practice.

However, for nurses' behaviors to change, they must first alter or modify their beliefs about involving families in health care. We have discovered that, when nurses do not include family members in their practice, some very constraining beliefs usually exist (Wright & Bell, in press). Some of these beliefs are:

- "If I talk to family members, I will not have time to complete my other nursing responsibilities."
- "If I talk to family members, I may open up a can of worms and I will have no time to deal with it."
- "It is not my job to talk with families; that is for social workers and psychologists."
- "I cannot possibly help families in the brief time I will be caring for them."
- "If the family becomes angry, what would I do?"
- "What if they ask me a question and I do not have the answer? What would I do? It is better not to start a conversation."

Uncovering these constraining beliefs makes it more comprehensible why nurses may shy away from routinely involving families in nursing practice. We postulate that if nurses were to embrace only one belief, that "illness is a family affair" (Wright & Bell, in press), it would change the face of nursing practice. Nurses would then be more eager to know how to involve and assist family members in the care of loved ones. They would appreciate that everyone in a family experiences an illness and that no one family member "has" diabetes, multiple sclerosis, or cancer. By embracing this belief, they would realize that, from initial symptoms through diagnosis and treatment, all family members are influenced by and reciprocally influence the illness. They would also come to realize that our privileged conversations with patients and their families about their illness experiences can contribute dramatically to healing and the softening or alleviation of suffering (Wright, 2005; Wright & Bell, in press). Our evidence for this belief comes from our clinical and personal conversations as well as from reading numerous blogs in which stories of healing are often poignantly told.

We also believe that nurses will increase their caring for and involvement of families in their practice, regardless of the practice context, if such behavior is strongly supported and advocated by health-care administrators. One powerful and visual way for health-care administrators to show their commitment to family-centered care is to involve nurses in the creation, development, and implementation of family-friendly policies and services (International Council of Nurses, 2002). Examples of family-friendly policies and actions at the larger system level could include having family members as advisory board or task force members, focus group participants, program evaluators, and participants in quality and safety initiatives. Ensuring that parking is available at health-care facilities for families with limited income is another strategy. At the department or unit level, examples can include providing family-friendly visiting hours and space, such as a play area for children; offering a quiet room for retreat or for family discussion of difficult situations or moments; and lobbying for routinely providing family nursing therapeutic conversations when families are suffering. Inviting family members to participate in new staff orientation or volunteer to orient new families to the inpatient unit and mentor other families are additional options. At the front line, nurses can invite families to patient conferences, accompany patients to tests, support patients during procedures, assist patients with personal care, and so forth. A combination of administrative support, family-friendly facilities, and nurses who have the commitment, knowledge, and skills to routinely involve families in their practice is necessary for nurses to be able to maximize their time with families.

We would like to offer some very specific ideas for conducting a 15-minute (or shorter) family interview. These ideas are the condensed or "Reader's Digest" version of the core elements previously presented in Chapters 5 to 7 about conducting family interviews. The ideas honor the theoretical underpinnings of the Calgary Family Assessment Model (CFAM) (see Chapter 3) and Calgary Family Intervention Model (CFIM) (see Chapter 4) and highlight some of the most critical elements of these models.

KEY INGREDIENTS

What are the key ingredients of a 15-minute family interview? From our observations and experience, the key and essential ingredients to a successful, productive, and effective 15-minute family interview are therapeutic conversations, manners, family genogram (and in some situations an ecomap), therapeutic questions, and commendations. Of course, all of these ingredients can take place only within the context of a therapeutic relationship between the nurse and family.

We are heartened that research on and clinical evidence for the usefulness of the 15-minute family interview is now appearing in family nursing's primary journal, the *Journal of Family Nursing*. Holtslander (2005) described how the 15-minute family interview was successfully applied to the needs of families in a postpartum unit. Martinez, D'Artois, & Rennick (2007) conducted research to explore nurses' perceptions of the impact of the 15-minute interview on the hospital admission process and on their family nursing practice. They found that practicing pediatric hospital nurses perceived the genogram, therapeutic questions, and commendations as having a positive impact on their ability to conduct family assessments and family interventions.These nurses felt that a 15-minute interview should be routinely incorporated into practice at the time of a child's admission.

Key Ingredient 1: Therapeutic Conversations

All human interaction takes place in conversations. Nurses are always engaged in therapeutic conversations with their clients without perhaps thinking of them as such. No conversation that a nurse has with a patient or family member is trivial (Wright & Bell, in press). Each conversation in which we participate affects change in our own and in patients' and family members' biopsychosocial-spiritual structures.

The conversation in a brief family interview is therapeutic because right from the start it is purposeful and time-limited, as are the relationships. Therapeutic conversations between a nurse and a family can be as short as one sentence or as long as time allows. All conversations between nurses and families, regardless of time, have the potential for healing through the very act of bringing the family together (Robinson & Wright, 1995; Hougher Limacher & Wright, 2003, 2006; McLeod, 2003). However, it is not the length of the conversation or time that makes the most difference. Rather, it is the opportunity for patients and family members to be acknowledged and affirmed that has tremendous healing potential (Hougher Limacher, 2003; Hougher Limacher & Wright, 2003, 2006; Moules, 2002). Nurses are socially empowered and privileged to bring forth either health or pathology in their conversations with families.

The art of listening is also paramount. The need to communicate what it is like to live in our individual, separate worlds of experience, particularly within the world of illness, is a powerful need in human relationships (Wright, 2005). Frank (1998) suggests that listening to families' illness stories is not only an art but an ethical practice. Nurses commonly believe that listening also entails an obligation to do something to "fix" whatever concerns or problems are raised. However, in many cases, the most therapeutic move, intervention, or action the nurse can perform is showing compassion and offering commendations (Bohn, Wright, & Moules, 2003; Hougher Limacher, 2003; Hougher Limacher & Wright, 2003; Moules, 2002).

It is the integration of task-oriented patient care with interactive, purposeful conversation that distinguishes a time-effective 15-minute (or shorter) interview. The nurse makes information giving and patient involvement in decision making integral parts of the delivery process. He or she takes advantage of opportunities and searches for opportunities to engage in purposeful conversations with families. These practices differ from social conversations and can include basic ideas such as:

- Families are *routinely* invited to accompany the patient to the unit, clinic, or hospital.
- Families are *routinely* included in the admission procedure.
- Families are *routinely* invited to ask questions during the patient orientation.
- Nurses acknowledge the patient's and family's expertise in managing health problems by asking about routines at home.
- Nurses encourage patients to practice how they will handle different interactions in the future, such as telling family members and others that they cannot eat certain foods.
- Nurses *routinely* consult families and patients about *their* ideas for treatment and discharge.

Key Ingredient 2: Manners

Good manners have always been the core of common, everyday social behavior. However, in the last two decades in North America, our social behavior has dramatically shifted from formal to casual social interaction; some would say it has even progressed to being rude or occasionally abusive. Even our style of dress has been altered from "Sunday Best" to "Casual Friday." Martin and Kanen's (2005) *Miss Manners' Guide to Excruciatingly Correct Behavior* offers their perspective and humor on manners. Miss Manners, as Martin is known, provides thoughtful commentary on what is missing in the core of our interactions with one another and thus what is missing in our society. Manners are simple but profound acts of courtesy, politeness, respect, and kindness. Unfortunately, our culture as a whole seems to be undergoing an erosion of manners and thus civility. This erosion has sadly spilled over into the nursing profession.

Nursing has not been immune to the changes in social behavior. In some situations, we can argue that formal nursing behaviors (such as dressing in starched uniforms and caps) perhaps inhibited our relations with clients and families. Countless nurses still maintain respectful, polite, and thoughtful relations with their clients. However, we have witnessed and listened to far too many professional and personal encounters between nurses, patients, and families in which manners were pitifully absent.

One of the most glaring examples of the absence of manners in nursing is in the basic social act of an introduction. Numerous stories have been told of nurses who do not introduce themselves to their patients, let alone the patients' family members. For example, Jorge, a 23-year-old Hispanic man was seen in an outpatient clinic in a large metropolitan hospital after open-heart surgery. He reported that the nurse did not introduce herself but began touching his body and adjusting his intravenous pic line without telling him what she was doing or why. He found this experience very invasive, frightening, and rude.

This clinical anecdote is consistent with what nurses have told us about nurse–family relationships in the intensive care unit. We believe that one of the nursing strategies that inhibits the establishment of therapeutic relationships is depersonalization of the patient and family. Examples include not referring to the patient by name, labeling the patient or family difficult, providing care without encouraging participation by the patient or family, and not talking or making eye contact.

Therefore, introduction is obviously an essential ingredient of a successful family interview and relational family nursing practice. However, introductions by nurses have changed from overly formal to overly casual. Just a few years ago, nurses would introduce themselves as "Miss Garcia," whereas now a more typical introduction is "Hello, my name is Sasha and I'm your nurse today." Any introduction is better than no introduction but, as one client remarked to us, "Nurses don't introduce themselves any differently from a waiter who says 'Hi, my name is Josh and I'm your waiter tonight.'" We encourage nurses always to introduce themselves by their full names, except in unique circumstances when there might be concerns for safety.

Sadly, the most serious sin of omission is the lack of introduction by nurses to their patients' family members. What inhibits or prevents nurses in hospitals, community health clinics, and home care from introducing themselves to the people at a patient's bedside? What prevents nurses from inquiring about their relationships to the patient? Worse yet, what precludes nurses from making eye contact with family members or friends, one of the most expected social norms in our culture? We have discussed this phenomenon with our nursing students and professional nurses. It has been revealed to us that the belief of "lack of time" constrains many nurses from talking with anyone but their patients for fear that family members or close friends may "ask questions" or "require time from me that I just don't have." We would like to counter this belief by offering the suggestion that, in the end, nurses would *save* time if they would use a few manners with family members or friends. Nurses who did so would not be pursued at even more inopportune times by family members or friends inquiring about their loved ones. Nurses who have involved family members in their practice have reported that they have enjoyed greater rather than less job satisfaction (Leahey, et al, 1995).

Good manners also have the effect of instilling trust in family members. Examples of good manners that invite a trusting relationship are:

1. Always call patients and family members by name.
2. Always tell the patient and family members your name.
3. Explain your role for that shift or meeting.

4. Explain a procedure before coming into the room with the equipment to do it.

5. If you tell the patient or a family member that you will be back at a certain time, attempt to keep to that time or provide an explanation about why it didn't occur.

Key Ingredient 3: Family Genograms and Ecomaps

Nurses need to make it a priority to draw a quick genogram (and sometimes, if indicated, an ecomap) for *all* families, but particularly for families who will likely be part of their care for more than 1 day. Extensive details for the collection of genogram and ecomap information were given in Chapter 3 in the discussion about the "Structural Assessment" category of the CFAM. In a brief interview, the collection of genogram and ecomap information needs to be brief also. This information can be gleaned from family members in about 2 minutes.

The most essential information to obtain includes data about ages, occupation or school grade, religion, ethnic background, immigration date, and current health status of each family member. Begin by asking "easy" questions (e.g., ages, current health) of the household family members. Drawing out information relating to, for example, siblings' divorces or grandchildren is not necessary or time-efficient unless this information immediately relates to the family and health problem. Once the genogram information is obtained, if indicated, expand the data collection to obtain external family structure information in the form of an ecomap. It may be useful to ask questions such as, "Who outside of your immediate family is an important resource to you or is a stress for you?" and "How many professionals are involved in treating your husband's current heart problems?" Obtaining structural assessment data through the genogram and ecomap also serves as a quick engagement strategy because families are usually very pleased that a nurse is asking about their entire family rather than just the person experiencing the illness. It quickly acknowledges to the family the nurse's underlying belief that illness is a family affair.

Ideally, the genogram should become part of the documentation about the family and patient. In one cardiac unit, genogram information is collected on admission and the genogram is hung at the patient's bedside. Emergency telephone numbers for family members are listed on the genogram. In this way, the genogram acts as a continuous visual reminder for all health-care professionals involved with the patient to "think family."

Key Ingredient 4: Therapeutic Questions

Therapeutic questions are a key, defining element in a therapeutic conversation. Many ideas about and examples of linear, circular, and interventive questions were given in the presentation of the CFIM (see Chapter 4) and in the discussion of family nursing skills (see Chapter 5) and will be given in the vignettes demonstrating the use of questions (see Chapter 9). Wright and Leahey's DVD (2006) provides clinical examples of the authors interviewing clients and asking questions. When nurses are attempting to have a very brief family meeting, they can ask key questions of family members to involve them in family health care. We encourage nurses to think of at least three key questions that they will routinely ask all family members. Of course, these questions need to fit the context in which the nurse encounters families. For example, the questions that a nurse may ask family members in an emergency or oncology unit in a hospital might differ from the questions that a nurse might routinely ask family members in an outpatient diabetic clinic for children or in primary care. However, some basic themes need to be addressed, such as the sharing of information, expectations of hospitalization, clinic or home care visits, challenges, sufferings, and the most pressing concerns or problems. The following are some examples of questions that address these particular topics:

- How can we be most helpful to you and your family (or friends) during your hospitalization? (Clarifies expectations and increases collaboration)
- What has been most and least helpful to you in past hospitalizations or clinic visits? (Identifies past strengths and problems to avoid and successes to repeat)
- What is the greatest challenge facing your family during this hospitalization, discharge, or clinic visit? (Indicates actual or potential suffering, roles, and beliefs)
- With which of your family members or friends would you like us to share information? With which ones would you like us not to share information? (Indicates alliances, resources, and possible conflictual relationships)
- What do you need to best prepare you or your family member for discharge? (Assists with early discharge planning)
- Who do you believe is suffering the most in your family during this hospitalization, clinic visit, or home care visit? (Identifies the family member who has the greatest need for support and intervention)
- What is the one question you would most like to have answered during our meeting right now? I may not be able to answer this question at the moment, but I will do my best or will try to find the answer for you. (Identifies most pressing issue or concern [Wright, 1989])
- How have I been most helpful to you in this family meeting? How could we improve? (Shows a willingness to learn from families and to work collaboratively)

Key Ingredient 5: Commending Family and Individual Strengths

The important intervention of offering commendations (Hougher Limacher, 2003; Hougher Limacher & Wright, 2006; Wright, 2005; Wright & Bell, in press) was fully discussed in the presentation of the CFIM (see Chapter 4). We wish to restate that we routinely commend families in each session the strengths observed during the interview. In a brief family interview of 15 minutes or less, we still endorse the practice of offering at least one or two commendations to family members of individual or family strengths, resources, or competencies that the nurse directly observed or gathered from another source. Remember that commendations are observations of behavior that occur across time. Therefore, the nurse is looking for patterns rather than a one-time occurrence that is more likely to be the offering of a compliment. An example of a commendation is: "Your family is showing much courage in living with your wife's cancer for 5 years." A compliment would be "Your son is so gentle despite feeling so ill today."

Families coping with chronic, life-threatening, or psychosocial problems commonly feel defeated, hopeless, or failing in their efforts to overcome the illnesses or live with them. In our clinical experience, we have found that most families who are experiencing illness, disability, or trauma also suffer from "commendation-deficit disorder." Therefore, nurses can never offer too many commendations.

Immediate and long-term positive reactions to commendations indicate that they are powerful, effective, and enduring therapeutic interventions (Bohn, Wright, & Moules, 2003; Hougher Limacher, 2003; Hougher Limacher & Wright, 2003, 2006; Moules, 2002). Robinson's (1998) study explored the processes and outcomes of nursing interventions with families experiencing difficulties with chronic illness. The families reported the clinical nursing team's "orientation to strengths, resources, and possibilities to be an extremely important facet of the process" (p. 284). Hougher Limacher's (2003) study, which specifically focused on understanding more about the intervention of commendations, lends even further validation to the power of commendations. Families who internalize commendations offered by nurses appear more receptive and trusting of the nurse–family relationship and tend to readily take up ideas, opinions, and advice that are offered.

By commending families' resources, competencies, and strengths, nurses offer family members a new view of themselves. When nurses change the view families have of themselves, families are commonly able to look at their health problem differently and thus move toward more effective solutions to reduce any potential or actual suffering. Additional ideas for interventions can be found in Wright and Leahey's DVD (2003) How to Intervene with Families with Health Concerns.

PERSONAL EXAMPLE OF INVOLVING FAMILY IN NURSING PRACTICE (LMW)

To poignantly illustrate how involving family members in health care can be both effective and healing, or ineffective and resulting in a needless increase of suffering, Lorraine M. Wright offers a personal story to illustrate the best and worst of family nursing. These experiences occurred during two very brief interactions with nurses in the emergency unit of a large city hospital while Dr. Wright accompanied her mother for a possible admission:

> Over the last 5 years of my mother's life, she experienced several major exacerbations of multiple sclerosis (MS), with frequent hospitalizations. Each exacerbation left my mother more physically disabled. The extreme exacerbations of the last year of her life left her a quadriplegic. With each exacerbation, she never returned to the level of either physical or cognitive functioning that she previously enjoyed. Despite all of these setbacks, there was tremendous courage on the part of both my mother and my father. Amazingly, my mother's moments of complaining, sadness, or grief were minimal, which of course buffered other family members' suffering. I saw my father become a very caring caregiver and "nurse" while his own life became very constrained.
>
> On one of my mother's admissions to the hospital, I encountered two very brief but powerful conversations with nurses in the emergency department (ED). One I prefer to call "Naughty Nurse" and the other "Angel Nurse." Both of these nurses had a profound impact on my emotional suffering. Both of these nurses interacted with me for a very brief time, not more than 5 minutes each.
>
> Before our arrival at the hospital ED, I spent a few very exhausting hours with my mother. My father, mother, and I were enjoying a day at our cottage about an hour out of the city. As the afternoon unfolded, it became apparent that my mother was becoming more wobbly when walking (at that time she was still able to walk a few steps with assistance). As we were packing to leave, she became unable to bear weight. With great difficulty, my father and I lifted her into her wheelchair and headed down the ramp of our cottage to the car. The greater challenge lay ahead of us: to get her from the wheelchair into the car. It took all of our strength and ingenuity to accomplish this task, with my mother, of course, frightened that we would drop her. After some 30 minutes and lots of perspiration, we realized our goal with my mother safely in the car. On the way into the city, we made a mutual decision to take her to the hospital where she had been admitted on previous occasions

to have her assessed for possible admission. We all believed that she was having another severe exacerbation.

When we arrived at the ED, I was very relieved. It had been a very worrisome and arduous few hours. I now looked forward to my mother's receiving nursing and medical assessment and treatment to assist her and us. My father waited with her in the car at the curb of the ED while I entered to seek assistance to lift my mother out of the car. On arriving at the nursing station, I encountered "Naughty Nurse." I explained the current situation to her and requested assistance to lift my mother out of the car and into the ED. "Naughty Nurse" responded in a curt, mistrusting tone by saying, "How did you get her into the car?" This initial brief interaction was shocking to me; it was accusatory, blaming, and mistrusting of one another. No therapeutic relationship was being developed. This nurse's response invited me to counter with an equally rude, impolite response. I said, "With great [difficulty], so we will need help to lift her out of the car." Our conversation now escalated in terms of accusations and recriminations as "Naughty Nurse" retorted, "Well, I can't lift her out of the car." I suggested that perhaps one of her male colleagues could assist us. As "Naughty Nurse" and a male colleague approached the car to assist my mother, they did not introduce themselves to my mother nor did they discontinue their conversation with each other. This was an extreme example of what family nursing should not be. By now, I was very distressed and upset about our treatment by this particular nurse. Of course, she was completely unaware that, in my professional life, I teach, practice, research, and write about family nursing.

However, all was not lost. Within a short while, we were placed in a room in the ED and, after a brief wait, "Angel Nurse" appeared. First, she introduced herself to my mother, explained that she would be taking her blood pressure and temperature and that "blood work" had been ordered. This "Angel Nurse" competently and kindly attended to my mother, inquiring about both her medical history and her illness experiences with MS. In a very impressive manner, she reassured my mother that she would probably be admitted for another round of intravenous steroids and that everything would be done to keep her comfortable. Then she came to me, reached out her hand to shake mine, introduced herself, and warmly inquired about the nature of my relationship to the patient.

I was softened by this nurse's kind and competent approach. I offered the information that I was the patient's daughter and that I was visiting from another city. Then the nurse offered a possible hypothesis in the form of a statement, "This must be very upsetting for you." In that one sentence, this nurse assessed and acknowledged my suffering. "Angel Nurse" provided comfort and understanding through her very brief interaction with me in probably less than 2 minutes. However, in just those 2 minutes, she had involved me in her practice and some of my emotional suffering had healed.

Later, on reflection, I realized that my reaction to this nurse's encounter with me was to make every effort to assist her in caring for my mother because I could see that she was overloaded with patients in the ED. "Angel Nurse's" particular nursing approach had encouraged me to want to be more helpful to her. Kindness invites kindness; accusations invite accusations. In this very brief interaction, "Angel Nurse" had entered into a therapeutic conversation with me, my mother, and my father. She also showed good manners by shaking my hand, introducing herself, eliciting some genogram information, and validating my suffering. Perhaps not all the key ingredients that we have suggested for a brief family interview are evident in this interaction with "Angel Nurse;" however, it exemplifies how the context and the appropriateness of the situation determine how much family members can be involved. This nurse beautifully demonstrated that family nursing can be done, even in busy EDs, in just 2 minutes and still effect healing.

PROFESSIONAL EXAMPLE OF A BRIEF FAMILY INTERVIEW WITHOUT FAMILY MEMBERS PRESENT

Dr. Maureen Leahey offers an example of a situation she was involved in while consulting with staff nurses on a medical unit:

> Greta, a 32-year-old woman, was admitted to a medical unit with a questionable diagnosis of influenza. Her weight had dropped to 82 lb, a loss of 10 lb in the week before admission.
>
> Greta also had a genetic disease involving weakness and wasting of skeletal muscles. The nursing staff perceived her to be angry and abrupt; they also wondered what the medical problem was. They felt sorry for Greta and

thought of her as "very dependent." A brief interview was scheduled to explore Greta's expectations, beliefs, and resources. Her family was invited to the meeting, which was held on the unit, but they did not come.

In a 15-minute interview with Greta alone, the nurse initially drew a quick genogram. She learned that Greta lived with her two younger brothers and their mother, all of whom had what Greta called "the disease" (wasting of the muscles). She was the only family member who was able to drive, and this was why the others did not attend the meeting. (This was new information for the nurse.)

The nurse then asked Greta about her expectations for the hospitalization and how the nurses could be most helpful. Greta responded to the circular questions by saying that she would know how the staff would care for her "by how they talk with me and other patients, show me respect and trust, and treat me independently." She stated that she needed to be strong to care for her brothers and mother "who depend on me."

The nurse asked Greta what hopes and expectations the other family members had for Greta's hospitalization. She replied that, when her mother had previously been hospitalized, the staff had "pushed her to eat." Greta found this very disrespectful. The nurse asked how the current staff was treating Greta's reluctance to eat. Greta described that they offered her food choices and reported that she found this quite satisfactory. The interview concluded with the nurse inviting Greta to talk more with her if she had any concerns about her care.

From this interview, the nurse revised her opinion of Greta being "very dependent" to thinking of her as someone who needed to be commended for her independence and caregiving. She now saw Greta as a "strong person" and passed this message on to her nursing colleagues.

A few days after the 15-minute interview, Greta commented to the nurse during morning care, "Remember when you told me to tell you if something wasn't going right?" She then related that the evening staff was "pushing me to eat and not respecting my choices." She had lost 1 lb. The nurse listened and remembered that, in the morning report, Greta was talked about as being "manipulative." The staff members were concerned with her weight loss and therefore "pushed her" to eat more. In turn,

Greta ate less. The nurse conceptualized the problem as a vicious circular interaction (see Chapter 3) between the patient and the evening staff. She decided to intervene by:

■ Inviting the dietitian to talk with the staff regarding food groups and choices

■ Putting a note in the record system that Greta could "eat on demand"

■ Encouraging individual members of the nursing staff to give Greta more choices of various types of food

The outcome of this brief, family-oriented interview and interventions was that Greta gained some weight over the course of hospitalization. The other staff nurses said that they felt "less responsible for making Greta eat" and more responsible for offering her choices and promoting her independence. Most significant to the primary nurse was the intervention used in the unit documentation system in which she identified the problem, provided a rationale, and recommended direction for other staff members.

From our perspective, an important outcome was that Greta's skills and competencies to manage and live with her chronic illness were reinforced. She went home stronger, both physically and emotionally. In addition, she was able to assist herself and other family members with ongoing health issues. This 15-minute interview also indicates how nurses can include other family members in the therapeutic conversation even if the members are not present. Involving family members in relational nursing practice includes inquiring about them whether they are present or not.

CONCLUSION

In conclusion, an overall framework for ritualizing a 15-minute (or shorter) family interview is:

1. Begin a therapeutic conversation with a particular purpose in mind that can be accomplished in 15 minutes or less.

2. Use manners to engage or reengage. Introduce yourself by offering your name and role. Orient family members to the purpose of a brief family interview.

3. Assess key areas of internal and external structure and function—obtain genogram information and key external support data.

4. Ask three key questions of family members.

5. Commend the family on one or two strengths.

6. Evaluate usefulness and conclude.

We generally find this framework to be a useful guide when conducting 15-minute (or shorter) family interviews. However, these key ingredients of a brief family interview need to be adapted according to the competence of the nurse, the practice context in which nurses and families encounter one another, and the appropriateness and purpose of the family meeting. We are confident that, if the interview is suitably implemented, both nurses and families will be satisfied with the usefulness of a brief family interview. Nurses can and do reduce families' physical, emotional, and spiritual suffering by engaging in therapeutic conversations with family members. This can occur in 15 minutes or even in one sentence!

References

Bohn, U., Wright, L.M., & Moules, N.J. (2003). A family systems nursing interview following a myocardial infarction: The power of commendations. *Journal of Family Nursing, 9*(2), 151–165.

Frank, A.W. (1998). Just listening: Narrative and deep illness. *Families, Systems and Health, 16*(3), 197–212.

Holtslander, L. (2005). Clinical application of the 15-minute family interview: Addressing the needs of postpartum families. *Journal of Family Nursing, 11*(2), 5–18.

Hougher Limacher, L. (2003). *Commendations: The healing potential of one family systems nursing intervention* [Unpublished doctoral thesis]. Calgary, Alberta, Canada: University of Calgary.

Hougher Limacher, L., & Wright, L.M. (2003). Commendations: Listening to the silent side of a family intervention. *Journal of Family Nursing, 9*(2), 130–135.

Hougher Limacher, L., & Wright, L.M. (2006). Exploring the therpeutic family intervention of commendations: Insights from research. *Journal of Family Nursing, 12*(8), 307–331.

International Council of Nurses (2002). Nurses always there for you: Caring for families. *Information and Action Tool Kit.* Geneva: Switzerland.

Leahey, M., et al. (1995). The impact of a family systems nursing approach: Nurses' perceptions. *The Journal of Continuing Education in Nursing, 26*(5), 219–225.

Martin, J., & Kanen, J. (2005). *Miss Manners' guide to excruciatingly correct behavior, freshly updated.* New York: WW Norton.

Martinez, A., D'Artois, D., & Rennick, J.E. (2007). Does the 15 minute (or less) family interview influence nursing practice? *Journal of Family Nursing, 13*(2),1–22.

McLeod, D.L. (2003). *Opening space for the spiritual: Therapeutic conversations with families living with serious illness* [Unpublished doctoral thesis]. University of Calgary, Alberta, Canada.

Moules, N.J. (2002). Nursing on paper: Therapeutic letters in nursing practice. *Nursing Inquiry, 9*(2), 104–113.

Robinson, C.A. (1998). Women, families, chronic illness, and nursing interventions: From burden to balance. *Journal of Family Nursing, 4*(3), 271–290.

Robinson, C.A., & Wright, L.M. (1995). Family nursing interventions: What families say makes a difference. *Journal of Family Nursing, 1*(3), 327–345.

Wright, L.M. (1989). When clients ask questions: Enriching the therapeutic conversation. *Family Therapy Networker, 13*(6), 15–16.

Wright, L.M. (2005). *Spirituality, suffering, and illness: Ideas for healing.* Philadelphia: F.A. Davis.

Wright, L.M., & Bell, J.M. (in press). *Beliefs and illness: A model to invite healing.* Calgary, AB: 4th Floor Press.

Wright, L.M., & Leahey, M. (Producers). (2000). *How to do a 15 minute (or less) family interview.* [DVD]. Calgary, Canada. www.familynursingresources.com.

Wright, L.M., & Leahey, M. (Producers). (2003). *How to intervene with families with health concerns* [DVD]. Available from www.familynursingresources.com.

Wright, L.M., & Leahey, M. (Producers). (2006). *How to use questions in family interviewing.* [DVD]. Calgary, Canada www.familynursingresources.com.

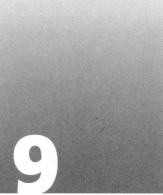

Chapter **9**

How to Use Questions
in Family Interviewing

Throughout this book we have discussed the usefulness of asking questions in family interviewing. We believe questions are not just useful for assessment; they are also one of the most helpful interventions nurses can offer to families. We would like to demonstrate, through the use of clinical examples, how questions are used in relational practice. These clinical interviews can be viewed in our DVD (Wright & Leahey, 2006) *How to Use Questions in Family Interviewing* (www.familynursingresources.com). We will discuss the application of questions in various clinical settings and contexts to:

- Engage all family members and focus the meeting
- Assess the impact of the problem or illness on the family
- Elicit problem-solving skills, coping strategies, and strengths
- Intervene and invite change
- Request feedback about the meeting

QUESTIONS IN CONTEXT

First, we would like to discuss a few ideas about asking questions in the context of clinical practice, specifically, in the context of a therapeutic conversation between a nurse and a family. So what *is* a useful or helpful question when interviewing families? We believe that useful or helpful questions have the potential to provide information to *both* the family and the nurse, invite family members to reflect on their illness experience, and can even be potentially healing when the nurse asks them in a manner of sincere inquiry or curiosity. Questions are not effective in and of themselves; rather, it is only through a therapeutic conversation that questions help nurses be effective. (See Chapter 8 for more ideas about therapeutic conversation.) Questions also enhance a nurse's understanding of family members' experience with a particular illness or problem. Answers to questions can help both the nurse and the family appreciate the family's coping strategies, unique strengths, and resources. These types of conversation are very different than one that a family may have with an intake worker or data clerk.

There are numerous and various types of questions such as difference questions, triadic questions, hypothetical questions, and behavioral-effect questions (see Chapter 4). In this chapter, we offer a simple dichotomy of questions that a nurse can ask: assessment and interventive questions.

- Assessment or linear questions are meant to inform the nurse; these are often investigative questions such as asking for a family member's description of the illness experience or problem. We have found that the telling of the story can frequently in itself be therapeutic. For example, telling of developmental transitions, such as the birth of a child or the placement of a parent in a nursing home can draw forth remembrances of strength and meaning that may have been overlooked or forgotten.

- Interventive or circular questions are meant to invite a reflection and effect change; these questions may encourage family members to see their problems in a new way and subsequently to see new solutions. They introduce alternative possibilities, theories, beliefs, and views, simply in their posing (McGee, Del Vento, & Bavelas, 2005).

The important difference between these two categories of questions is in their *intent*. Thus, as the family's answers provide information for both the family and the nurse, the nurse's questions may provide information for the family.

It can be helpful for the nurse at the start of the family meeting to explain to the family that she will be asking various kinds of questions to obtain a thorough understanding of their situation. Also, it gives the family an opportunity to familiarize themselves with the nurse. In a social conversation, it is often considered rude to interrupt someone who is speaking with a question. However, in a time-limited family interview, it could be considered rude not to obtain each family member's perception of the health concern. Sometimes interrupting one family member to include the perspective of another is most appropriate.

It is also appropriate in therapeutic conversation for nurses to understand they are not invading a family's privacy when asking questions. In training our students to overcome such a mental barrier, we have found it helpful to teach them to say to clients, "I don't know you very well, so can I trust that if I ask you something too sensitive, or something you would prefer not to talk about, that you will let me know?" In this way, the student obtains the family's permission to have a wide-ranging discussion. If conflict among family members erupts as a result of the nurse's questions, we encourage our students not to be frightened or intimidated by this. Rather, the nurse could say for example, "Is this typically what happens when the two of you do not agree on an issue?" The nurse's tone is also vitally important when asking questions so as not to convey judgment or criticism, but rather to convey a message of the nurse's desire to seek a sincere understanding of the illness or issue and invite the family to a reflection that hopefully would result in a new perspective and new behaviors. (See Chapter 7 for additional ideas about engagement and assessment.)

In summary, useful, effective, and time-efficient questions are part of relational practice in that they aid in relationship building and collaboration between nurses and families. Most importantly, questions can be very effective in creating a safe context for the family to describe their illness experience and hopefully glean ideas for how to soften or diminish their suffering. Through the asking of interventive questions as well as other useful interventions, the nurse can invite, encourage, and support families to change.

Example #1: Engage All Family Members and Focus the Meeting

In this first example, Lorraine is meeting with a couple, Nicholas and Bev. Nicholas had a heart attack recently, and this is a follow-up clinic visit. Lorraine asks "the one question question": "What one question would you most like to have answered during our meeting together?" "The one question question" is a term that Lorraine coined (Wright, 1989), and themes of answers to this question have been explored in a recent study (Duhamel, Dupuis, & Wright, in press). This question emphasizes a *specific* concern and also asks the couple to prioritize their concerns; she asks what they would *most* like to have answered. The question also includes a timeframe (i.e., "during our meeting together").

In this first clinical vignette, Lorraine asks the "one question question" of both Nicholas and Bev. She does not ask Bev to comment on Nicholas' answer. Rather, she engages *each* family member to elicit their primary concern. Lorraine paraphrases and clarifies each person's response so that both she and the person are in agreement about what has been said. The following is an example of relational practice, the nurse and the client collaborating in setting the focus for the meeting:

> **Dr. Lorraine Wright:** I'm wondering then in the brief time we have, is there any particular question you would most like to have answered during our meeting today?
>
> **Husband:** I'd like for her (*looking at his wife*) to deal differently with her anxiety. Me ... I'm fine.
>
> **Wife:** Hmm ... Oh yes, he wants me to go on tranquilizers. So ... sure ... (*Turning away*)
>
> **Dr. Lorraine Wright:** (*Looking at the husband*) So you want to know how to help your wife deal with her anxiety?

Husband: Oh yeah …

Dr. Lorraine Wright: And for you, Bev, what is the one question you would most like to get answered?

Wife: I would like to get him to start exercising more, watch his diet, spend some time with the family, and stop worrying so much about work ….

Husband: (*Looking down*)

Dr. Lorraine Wright: Is there one question you'd like, Bev …

Wife: Well, how can we get him to change his lifestyle?

Dr. Lorraine Wright: Okay …

In reading the transcript of the actual interview, did you notice how the nurse, Lorraine, persisted in obtaining an answer from Bev? Gentle persistence can be an important skill in establishing a focus.

There are many other kinds of questions that could also be used in focusing a conversation. For example, a nurse could ask, "What would you like to see happen today so that you would know our meeting has been helpful for you"? We want to emphasize that there is no single, "correct" question to ask. Rather, by engaging in purposeful conversation with patients and their families, nurses will choose and select the most helpful questions in the context of each particular family along with their unique concerns and issues.

Example #2: Use Questions to Assess the Impact of the Problem/Illness on the Family

Asking questions about the impact of the illness or problem is essential to understanding the effect, impact, and changes caused by illness in family members' lives and relationships. By inquiring in this manner, we are giving the family an opportunity to talk about their illness experience or illness story. Families have reported to us that often telling their illness story or narrative was helpful in their emotional, physical, or spiritual healing as the illness is understood, listened to, acknowledged, and witnessed. Too often families have not been given this opportunity to tell their illness story through useful and skillful questions posed by a caring nurse.

In the next clinical vignette, Maureen is meeting with a middle-aged couple who are experiencing multiple chronic illnesses. In particular, Phyllis is coping with osteoarthritis and uses a scooter for mobility. Both Ken and Phyllis are 59 years old. They have two sons: the eldest, age 26, is married while the youngest, age 22, lives in the family home.

In this interview, the nurse is Maureen, and she explores the impact of the osteoarthritis upon the couple. Notice how initially the husband says it has not had an impact on them but then does talk about the impact of his wife's pain upon him. Phyllis commends her husband for his support and assistance with household chores, but then offers, with sadness, her decision to leave the teaching profession, which she loved, as her energy was being depleted by her illness. Phyllis believed she needed to save her energy for her family but openly admits that it was a huge adjustment to being a full-time homemaker.

This one question about the impact of the illness upon them as a couple opened up a very useful discussion about how osteoarthritis has dramatically changed their lives, careers, and relationships and offered a window into their suffering, coping, and healing experiences.

Dr. Maureen Leahey: What has been the impact of these illnesses on the two of you?

Husband: I don't know if there has really been an impact ... I know that I feel at times ... I wish I could take some of the pain away. It is very hard on me to see ... especially someone I love so much, suffering with pain.

Wife: (*Looking at husband*)

Dr. Maureen Leahey: (*Nodding*)

Husband: ... And it's a continual, chronic pain ...

Dr. Maureen Leahey: Yes (*Nodding*)

Husband: But I try to be as supportive as I possibly can, but ...

Wife: He is just so helpful and so wonderful ... When I think about the impact ... I was a teacher, an elementary teacher, and when my arthritis got to bother me so badly, I decided to take a leave of absence because at school, I had to be cheerful and bubbly. I had to put myself forward, but when I came home I was not (*Turning toward husband and laughing*) quite as bubbly. I thought this is not really fair to my own children. So I thought if I am at home, I will be able to do more for them with less effort. So actually, it did impact our lives because I stopped teaching ... and when I was teaching I was really quite independent, I think ...

Husband: (*Nodding*) You were ... It took you a long time to adjust ...

Wife: It did. Away from school, from being a teacher at school to just being at home, it was really difficult for me, but Ken adjusted really quickly with helping me with things I needed help with. Also, our boys, I think, were very aware of the change in our family ... how things changed, because truly they were different.

Dr. Maureen Leahey: It sounds like the two of you made tremendous changes.

Other kinds of interventive questions that can assess the impact of an illness are:

■ What changes, if any, have there been in your life since you were diagnosed with serious illness?

■ What has been the effect of this illness on your family? Your sexual relations? Your work life?

These types of questions address the suffering the family may be enduring and the systemic effects of that suffering. We find it helpful to remember that talking can be healing, and these kinds of questions have the potential for simultaneously assessing and intervening! If the couple in the above example expressed a desire to work on changing or modifying a particular coping strategy, Maureen could then have asked them a variety of other questions to foster change. Some examples might include:

■ What has been most helpful for you in adjusting? What do you think your sons noticed?

■ What has been least helpful?

■ What advice have you been given by family members? Friends? Health care providers? Did you try it? What did you discover?

■ What ideas for change have you been considering? What would be a first step in trying out these ideas? Who would support you in this change? Who might not support you? How might you resist the temptation to fall back into old habits? How might you reward yourself for developing new habits?

It can be seen that these kinds of questions about possible ideas and ways to change are ones that invite families to reflect on what has and has not been useful in the past and to develop new ideas for the future.

Example #3: Use Questions to Elicit Problem-Solving Skills, Coping Strategies and Strengths

Families coping with chronic or life-threatening illness or psychosocial problems can commonly feel defeated, hopeless, or failing in their efforts to overcome the illness or live alongside of it. Asking questions about the family's problem-solving abilities and their coping strategies and strengths not only serves as assessment but also can be considered interventive.

Exploring theses areas of problem-solving skills and coping strategies can remind families of often forgotten or suppressed skills and strengths. Through interventive questioning, families can rediscover and reclaim their own abilities to solve problems and bring back to their hearts and minds their inherent strengths.

Now we would like to turn to a vignette of a biracial family with young children: Chris, age 36, Carleen, age 28, Reuben, age 5, Mariah, age 2, and

Rebecca, 9 months. Chris, an immigrant from Zimbabwe, is employed full-time; Carleen, who grew up in a small, rural town in western Canada, is the resident manager in their building. The health concern for this family is the mother's thyroid condition.

In the first section of the example, the husband and father Chris comments on the many changes in his life with three pre-schoolers, in addition to his working full time and taking evening courses. Notice how Lorraine empathizes with the many demands upon Chris but then asks the couple an interventive question: "What have you learned that works to assist you with all of these demands"?

This interventive question invites Carleen to talk about how things are more organized for her family when she mobilizes resources such as friends to assist them. This solution gives her an opportunity to do her own work as resident manager plus gives her husband more time for his studies.

> **Husband:** The accounting program is very demanding time wise ... and then the kids ... I'm finding it ... I am having a hard time finding time to study because we have three of them ... to feed them, get them ready for bed sometimes and then to help clean up the house. By the time ... I am so tired ...
>
> **Wife:** (*Looking over at him*)
>
> **Dr. Lorraine M. Wright:** Well, sure ... you are pooped yourself.
>
> **Husband:** I do not put in as much time as I should into studying. This has been one of the biggest changes from my point of view.
>
> **Dr. Lorraine M. Wright:** So many demands upon yourself ... and so what have you learned to handle this? What have you learned that works, does not work?
>
> **Husband:** Mmm ...
>
> **Wife:** If I can get things ready, have them all fed, have the place cleaned, have my work done...'cause often when he comes home I have to go out and do some of my work. I have friends who help me out and I help them out. We baby sit for each other.
>
> **Dr. Lorraine M. Wright:** Oh really ... that is good ...
>
> **Wife:** That allows me to get work done during the day.
>
> **Dr. Lorraine M. Wright:** That's a good idea ... a good arrangement.
>
> **Wife:** It gives me more time in the evening.

Did you notice that, after Carleen shared her thoughts about "what works" in the family to assist with all of their demands, Lorraine commended the couple for their very good idea of friends taking turns caring for each other's children?

In this next section of the vignette, Lorraine normalizes the difficulty of time pressures for mothers and fathers; she asks if Carleen has been able to work out finding any time for herself. An important conversation unfolds with Carleen illustrating her problem-solving skills. She talks about involving her son to watch the youngest child while she does yoga in their home. This sparks the father to remember how he gives his wife some time for herself when he takes all three children to the park. Once again, Lorraine is able to commend the family for these efforts.

> **Dr. Lorraine M. Wright:** (*To wife*) Have you been able to find any time for yourself?
>
> **Wife:** Yeah, I have. I try to get up before the kids ... that does not always work though. This one (*Turning toward 5-year-old Reuben*) gets up, and then the baby is up ... I'll go downstairs and I'll do yoga, and Reuben will just watch me. Or I'll do aerobics ...
>
> **Dr. Lorraine M. Wright:** (*Looking at Reuben*) So you watch Mommy do yoga...Do you ever join in and do it with her?
>
> **Reuben:** (*Looking at Dr. Lorraine M. Wright*) ... when the baby's awake ... watching her ...
>
> **Wife:** He watches the baby.
>
> **Dr. Lorraine M. Wright:** Very nice.
>
> **Husband:** Sometimes what I do is take the kids out to the park so she can have the day to herself. I still try to do it, but some days she'd rather be doing her work.

Asking about a family's problem-solving skills, coping, and strengths can set the stage for further interventions, if needed. For example, if Carleen had stated she wanted to increase her problem-solving skills, Lorraine could have pursued this with her. For example, they could have discussed possible play groups in the area, available community resources, and so forth. Other questions that could be asked to bring forth a family's problem-solving skills and strengths include:

- Asking the husband in his wife's presence: "What do you think your devotion and caring for your wife during her illness does for your marriage"?
- Asking the teenagers in a family meeting: "What do you think other families could learn from your family about coping with a chronic illness"?

Example #4: Use Questions as Interventions and to Invite Change

The intervention process represents the core of clinical practice with families. Myriad interventions are possible, but nurses need to tailor their interventions to each family they encounter. Openness to certain interventions is profoundly influenced by the relationship between the nurse and the family and the nurse's ability to help the family reflect on their health problems.

Questions in and of themselves can provide new information and answers for the family; thus, they become interventions. Interventive questions can encourage family members to view their problems or illness experience in a new way or to change their beliefs and subsequently discover new solutions.

The next clinical example is with a couple, Al and Benz. She is a documented Chinese immigrant, and this is her first marriage. Al is a native Canadian, and this is his second marriage. Benz is close to being discharged from the hospital following surgery for breast cancer. The first interventive question in this clinical vignette is, "Who between the two of you was the most upset with the news of the diagnosis?" This leads to a very poignant therapeutic conversation about Benz's future.

> **Dr. Lorraine M. Wright:** (*Looking at the wife*) Have there been any other kinds of cancer in your family?
>
> **Wife:** No ... we are all pretty healthy.
>
> **Dr. Lorraine M. Wright:** (*Looking at the husband*) ... and what about for you, Al, has there been any history of cancer in your family?
>
> **Husband:** No ... I cannot think of any ... I had an aunt and uncle who got lung cancer. Both were heavy smokers.
>
> **Dr. Lorraine Wright:** So this was something very new for both of you dealing with cancer. And who would you say, between the two of you, was most upset about this diagnosis and news when you got it?
>
> **Husband:** Oh Benz was, I think.
>
> **Wife:** I would say so, too. I cried and cried. I just could not handle it.
>
> **Dr. Lorraine Wright:** Yes ...
>
> **Husband:** ... and I just don't see what a lot of crying accomplishes. I think you have to really think positively and know in your heart that you can beat this thing.
>
> **Dr. Lorraine Wright:** That's how you've been trying to encourage Benz?

Wife: Yeah, he kept telling me that. I just felt I needed to cry. That's the only thing I needed to do ...

Dr. Lorraine M. Wright: Yes ...

Husband: Well, a certain amount of this is understandable, and I have tried to be sympathetic, but you have got to get onto the positive thinking path and really believe you're going to beat this thing.

Dr. Lorraine M. Wright: (*Nodding*)

Husband: I really do believe that. I really do believe that.

Dr. Lorraine M. Wright: (*Looking at husband*) ... You do. (*Looking at wife*) And what are your thoughts for the future? Because I've met other women with breast cancer that worry ... What are your thoughts?

Wife: Some days I am pretty good about it. I am in good hands; my doctor is good. And some days, I just do not know. It fluctuates. Some days are good and some are bad.

Dr. Lorraine M. Wright: So some days you are more optimistic about your future and other days you ...

Wife: I think the worst.

Dr. Lorraine M. Wright: And what do you think about when you think the worst?

Wife: That Al and our child, Bryan, would be alone without me. I care about them so much.

Husband: And this is the kind of thinking I try to discourage. I do not think it is good.

Dr. Lorraine M. Wright: So when you hear your wife talking this way and I am not here, do you try to cheer her up and get her off of this topic?

Husband: Oh yeah. I allow her a little bit of it. She has to express herself and express her feelings, but once she has got that out, she has to get back to being hopeful.

Dr. Lorraine M. Wright: (*Looking to wife*) And do you like that approach Al takes? He tries to get you off of this topic and to think optimistically. Or do you want to be able to say more about the other side, the 'worry side' ...

Wife: Well, I know he is being kind and wants me to do well. But sometimes, that is just the way I feel. Maybe if he would just listen to me ...

In this very heart-rending, therapeutic conversation, Benz was very concerned about her prognosis. Lorraine had asked about Benz' beliefs about her prognosis when she said to Benz, "What are your thoughts about your future?"

These are not easy conversations when a nurse "speaks the unspeakable" by introducing a conversation about their beliefs about prognosis (Wright & Bell, in press). Knowing the family's beliefs about various aspects of their illness assists the nurse in knowing if their beliefs are constraining or facilitating. We believe that nurses have a socially sanctioned role and thus can talk about such delicate and intimate topics with families. In our clinical experience, we have found that families rarely mind any question if it is asked in a kind and thoughtful manner. We have encouraged our students to be curious and pursue hard topics with families. If the nurse working with the family cannot address potentially difficult areas with the family, then we encourage the nurse to transfer the family to another nurse if possible or request that another nurse continue the conversation.

Lorraine's question invited a very useful disclosure about this couple's differences in beliefs about how to cope with worries and face the future. Benz wanted to talk about her fears for the future, whereas Al's preferred way to deal with worry was to be optimistic. Instead of Lorraine taking sides with either Al or Benz about the best way to handle fears, she asked Benz: "Do you like this approach (her husband's optimism), or do you want to say more about the 'worry side'?"

This simple, but powerful interventive question had the potential for inviting healing change in one or both spouses. Benz offered very clearly that she would prefer that her husband listen to her. It is very understandable that Al wanted to cheer her up, but it was not Benz' preferred way for her husband to comfort her.

In this clinical example, interventive questions invited family members to explore and reflect on their beliefs about the illness experience, the prognosis, and how best to manage their illness. Reflections are invited through very deliberate, thoughtful, and purposeful interventive questions.

Examples of other interventive questions are:

- How do you make sense of your suffering?

- In 6 months from now, how do you think your family will have adjusted to this illness?

In our therapeutic conversations with families, we hope that healing will be enhanced as new thoughts, ideas, or solutions come forth, are pondered, and acted upon. As family members consider how to best live their lives with illness, change may occur.

Example #5: Use Questions to Request Feedback About the Family Meeting

We seek to ask questions that are in keeping with our philosophy of fostering collaborative relationships between nurses and families. These kinds of questions imply to family members that their satisfaction with the meeting, or lack thereof, matters and that we want to improve our care to families. Collaborative questions also open space for the family to voice concerns about what specifically was helpful to them.

In the following vignette, at the end of the meeting with Al and Benz, Lorraine asks if the conversation has been helpful to them. Benz gives a short answer and comments on the relationship with Lorraine by saying, "You are kind."

But notice how Lorraine's question invites much more pondering from Al. He reflects back on Benz' suggestion about wanting him to listen more. This is a lovely example of how an interventive question invited a reflection and how Al decides on his *own* that he could make a behavioral change that would be more his wife's preferred way to be comforted. This is always the most desirable and sustaining kind of change, that is, when a family member initiates the change rather than being instructed to do so.

> **Dr. Lorraine M. Wright:** (*Looking at the couple*) Well, just before we end, was there anything about this conversation that has been useful or helpful for you or not helpful?
>
> **Wife:** ... I think you are very kind.
>
> **Dr. Lorraine M. Wright:** (*Nodding to the wife and then looking to the husband*) Anything that was helpful for you, Al?
>
> **Husband:** Yeah ... it made me think. It made me think. Perhaps I need to listen a little bit more and not be so free with the advice.
>
> **Dr. Lorraine M. Wright:** (*Looking at the wife*) I think it is wonderful to have a husband who wants to cheer you up and make you feel better ...
>
> **Wife:** I'm lucky.
>
> **Dr. Lorraine M. Wright:** But there are times when you want him to hear you out about what you are thinking and feeling.

Other questions that can invite feedback about the usefulness of the therapeutic conversations that nurses have with families are:

- In what ways was our discussion useful to each of you, or not useful?
- On a scale of 1 to 10 (with 1 being very low and 10 being very high), how well do you think I understood your situation?
- Is there anything you were hoping for in this meeting that did not happen?

Of course, families do not always convey positive feelings about the meeting with the nurse. If the family expresses dissatisfaction, we encourage the nurse to explore their reasons for being dissatisfied and accept the feedback nondefensively. The nurse can thank the family for their insights and ask their suggestions for how she could be more helpful to other families. If the nurse takes a sincere "one-down" position when receiving feedback, it encourages the family to maintain a collaborative relationship. It also permits the nurse to reflect on her practice and potentially alter her actions for future family meetings.

CONCLUSIONS

We hope this chapter has given you ideas on how to use questions in family interviewing—questions that invite possibilities for healing and change. Of course, there is an unending number of questions that nurses could ask families. But we hope that this sample roadmap for the interview will assist you to be more selective and time-efficient when asking your questions. We hope you will find that asking families questions will give you an increased understanding and appreciation of their illness experience or concerns and that this will soften suffering and invite more hope and healing.

References

Duhamel, F., Dupuis, F., & Wright, L.M. (2009). Families and nurses answers to the 'One Question Question': Helpful directions clinical practice, education, and research in family nursing. *Journal of Family Nursing, 15*(4), 420–428.

McGee, D., Del Vento, A., & Bavelas, J.B. (2005). An interactional model of questions as therapeutic interventions. *Journal of Marital and Family Therapy, 31*(4), 371–384.

Wright, L.M. (1989). When clients ask questions: Enriching the therapeutic conversation. *Family Therapy Networker, 13*(6), 15–16.

Wright, L.M. & Bell, J.M). (in press). *Belief and illness: A model to invite healing.* Calgary, AB: 4th Floor Press.

Wright, L.M., & Leahey, M. (Producers). (2006). *How to use questions in family interviewing.* [DVD]. Calgary, Canada

10

How to Avoid the Three Most Common Errors in Family Nursing

Nurses working with families want to be helpful and to soften or alleviate emotional, physical, or spiritual suffering whenever possible (Wright, 2005). However, despite nurses' best efforts, errors, mistakes, or misjudgments sometimes occur. Whether nurses are beginners or experienced clinicians in family nursing, they can benefit from knowing the most common errors and how they might avoid or sidestep them. We have identified three errors that we believe occur most frequently in relational family nursing practice. They are:

1. Failing to create a context for change
2. Taking sides
3. Giving too much advice prematurely

We, ourselves, have committed, experienced, or witnessed these errors in our own practice and in the supervision of our students.

For each error, we will explain in what way we believe it is a mistake and how it can have a negative impact on the family. We also suggest practical ways for avoiding these errors and offer a clinical vignette for each error. It is our hope that by sidestepping the most prevalent mistakes, nurses cannot only sustain but improve their nursing care of families. Also, nurses will have more confidence and competence in their nursing practice if they can offer a context for healing that is more likely to be helpful.

ERROR 1: FAILING TO CREATE A CONTEXT FOR CHANGE

Every nurse in every encounter and experience with a family, whether for 5 minutes or over 5 years, has the responsibility to create a context for healing and learning. "Creating a context for change is the central and enduring foundation of the therapeutic process. It is key to the relationship between the clinician and family. It is not just a necessary prerequisite to the process of therapeutic change, it is therapeutic change in and of itself" (Wright & Bell, in press). In creating this context for change, both the nurse and family undergo change. From the first meeting, the nurse and family co-evolve together, with both the family and the nurse changing in response to the other and according to their own individual biopsychosocial-spiritual structures, which have been influenced by their history of interactions and their genetic make-up (Maturana & Varela, 1992).

What must happen in order to create a healing context for change? Empathy, mindfulness, and empathic responding are all necessary ingredients for creating a healing context (Block-Lerner, et al, 2007). Wright and Bell (in press) suggest that before a context for change can be created, all obstacles to change must be removed. Such obstacles can include: a family member who does not want to be present or attends the session under duress, a family member who is dissatisfied with the progress of the clinical sessions, a family that has had previous negative experiences with health-care professionals, or a situation in which there are unclear expectations for the meetings.

At the Family Nursing Unit, University of Calgary, a hermeneutic research study was conducted by Drs. Janice M. Bell and Lorraine M. Wright to explore the process of therapeutic change (Bell, 1999). The focus of this study was to analyze the clinical work with three families who reported negative responses. These families suffered from serious illness and were seen in an outpatient clinic by a clinical nursing team of faculty and graduate nursing students. Preliminary results of this study provided helpful feedback that can be used to improve family interviews. The most informative learning was that creating a context for change was either ignored or neglected among families that were dissatisfied with the nursing team's clinical work. Curiosity was absent on the part of the nurse interviewer. For example, the nurse interviewer did not seek clarification of the presenting problem or concern. Also, the nurse interviewer paid no attention to how the intervention "fit" the family's functioning. The nurse interviewer did not ascertain from the family if the intervention ideas offered were useful. Another example of not creating a context for change was the error of commission of the clinical nursing team becoming too "married" to a particular way of conceptualizing the family's problems or dynamics that was not in harmony with the family's conceptualization.

These findings draw attention to the importance of the "common factors" Hubble, Duncan, and Miller (1999) discovered were associated with positive clinical outcomes. These included:

- Extratherapeutic factors, including client beliefs about change, strengths, resiliencies, and chance-occurring positive events in clients' lives (40%). Such events could include obtaining a new job, moving to a new city, etc.

■ The client–therapist relationship experienced as empathic, collaborative, and affirmative in focusing on goals, methods, and pace of treatment (30%)

■ Hope and expectancy about the possibility of change (15%)

■ Structure and focus of a model or approach organizing the treatment (15%)

In more recent work, Blow, Sprenkle, and Davis (2007) argue that the clinician is a key change ingredient in most successful therapy and that it is the "fit" between the model and the clients' worldviews that is important.

HOW TO AVOID FAILING TO CREATE A CONTEXT FOR CHANGE

1. **Show interest, concern, and respect for each family member.** The most useful way to do this is to ask anyone who is involved with or concerned about the problem or is suffering as a result of it to come for a family meeting. After introducing oneself and meeting each family member, the nurse should express his or her desire to learn from the family how this problem or illness has affected their lives and relationships. This articulation can convey to the family that the nurse is interested and willing to learn about them and their most pressing concerns. A nurse will find this task easier to accomplish if he or she embraces the belief that all families have strengths that are often unrealized or unappreciated (Wright & Bell, in press).

2. **Obtain a clear understanding of the most pressing concern or greatest suffering.** Seek each family member's perspective on the problem/ illness and how it affects the family and their relationships. Even if the perspectives vary, each perspective offers the nurse the best understanding of the family's challenges and sufferings.

3. **Validate each member's experience.** Remember that no one view is the correct or right view or the truth about the family's functioning but is each family member's unique and genuine experience. Be open to all perspectives about the family's concerns. To bring understanding to the nurse and family, not only must each member's perspective be elicited, but each member's perspective must also be valued and considered important.

4. **Acknowledge suffering and the sufferer.** Health providers' acknowledgment of clients' suffering can be a powerful starting point to begin understanding the family's situation and for healing to occur (Wright, 2005). Through these efforts to understand, the nurse–family relationship is enhanced and strengthened. When nurses acknowledge their clients' suffering and are compassionate and nonjudgmental, families are often more willing to disclose fears and worries. As a result, the potential for healing, growth, and change increases.

Clinical Example

Creating a context for change is often begun in the same manner as meeting a stranger for the first time. However, in the clinical example that follows, the nurse excludes an introduction which is usually part of the greeting ritual with strangers. She also neglects to determine the goals for this meeting. Therefore, some of the important aspects of establishing a new relationship are omitted and the therapeutic relationship starts down a slow, slippery slope to the point where the family is not interested in any further meetings.

The nurse first met the family at the bedside on a busy medical unit in a large, urban hospital. Mr. Garcia had been admitted to the hospital because of his chronic obstructive pulmonary disease. A woman visited frequently and was usually crying during visits. On one occasion, the primary nurse asked the husband, "Do you know why your wife is crying?" Unfortunately, the nurse did not introduce herself to the woman who was visiting and made the assumption that it was the patient's wife. He responded: "No, this is not my wife. My wife and I are divorced; this is my sister." The nurse was somewhat embarrassed but responded: "Oh, I'm sorry. Well, do you know why your sister is crying? She cries on every visit." Mr. Garcia responded: "I'm not sure". At that point, his sister stopped crying and looked up but did not speak.

The nurse then made a premature conceptualization and offered her assessment by saying: "Well, I think she is crying because she is worried that you are not going to get better if you don't stop smoking, isn't that right?" The sister shook her head to indicate "no."

At this point, Mr. Garcia stated, "Well, it's too late even if I do stop smoking." The nurse then said she would like to come back at another time to discuss the issue with them more fully, at this point addressing the sister for the first time. However, the sister replied that she did not want to meet because this was her brother's problem. The nurse accepted this response and did not have any further discussions with this family.

This encounter illustrates many missed opportunities to create a context for change. First, the nurse should have introduced herself to the sister; clarifying the sister's relationship to the patient. By acknowledging the sister right at the start, the nurse may have encouraged the sister to be more forthcoming and more willing to have another meeting. In addition, the nurse could have asked Mr. Garcia and his sister if they had any questions about the patient's condition or if they had any worries or concerns. This would have given the nurse an opportunity to validate any concerns or sufferings they might have. The sister's weeping on each visit indicates that she may be suffering; however the nature of her suffering and its cause is unclear. Finally, the nurse offers a quick conceptualization of the problem by assuming that the sister is worried about the brother's smoking habit and its relationship to his recovery. However, the sister denies this conceptualization of her suffering and, unfortunately, the nurse does not ask any therapeutic questions to ascertain the nature of her suffering.

The findings of the previously mentioned study by Bell and Wright (Bell, 1999) are clearly evident in this clinical example. There was no clear identification of the presenting concern or suffering, and a conceptualization of suffering was offered too quickly without obtaining the perspective of each family member. Without these ingredients to create a context for change, there was no opportunity for healing to occur. Sadly, good manners were also missing.

ERROR 2: TAKING SIDES

One of the most common errors in family work is for the nurse to take sides or form an alliance with one family member or subgroup of the family. Although this is commonly done unintentionally, at times the nurse may do so deliberately, usually with a benevolent intent. However, aligning with one person or subgroup can often result in other family members feeling disrespected, disempowered, and noninfluential as the family pursues its goals with the nurse.

How to Avoid Taking Sides

1. **Maintain curiosity.** Be intensely interested in hearing each person's story about the health concern or problem. When each family member's perspective has been revealed, the nurse can generally come to an understanding of the multiple forces interacting together to stimulate or trigger the problem. Families are always very complex, and the complexity is increased when an illness or problem emerges. Be open to experiencing an altered view of any family member and/or situation as more information is revealed. This is particularly important when nurses work with the elderly, because there can be a temptation to take the side of the 55-year-old son (who is dressed in a suit) and not listen sufficiently to his 83-year-old mother lying passively in a bed in an extended care facility.

2. **Remember that the glass can be half full and half empty simultaneously.** There are multiple truths and therefore many ways to view a problem. The more all-inclusive an understanding from as many family members as possible, the more possible options for resolution. However, we wish to emphasize that we do not condone violence and we do not fail to act in dangerous, illegal, or unethical situations.

3. **Ask questions that invite an exploration of both sides of a circular, interactional pattern.** (See Chapter 3 for more explanations about circular interactional patterns and the Calgary Family Assessment Model [CFAM].)

4. **Remember that all family members experience some suffering when there's a family problem or illness.** Invite family members to describe their suffering and the meaning they give to it. The nurse can also ask,

"Who in the family is suffering the most?" Often it is surprising to find that the family member suffering the most is not the person with the illness diagnosis, but rather another family member (Wright, 2005).

5. **Give relatively equal "talk time" and interest to each family member.** This of course may vary with very young children or family members who are only able to minimally contribute verbally, such as those who are disabled or have dementia.

6. **Remember that information is, as Bateson (1972) described it, "news of a difference."** Treat all information as new discoveries; maintain a systems or interactional perspective regarding your understanding of the illness and family dynamics.

7. **Try not to answer phone calls or have "side conversations" involving one family member "telling on" another family member.** Instead, invite the person to bring the issue to the next family meeting. Alternatively, invite one parent to ask the other parent to join in the phone conversation. In this way, the conversation is transparent for all. Sometimes, emailing all parties participating in the family interviews also facilitates transparency.

Clinical Examples

A clinical example often encountered by community health nurses and nurse practitioners involves families and the eating habits of children. In our culture and worldwide, we know there is a tremendous concern about obesity, and in particular, childhood obesity. Given this situation, it is not uncommon for the nurse to believe wholeheartedly a mother's report about a school-age child's poor eating habits. In particular, the mother describes how the father is laid back about their son's eating habits. "It is like I have two children!" referring to her husband's behavior as child-like. However, listening to the father's viewpoint, the nurse hears an entirely different story about how his son readily eats in his presence. He describes how his wife becomes tense, screams, and gets "stressed out" by the boy's continuous eating of what she calls junk food.

The nurse then asks herself, "Who should I believe? Who is telling the truth?" If she sides with one parent, then she alienates the other. She misses opportunities to work with the entire family on helping them adjust to normal developmental child-care issues. This trap is especially easy to fall into if one parent negatively labels the other. For example, the husband may say, "You know my wife gets hysterical" or the wife may say, "My husband is so irresponsible; he struggles with depression. And furthermore, I think he may be addicted to watching porn. I can never get him away from the computer."

To address this situation, the nurse practitioner could: (1) ask the mother, "When your husband shows you indifference, what do you find yourself doing?" (2) ask the father, "When your wife starts to scream at your son, what do you do?" (3) invite both parents to a meeting together to talk about the challenges involved in raising a child to have healthy eating habits. Having obtained a circular view of the interaction, the nurse can look at them both and ask, "Which do you think would be harder: for your wife to give up screaming or for your husband to show more responsibility? Who, between the two of you, would find it easier to believe the other might change?"

Another example concerns a family with a teenager dealing with anorexia. Sheena, aged 16, is being seen by the unit nurse Karin Johnson, age 51, to receive help developing more appropriate eating habits and to increase her socialization. Sheena has begun successfully to conquer the grip of anorexia and is very appreciative of Karin's assistance. She looks forward to individual meetings with Karin and compliments Karin frequently on wearing "fashionable clothes my mother never would wear." Karin believes she and Sheena have an "excellent" working relationship and is pleased that Sheena likes her taste in clothes.

Karin has agreed to alternate individual meetings with Sheena with family interviews including both parents. During a family meeting in which Karin proudly described Sheena's recent accomplishments on the unit, Sheena's mom starts to downplay her daughter's successes. She tells Karin of the various "bad behaviors" Sheena engaged in during a recent pass home. Following this, Sheena bursts out to her mother, "How come you do not treat me as an adult like Karin does?"

By inadvertently aligning too much with Sheena (for example, around clothes and a special relationship) and not sufficiently aligning with Sheena's parents (e.g., never seeing them as a couple alone to appreciate their challenges in raising a daughter who is in the grip of anorexia), Karin has sacrificed her ability and therapeutic leverage to be multipartial in the family meetings. Rather, the nurse is now perceived by both mother and daughter to be on the teen's side. This makes it difficult for the mother–daughter relationship to flourish and for Sheena's changes to be acknowledged by her mother. Rather, Sheena's mom may feel inadvertently competitive or usurped by the nurse. Indeed, nurses who take the side of one or more family members most often are not consciously trying to alienate, compete, or usurp any particular family member. In fact, they are usually unaware of doing so and thus it comes as a shock when other family members express dissatisfaction or begin to disengage or discontinue family meetings.

ERROR 3: GIVING TOO MUCH ADVICE PREMATURELY

Nurses are in the socially sanctioned position of offering advice, information, and opinions about matters of health promotion, health problems, illness suffering, illness management, and relationship issues. We believe, similar to Couture and Sutherland (2006), that advice can have generative and healing potential when it is offered collaboratively. Families are often keen and receptive to nurses' expertise concerning health issues. However, each family is unique, as is each situation. Therefore, timing and judgment are critical for nurses to determine when and how to offer advice.

How to Avoid Giving Too Much Advice Prematurely

1. **Offer advice, opinions, or recommendations only after a thorough assessment has been done and a full understanding of the family's health concern or suffering has been gained.** Otherwise, advice and recommendations can appear too simplistic, patronizing, or lacking an in-depth understanding. Of course, in crisis situations or in a busy emergency or intensive care unit, a full family assessment may not be possible. When families are in shock, numb, or overwhelmed, they can benefit from clear, direct advice from a nurse, who through professional experience and knowledge, can bring calm and structure in a time of crisis.

2. **Offer advice without believing that the nurse's ideas are the "best" or "better" ideas or opinions.** "Often there is a tendency and temptation among health-care providers to offer their own understandings, their own 'better' or 'best' meanings or beliefs for clients' suffering experiences with serious illness. One way to avoid this trap of prematurely offering explanations or advice to reduce suffering is to remain insatiably curious about how clients and their families are managing in the midst of suffering" (Wright, 2005, p. 102). Specifically, nurses should ask themselves: What do family members believe, and what meaning do they give to their suffering? (Wright & Bell, in press) In working with the elderly this is particularly important. Nurses should examine their own beliefs about whether they think seniors can change or whether they hold the belief that "old dogs can't learn new tricks." Health professionals who are insatiably curious put on the armor of prevention against blame, judgment, or the need to be "right."

3. **Ask more questions than offering advice during initial conversations with families.** Asking therapeutic or reflexive questions (Tomm, 1987; Wright & Bell, in press) invites a person to explore and reflect on their own meanings of their health concerns or suffering, not the nurse's. Everyone, especially the elderly, has accumulated over the years a vast reservoir of personal local wisdom and knowledge about health and wellness. Hopefully, through reflections that happen in the therapeutic conversations we have with families, healing may be triggered as new thoughts, ideas, or solutions are brought forth about how a family can best live with illness (Wright, 2005).

4. **Obtain the family's response and reaction to the advice.** After offering advice, it is essential to obtain family members' reactions to the information. Specifically, does this information "fit" for the family with their own biopsychosocial-spiritual structures? We believe it is the manner in which advice is delivered, received, interpreted, and refined

that is most critical in our clinical work. Therapeutic conversations that include advice-giving are ongoing, collaborative, clarifying, and meaningful. There is a forward process to the conversation; advice-giving is not just a prescription of a particular course of action for the family to follow. (See Chapter 4 for an in-depth discussion about "fit" and matching information offered to families with family functioning.)

Clinical Examples

Nurses commonly encounter families who are experiencing deep suffering and grief due to the anticipated or recent loss of a family member. One such family had recently experienced the loss of their 88-year-old father, William Li, who had lived with them for 10 years. Mr. Li had left Hong Kong after the death of his wife and moved to Canada to live with his son and son's family. Just 3 weeks after the death of the elderly father, his daughter-in-law, Ming-mei, presented with her husband, Shen, at a walk-in medical clinic with abdominal pain. Upon concluding a medical exam, a doctor determined that there were no physical reasons for her pain. A nurse was asked to meet with the husband and wife. Shen told the story of the recent loss of his father, explaining that his wife had been the primary caregiver and had given up her employment to care for her father-in-law. He then offered his belief that his wife's pain was due to her extreme grief at the loss of her father-in-law. The nurse, upon hearing this story, but without inquiring about the wife's extreme grief or the meaning of her loss and suffering, prematurely offered the following advice to the couple. To the husband she said: "You need to take your wife on a holiday. She is very tired after caring for your father." To Ming-mei, she said: "Your father-in-law was an elderly man and his time had come. And since he was not your father, you will get over this quickly."

Understandably, the Li family did not find this advice helpful or comforting. If the nurse had asked a few assessment questions, even some structural assessment questions within the CFAM (see Chapter 3), she would have learned that Shen owns a small coffee shop and is unable to take holidays because he is the sole provider and works 7 days a week. Ming-mei also did not find the nurse's words healing, particularly because the nurse ignored the very close relationship she had with her father-in-law.

By offering premature albeit well-intentioned advice, the nurse missed the opportunity to offer opinions and recommendations that would have been more healing. By not being more curious (through the asking of pertinent questions) and more interested in understanding the daughter-in-law's beliefs about the loss of her father-in-law, the nurse offered her own "best" ideas and advice, but the recommendations did not "fit" with this couple. Also, the nurse did not recognize the Chinese culture of the Li family and their sense of honoring and caring for their elderly family member. Sadly, this nurse also missed a golden opportunity to commend the daughter-in-law for the care of her father-in-law. (See Chapter 4 for a more in-depth discussion of the intervention of commendations.)

CONCLUSIONS

Working with families in relational practice offers nurses many opportunities for helping them to live alongside and manage illness and increase their sense of wellness. Similar to other professionals, at times we make errors in our practice and are less helpful than we desire. It is our hope that by describing what we consider the three most common errors in relational family nursing practice that nurses will either avoid the errors, or if they do make a mistake, will find ways to rectify the situation and recoup with the family. The process of collaborating with families is rich with opportunities for creative healing despite the making of errors. By sidestepping the most frequent mistakes, nurses can offer a context for healing that is more likely to be helpful than not.

References

Bateson, G. (1972). *Steps to an ecology of mind: Collected essays in anthropology, psychiatry, evolution, and epistemology.* New York: Ballantine Books.

Bell, J.M. (1999). Therapeutic failure: Exploring uncharted territory in family nursing. [Editorial]. *Journal of Family Nursing, 5*(4), 371–373.

Block-Lerner, J., et al. (2007). The case for mindfulness-based approaches in the cultivation of empathy: Does nonjudgmental, present-moment awareness increase capacity for perspective-taking and empathic concerns? *Journal of Marital and Family Therapy, 33*(4), 501–516.

Blow, A.J., Sprenkle, D.H., & Davis, S.D. (2007). Is who delivers the treatment more important than the treatment itself? The role of the therapist in common factors. *Journal of Marital and Family Therapy, 33*(3), 298–317.

Couture, S.J., & Sutherland, O. (2006). Giving advice on advice-giving: A conversation analysis of Karl Tomm's practice. *Journal of Marital and Family Therapy, 32*(3), 329–344.

Hubble, M.A., Duncan, B.L., & Miller, SD. (1999) Introduction. In M.A. Hubble, B.L. Duncan, & S.D. Miller (Eds.) *The heart & soul of change: What works in therapy* (pp. 1–19). Washington, DC: American Psychological Association.

Maturana, H.R., & Varela, F.G. (1992). *The tree of knowledge: The biological roots of human understanding* (Rev. ed.). Boston: Shambhala.

Tomm, K. (1987). Interventive interviewing—part ii. Reflexive questioning as a means to enable self-healing. *Family Process, 26,* 167–183.

Wright, L.M. (2005). *Spirituality, suffering, and illness: Ideas for healing.* Philadelphia: FA Davis Co.

Wright, L.M., & Bell, J.M. (in press). *Belief and illness: A model to invite healing.* Calgary, AB: 4th Floor Press.

Chapter

11

How to Document Family Interviews

It is very important for the nurse to devise a workable, efficient system for integrating, recording, and documenting the large amount of complex data gathered in family interviews. Such a system provides the nurse with an organized and clear overview of work with the family to address their goals. Using this overview, the nurse can decide which issues are key and which ones are tangential. With an organized recording system, the nurse is able to move back and forth from macroscopic to microscopic data, and the family receives more holistic health care. Having an organized documentation system is particularly germane in today's health-care delivery climate of electronic health records (EHR), downsized hospital facilities, increased health-care networks, and proliferation of the many varieties of managed care and primary care ventures. Increased integration of health information through the EHR has been accompanied by greater emphasis on capitation, decreased financial resources, decreased number of beds, shorter hospital stays, and limited staff time. Therefore, efficient documentation and useful communication among nurses and between nurses and other health professionals are even more necessary to achieve helpful family nursing.

The purpose of this chapter is to discuss how to integrate and record data obtained from families and from the nurse's own interpretations and observations. The nurse's impression of a family interview is addressed first. How to examine the data and use both the Calgary Family Assessment Model (CFAM) and the Calgary Family Intervention Model (CFIM) are discussed. A list of strengths and problems, an initial assessment summary, and an intervention plan are also detailed. The use of progress notes for integrating and recording hypotheses, interventions, and family responses is addressed. How to record a discharge synopsis is presented. The issue of confidentiality of records is also discussed.

We are acutely aware of the vast variety of recording systems currently in use in health care and offer our ideas about documentation to stimulate local discussion of how family data might be recorded and used. Of course each context of nursing practice will dictate somewhat the extent and expansiveness of documentation of families involved in health care. Often the amount of documentation reflects the amount of time that was available to spend with families. If there is only a brief amount of time spent with families, then we strongly champion the idea that the amount of data on every chart or file should include *at least* the following: a family genogram; the answer to the "one question question"; the level of family suffering; and the family's goal or desire for assistance during the hospitalization or clinical visit (see Chapter 8 for how to conduct a 15-minute [or less] family interview).

The ideas for documentation that we offer in the remaining part of this chapter are suitable for contexts where nurses are working with families a substantial amount of time (weeks or months), such as in community health clinics, psychiatric settings, outpatient clinics addressing chronic illness, and/or nurse-managed family practitioner clinics. In any area though, documentation is not separate from care and is not optional (CARNA, 2006). High-quality documentation helps nurses provide skilled and safe care wherever they practice.

INITIAL IMPRESSIONS, OBSERVATIONS, AND RESPONSES

Several factors usually affect a nurse's first response to an initial family interview. External factors might include how cold or warm the interview room is, how dirty or clean it is, how noisy the surrounding area is, and so forth. Internal factors have an even more profound influence on the nurse's evaluation. Inherent within each nurse are his or her self-image, beliefs, mores, prejudices, attitudes, and past personal and professional experiences with families, as well as his or her unique way of perceiving other individuals. These internal factors strongly influence the nurse's response to a family and can be positive or negative.

The nurse's response must be recognized as important data. We have encouraged masters and doctoral students specializing in family nursing to consider their personal experience of a family session and to include these impressions in their documentation. Areas for consideration might include:

- One belief of mine that was challenged, reaffirmed, or altered as a result of this session was …
- The family taught me …
- One new learning for me was …
- What stood out for me in this session was …
- My personal goals for the next session are …
- (If this was the final session) Things I have learned from this family that will help me in my work with another family in the future were …

Encouraging graduate nursing students to record their reflections of the impact of their clinical work with families honors the principles of reciprocity, systemic interaction, and mutual influence between families and nurses. Nurses are also affected and changed by their interactions with family members. Too often in the past, nurses have striven for a purely clinical response to an individual or a family. They were either embarrassed or ashamed to admit, or more likely did not recognize, how their personal thoughts and feelings influenced their clinical functioning. We recommend that nurses consciously take a few minutes after an interview to blurt out (to themselves) personal initial reactions to a family interview. These quick "gut reactions" can be dealt with as the nurse formally starts to integrate the data and then to document it. In our experience, interviewers who are able to quickly acknowledge their personal reactions become more able to suspend any of their judgments, prejudices, biases, or constraining beliefs. They are much more able to integrate and conceptualize the data about the family in a manner that is the most collaborative and, hopefully, helpful to families. The unacknowledged initial hypotheses or responses, if not addressed, can be the most mischievous, disrespectful, and judgmental toward families; if addressed early, they can be a positive source of energy and inspiration for the nurse.

The following case scenario illustrates a nurse's initial reactions to a family interview. The family is composed of the husband, Leroy Hixon, age 28, who is a roofer; the wife, Melvina, age 27, who works part-time for a dry cleaner; and the children, Torrance, age 3, and Chloe, age 9 months. The couple have been married for 6 years. When Torrance was examined in the outpatient clinic, his speech was found to be approximately 8 months delayed, and it was noted that he was small for his age. The nurse also noticed that the mother had difficulty controlling Torrance when he was running up and down the halls. After the clinic session, the interdisciplinary team made the following plans: the physician would continue with the physical investigations, the nurse would arrange for a family interview to discuss Torrance's difficulties, and the team would reconvene for a conference with the parents in 2 weeks.

Mr. and Mrs. Hixon, Torrance, and Chloe attended the initial interview. During the interview, Mrs. Hixon revealed that Mr. Hixon's parents were interfering with the children's upbringing and that she was upset by this interference. More of the story will unfold throughout this chapter. Immediately after the initial interview, the nurse said to herself:

- So much crying! I would have been so frustrated with Chloe. I could never have been as nice to her as Mrs. Hixon was! Mr. Hixon never once offered to take the baby or help out.

- The poor parents, they have so many problems with their extended family. No wonder they feel "maybe we are doing something wrong as parents."

- They are awfully critical of Torrance and never had a good word to say about him.
- Torrance is friendly. He gave me a hug on the way out.
- They jump around a lot in their conversation. I am not really sure what the issue is: Torrance's misbehavior or his problem with eating. They never mentioned his delayed speech.

In voicing these initial impressions and reactions, the nurse was able to express her own anxiety and feelings of empathy, compassion, and frustration. She was also reminded of her own family and how her ex-husband, who was Iranian, worked excessively long hours and did little to support her when their infant was crying. The nurse also remembered that her Iranian mother-in-law was very controlling, although the mother-in-law called it "trying to be helpful." The nurse was aware, therefore, that she had to guard against a tendency to feel overly sympathetic toward the wife and overly critical toward the husband.

In summary, we recommend that nurses acknowledge their feelings and immediate reactions, impressions, and observations of family members. After doing so, they can decide either to discard these beliefs or feelings or use them appropriately. For example, the nurse used her own initial impressions of the Hixon family in the following methodical way:

- The baby's prolonged crying may stimulate frustration in the father and Torrance. I will explore this in the future.
- Given the relationship with their extended family, the parents are probably exquisitely sensitive to being blamed. I must watch my tone of voice and choice of words so that I do not inadvertently blame them.
- Torrance's hug may indicate that he is hungry for attention. It would be inappropriate for him to receive too much attention from me because I am not available to him consistently. Also, the parents may feel that I am usurping their position if I give him lots of praise. I will try to encourage the parents to do this.
- The parents are quite concerned but seem to be under a lot of stress. Maybe that explains why the conversation jumped around a lot. I will try to keep the next interview more focused.

Having acknowledged her initial impressions, the nurse can proceed to review the content and process of the interview by using the CFAM. The *content* of the interview refers to the concrete communication: "what" is stated. The *process* refers to the "how," implying movement. Process is a dynamic concept, whereas content is static. The process is not the activity per se, but the way in which the activity is carried out. An example of content from the Hixon interview is the description of the grandparents' interfering with the couple's management of the children. The process of the discussion was that Mrs. Hixon became sad and tearful and her husband tried to minimize the problem: "Ah, she gets too emotional with the folks all the time. The best thing is to forget about what they say and live your own life."

RECORDING SYSTEM

There are many different kinds of tools a nurse can use to record family interviews. These tools range from paper and pen notes to computer-generated checklists and personal digital assistant notes to an EHR. Some recording forms are fairly specific, whereas others are more general. The ideal recording tool should, above all, be consistent with the nurse's interviewing practice. That is, if the thrust of the family interview is to obtain information about medication compliance, then considerable space should be allocated for this data. Second, the record should provide an integrated picture of family strengths and problems. Too much emphasis on problems or constraints can lead to too much involvement and intrusion by the nurse. It can also foster dependency on the part of the family. Third, an assessment record should be a springboard for developing an intervention plan. Isolated bits of information, such as "the mother is experiencing depression" or "the father is unemployed," need to be drawn together into a composite picture. Strengths need to be linked to the problem so that they can be used as resources for problem solving. From this integrated picture, a plan of action emerges. Without this picture, the deficiencies and gaps in the data are obscured. Last, the recording system should be one that the nurse interviewer can easily use. Most nurses have heavy workloads and become frustrated if they have to fill out lengthy forms.

The recording system that we recommend is fairly general. It can be adapted to almost any agency's or hospital's philosophy and any style of nursing practice, and it can be computerized. The system consists of six parts:

1. Assessment—CFAM
2. List of strengths and problems
3. Family assessment summary
4. Intervention—CFIM
5. Progress notes
6. Discharge summary

Before dealing with each part separately, we would like to emphasize strongly the conceptual skills that are involved in integrating the data after an interview. Nurses must think in a critical, analytical, and interpretive fashion to integrate data; that is, they must sort through all the information and generate ideas about its meaning. They must distinguish between observation and inference and must be willing to entertain hypotheses and equally willing to discard them as new data emerge that are inconsistent with their first hypothesis. In deciding which information to include and which to discard, nurses engage in the processes of deliberation, judgment, and discernment. The task of integrating and recording the data is not an easy one. It requires intellectual discipline.

Assessment—How to Use the CFAM

As we discussed in Chapter 3, the CFAM is a "map of the family," an integrated conceptual framework consisting of three major categories: structural, developmental, and functional. Each category contains several subcategories. It is useful to conceptualize the three assessment categories and the many subcategories as a branching diagram (Fig. 11-1). As nurses use the subcategories on the right of the branching diagram, they collect more and more microscopic data. It is important for nurses to be able to

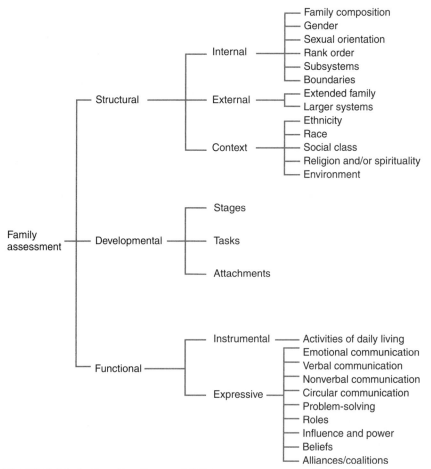

FIGURE 11-1: Branching diagram of CFAM.

move back and forth on the diagram to draw together all relevant information into an integrated assessment. For example, the nurse may explore boundary issues in depth with a family. The nurse thus obtains microscopic data within the structural category of the assessment model and needs to be able to integrate this data with other data within the diagram. Isolated microscopic statements such as "The parental subsystem has a diffuse boundary" have little meaning and are of limited help in devising an intervention plan. In combination with other data, however, this statement may become particularly rich and meaningful: "The parental subsystem has had a diffuse boundary since Chloe was born and the grandmother began to visit and care for her." In this example, structural, developmental, and functional data are combined:

- Structural: parental subsystem with diffuse boundary
- Developmental: stage of families with young children (stage 3)
- Functional: grandmother's assumption of parenting role

After an initial interview, it is important for the nurse to mentally review each category. In this way, the nurse gains a macroscopic view of the family.

After reviewing the family structure outline (the top branch of Fig. 11-1), the nurse should examine the family genogram and ecomap. This will help the nurse to conceptualize this particular family and how it differs from or is similar to other families. The Hixon family, for example, is a young, working-class family with the mother working part-time and the father working full-time. The family boundary seems fairly permeable, with much interface with the extended families. Subsystem boundaries are clear.

In addition to an understanding of the family structure, who is in it, and how they fit into their context, the nurse requires an understanding of how this family came to be at this stage in its developmental life cycle (Box 11-1). We recommend that the nurse review the stages and tasks appropriate to the family's specific developmental life cycle (Table 11-1). Also, we suggest that the nurse draw a diagram illustrating family attachments. The Hixon family attachment diagram is given later in this chapter.

While reviewing the developmental category, the nurse can identify the normative as well as the crisis issues that the family dealt with during each

---

Box 11-1 The Developmental Category of CFAM: Sample Family Life Cycle Variations

- Middle-class North American
- Divorce and postdivorce
- Remarried and stepfamily
- Adoptive
- Lesbian, gay, queer, bisexual, intersex, transgendered, and two-spirited families
- Other types

Table 11-1	Stages of the Family Life Cycle	
FAMILY LIFE CYCLE STAGE	**EMOTIONAL PROCESS OF TRANSITION: KEY PRINCIPLES**	**SECOND-ORDER CHANGES IN FAMILY STATUS REQUIRED TO PROCEED DEVELOPMENTALLY**
1. Leaving home; single young adults	Accepting emotional and financial responsibility for self	1. Differentiation of self from family of origin 2. Development of intimate peer relationships 3. Establishment of self regarding work and financial independence
2. The joining of families through marriage; the new couple	Commitment to new system	1. Formation of marital system 2. Realignment of relationships with extended families and friends to include spouse
3. Families with young children	Accepting new members into the system	1. Adjusting marital system to make space for child(ren) 2. Joining in childrearing, financial, and household tasks 3. Realignment of relationships with extended family to include parenting and grandparenting roles
4. Families with adolescents	Increasing flexibility of family boundaries to include children's independence and grandparents' frailties	1. Shifting of parent–child relationships to permit adolescent to move in and out of system 2. Refocus on midlife marital and career issues 3. Beginning shift toward caring for older generation
5. Launching children and moving on	Accepting a multitude of exits from and entries into the family system	1. Renegotiation of marital system as a dyad 2. Development of adult–adult relationships between grown children and their parents 3. Realignment of relationships to include in-laws and grandchildren 4. Dealing with disabilities and death of parents (grandparents)
6. Families in later life	Accepting the shifting of generational roles	1. Maintaining own and couple functioning and interests in face of physiological decline; exploration of new familial and social role options 2. Support for a more central role of middle generation 3. Making room in the system for the wisdom and experience of the elderly, supporting the older generation without overfunctioning for them 4. Dealing with loss of spouse, siblings, and other peers and preparing for own death; life review and integration

stage. For example, the Hixon family is currently in stage 3 (families with young children). They have adjusted the marital system to make space for children. During stage 2, they dealt with the unexpected death of Mrs. Hixon's brother. This event influenced their marital relationship by creating emotional distance between the couple. Also, the relationships with their families of origin were not adequately defined during stage 2. These past difficulties in stage 2 are having repercussions for task achievement in stage 3. Hence, they are of current significance.

After considering the CFAM structural and developmental categories, the nurse can review the family functioning category. (This third CFAM category is detailed in Box 11-2.) For the Hixon family, the nurse can

---

Box 11-2 Functional Category of the CFAM

A. Instrumental
  1. Activities of daily living

B. Expressive
  1. Emotional communication
    a. Types of emotions
    b. Range of emotions
  2. Verbal communication
    a. Direct versus displaced
    b. Clear versus masked
  3. Nonverbal communication
    a. Types
    b. Sequencing
  4. Circular communication
  5. Problem solving
    a. Identification patterns
    b. Instrumental versus emotional problems
    c. Solution patterns
    d. Evaluation process
  6. Roles
    a. Role flexibility
    b. Formal versus informal
  7. Influence or power
    a. Instrumental
    b. Psychological
    c. Corporal
  8. Beliefs
    a. Family expectations or goals
    b. Family beliefs about problems
    c. Family beliefs about change
  9. Alliances and coalitions
    a. Directionality, balance, and intensity
    b. Triangles

identify strengths as well as difficulties in the area of expressive functioning, particularly emotional and circular communication, influence and power, and coalitions.

The nurse need not be too microscopic in the review of CFAM categories. It may not be useful or relevant to assess each category of the functional domain. If the nurse uses too many subcategories, she may become overwhelmed by the complexity of the data. It is important for the nurse to maintain a macroscopic, integrated metaview of the family. After the nurse has used the CFAM several times, the categories will become more familiar. To cue nurses' awareness of the various categories to assess, some community- and hospital-based nurses carry with them small cards with the branching diagram and a few possible questions to assist them during meetings with families. The other cue for nurses is to integrate categories of family assessment into the charting system that will bring back those aspects of family functioning that were observed or reported in the interview. Family data become much more valued, visible, relevant, and utilized by nurses and other health-care providers when they are documented.

How to Develop a List of Strengths and Problems

Having reviewed the CFAM, the nurse should identify family strengths and problems in the structural, developmental, and functional categories. Using the interview data, the nurse should prepare a list of strengths and problems and indicate issues at whatever system level the nurse presently conceptualizes them. Thus, the nurse will have completed three steps in integrating the assessment data:

1. Reviewing the CFAM

2. Identifying strengths and problems

3. Listing strengths and problems according to system level

Various systems levels are indicated on the strengths and problems list. Community–whole-family system refers to the relationship between the family and its neighborhood or community. A problem at this system level might be, for example, that the family members are isolated and have been made scapegoats by the community because of their race. The professional–whole-family system level depicts the relationship between the family and health-care providers in particular but also with other professionals, such as teachers or clergy. A strength at this system level might be, for example, that the family and the home-care service have developed a cooperative working relationship.

The next system level is that of the nurse and the whole family. This level depicts the nature of the relationship between the nurse and the family. The relationship between families and nurses is more positive when nurses are educated about utilizing a family-focused approach (LeGrow & Rossen, 2005; Goudreau, Duhamel, & Ricard, 2006). The whole-family system level refers to interactions among all family members. The marital subsystem designates issues pertaining to the couple as marital partners or as parents. The parent–child system level refers to issues between the children and the parents. The sibling subsystem depicts the relationship issues among brothers and sisters. The individual systems level refers to the biological, psychological, and social issues pertaining to individual family members.

Family strengths are very important to note. They can be used effectively to enhance family life. More specifically, they can be linked to problems and used as effective resources in problem solving. It is crucial to ask the family what they believe their particular strengths are rather than arbitrarily categorizing a family's strengths. For example, if during the interview the nurse asked Leroy, in the presence of his family, what his wife did that was most helpful for him in coping with the stress of Torrance's problems, the nurse could note this in the documentation. Some typical family strengths include:

- The ability to provide for the physical, emotional, and spiritual needs of the family members
- The ability to be sensitive to the needs of the family members
- The ability to communicate thoughts and feelings effectively
- The ability to provide support, security, and encouragement
- The ability to initiate and maintain growth-producing relationships and experiences within and outside the family
- The capacity to maintain and create constructive and responsible community relationships
- The ability to grow with and through children
- The ability to perform family roles flexibly
- The ability for self-help and to accept help from others when appropriate
- The capacity for mutual respect for the individuality of family members
- The ability to use a crisis experience as a means of growth
- The concern for family unity, loyalty, and interfamily cooperation

In developing a list of strengths and problems, the nurse should acknowledge major structural, developmental, and functional issues that are presently affecting family interaction. The nurse should not try to make a perfect list but should strive to identify the major issues in collaboration with the family. Problems frequently overlap several system levels. It is often difficult, therefore, to differentiate whole-family problems from marital issues and from individual difficulties. Under which system level a problem is placed is quite arbitrary. It does have significance, however, in that it guides which interventions are chosen. For example, a nurse could identify Mrs. Hixon's sadness as an individual problem and list it as depression. Most likely, the intervention for this problem would then be medication or individual therapy. However, if the problem of sadness is identified as "difficulty with emotional communication" and is listed as a marital issue, the intervention would be different; it would probably involve marital intervention to help both partners meet their needs.

We strongly recommend that beginning nurse interviewers first attempt to identify as many family strengths and problems as possible. That is, they should initially restrain themselves from listing issues under the individual category level. We find that this helps nurses to "think family." Nurses are often very accustomed to thinking of individual issues, such as the father's alcoholism or the mother's anxiety. They need to reconceptualize these problems at a higher system level if they are to deal with the family. To assist in this conceptualization, we recommend that nurses ask themselves questions such as:

- Who is most affected by the problem (e.g., the father's drinking)?
- How does that person attempt to influence the father?
- Who supports that person in attempting to influence the father?
- Who does not support that person's attempts to influence the father?

By thinking through these questions, the nurse will start to conceptualize the father's individual issue as a whole-family system or marital system problem.

Although we strongly recommend family assessment and intervention, we do not subscribe to the view that all issues are family centered. Major physical, psychological, and social issues that are primarily personal in origin are listed under the individual category level. For example, Torrance Hixon's delayed speech and short stature are listed as individual problems. Mrs. Hixon's sadness, on the other hand, is conceptualized as a marital issue, "difficulty with emotional communication." It is therefore listed under the marital system level. Her interest and concern about being a good parent are also listed under the marital and parental system levels and not under the individual level. Table 11-2 shows a sample strengths and problems list for the Hixon family.

Once the nurse has identified the strengths and problems of the family, she can begin to analyze the relationship of the family's strengths to its problems. For example, in the Hixon family's list of strengths and problems, the unresolved conflict between the couple and the grandparents is identified. Thus, the nurse could think about the following questions: "What is the relationship between the strengths and the problems?" and "Is there a way that the strengths can be used to deal with the problems?"

With the Hixon family, the nurse hypothesized that the grandparents were genuinely concerned about Torrance and the family but demonstrated their concern in a way that exacerbated the problem rather than helped it. The grandparents tended to interfere by offering unsolicited advice, and the couple had not found ways to deal with this.

Table 11-2	Strengths and Problems List for the Hixon Family

FAMILY NAME: HIXON

SUBSYSTEMS	STRENGTHS	DATE PROBLEMS
Community–whole-family system	• Grandparents a possible support	• Unresolved conflict with both families of origin • Isolated (five moves in 3 years)
Professionals–whole-family system	• Engaged with pediatric clinic	• Reluctant to ask for information concerning Torrance's health problems
Nurse–whole-family system	• Guarded alliance	
Whole-family system	• Strong beliefs: "We're survivors" and "We're a special family"	
Marital/parental subsystem	• Care about each other • Concerned about being good parents	• Difficulty with emotional communication–Melvina sad, shows helplessness; Leroy disconfirms
Parent-child subsystem	• Able to bond with Chloe • Father can be positive with Torrance	• Difficulty with behavior controls • Unrealistic expectations of a 3$^1/_2$-year-old with new sibling • Isolation of Torrance
Sibling subsystem	• At clinic, Torrance can be positive with Chloe	• Intense rivalry reported
Individual system	• Torrance is determined; strives to learn new skills	• Torrance has speech delay of 8 months, small stature

In evaluating the list of strengths and problems, the nurse decided to leave the apparent conflictual data on the list. She reasoned that this would help her to maintain a neutral stance vis-à-vis the grandparents. Furthermore, it would help her to keep a metaperspective on the Hixon family situation. Should the nurse and the couple decide in the future to invite the grandparents for a joint family interview, the nurse would be aware of the boundary issue between the generations.

Having considered the relationship between family strengths and problems, the nurse should attempt to prioritize the concerns. The nurse and the family will have already collaborated on this during the interview. We recommend, however, that the nurse reflect again after completing the list of strengths and problems. In our experience, we have found that inexperienced family interviewers often become overly enthusiastic and change-oriented when they are integrating and recording data. Not every family needs intervention, and not all problems require resolution. Rather, some problems or illnesses require adjustment and others invite us to accept and "live with them." We therefore strongly urge nurses to concentrate on the presenting issue. With the Hixon family, the parents' primary concern was their difficulty controlling Torrance's behavior.

How to Summarize the Family Assessment

Although the list of strengths and problems is a useful working tool, it does not provide a sufficient summary of the family assessment. It would probably be too cryptic and fragmented for the rest of the nursing and health-care team to use in delivering service to a family. Instead, a family assessment summary should be completed to guide the delivery of care. Box 11-3 outlines a family assessment summary. Box 11-4 presents a sample family assessment summary of the Hixon family.

Box 11-3 Outline of a Family Assessment Summary

Family Name: _____   Date: _____
Family Members Present at Interview: _____
Interviewer: _____
Place of Interview: _____
  I. Referral Route and Presenting Problem
One or two sentences summarizing reason for referral and referral source.
  II. Family Composition
Draw a genogram. Include name, age, and occupation or school grade for each member of the family. Circle those currently living at home.
  III. Family Attachment
Draw an attachment diagram. Indicate the strength and nature of the bonding among family members.
  IV. Pertinent History (very brief and relevant to presenting problem)
     a. Chronological sequence of events leading to current presenting problem. Include previous solutions to cope with the problem and professional help sought.
     b. Developmental history of the family, including pertinent information regarding families of origin and significant personal, social, vocational, and health/medical events.
  V. Strengths and Problems
Identify family strengths. List family problems (structural, developmental, and functional) and individual problems (physical, psychological, and social) at their appropriate system levels.
  VI. Hypothesis/Summary
Summarize the connections between the initial hypothesis, presenting problems, pertinent history, and family strengths. If necessary, refine the hypothesis to provide directions for intervention.
  VII. Goals and Plans
Indicate plans for interventions, referral, or discharge. Indicate family's reaction and the outcome.
  VIII. Signature

Box 11-4	Family Assessment Summary: The Hixon Family

Family Name: Hixon _____   Date: _____

Family Members   Whole Family _____
Present at Interview:

Interviewer: Anne Marie Levac, RN, BS _____

Place of Interview: Children's Hospital _____

I. Referral Route and Presenting Problem

Torrance Hixon, age 3½, and his mother were identified at the Pediatric Outpatient Clinic by myself and Dr. Carpenter as needing a family assessment. The mother had difficulty controlling his behavior (running up and down the halls) and appeared extremely upset.

II. Family Composition

The family is composed of husband, Leroy, 28, a roofer; wife, Melvina, 27, who works part time in a dry cleaners; and children, Torrance, 3½, and Chloe, 9 months.

III. Family Attachment

IV. Pertinent History

Torrance: Normal pregnancy and delivery and milestones to age 34 months. Speech delay of 8 months and small stature. Complete history on Dr. Carpenter's report.

Family: When Torrance was approximately 1 year old, parents began to have difficulty controlling his behavior, that is, spreading feces, refusing to listen, and being a picky eater. Tried toilet training him at 13 months and have tried punishing him by sending to his room, getting him to help clean up the mess, and spanking. Have also visited two other pediatric clinics for the same complaints. Report these visits were "not helpful."

The couple have been married for 6 years, no separations, five moves within the past 3 years (two between cities). Mother's brother died when Torrrance was 1 year old. Both extended families are heavily involved in giving conflicting advice.

V. Strengths/Problems

  a. Community–Whole-Family System

    1. Strengths

    Extended family interested. The grandparents might be available as a source of support.

    2. Problems

      (a) Unresolved conflict with both families of origin. The paternal grandparents live outside of the city but see the family about once a month. They telephone frequently and, according to both parents, imply that the children are not being raised properly. Melvina in particular feels angry with them for interfering. The maternal grandparents live in the city and, although they do not interfere as much with regard to the children, seem to imply that Melvina is not a competent mother. She apparently was overprotected as a child and feels resentful that her parents now seem to favor her sister-in-law. The couple has not found helpful ways of dealing with their anger toward their parents.

      (b) Isolation. The family has moved five times in 3 years and has no close neighbors or friends.

  b. Professionals–Whole-Family System

    1. Strengths

    The family engaged readily with Pediatric Clinic. The father took time off work without pay to attend.

Continued

Box 11-4 Family Assessment Summary: The Hixon Family—*cont'd*

   2. Problems
   The parents lack information about Torrance's health problems.
   c. Nurse–Whole-Family System
      1. Strengths
      The parents asked about my qualifications and areas of expertise. They
      responded fairly quickly to a collaborative approach. We developed a guarded
      alliance given their feelings of mistrust with previous nurses.
   d. Whole-Family System
      1. Strengths
      Family believes they are "special." They have overcome adversity in the past
      (e.g., unemployment, automobile accident) and are proud of being "survivors."
   e. Marital/Parental System
      1. Strengths
      Concerned regarding good parenting. The couple cares a tremendous amount
      for each other and are concerned about being good parents.
      2. Problems
      Difficulty with emotional communication. Since the mother's brother's death,
      the couple has had difficulty communicating emotionally. Mrs. H. reports that
      her brother was "the only person we could talk to." She is sad, feels inadequate
      as a mother, and tends to share this by crying or expressing her helplessness.
      How this affects her husband is not clearly known at this time. He responds to
      his wife by overprotecting her, not confirming what she says, or trying to talk
      her out of it. This perpetuates her feelings of inadequacy. The couple report
      not having a satisfactory emotional relationship.
   f. Parent–Child System
      1. Strengths
      Ability to bond. The couple has been able to bond adequately with Chloe. The
      father can be positive with Junior and seems interested in him. The father is
      very concrete but seems willing to learn.
      2. Problems
      Difficulty with behavioral controls. Torrance seems confused about behavioral
      limits and tends to act up. When he does test, his father responds by
      becoming frustrated and ignoring him or withdrawing. His mother feels
      overwhelmed, and both parents focus on the negative rather than on the
      positive. They have limited knowledge of normal growth and development.
   g. Sibling Subsystem
      1. Strengths
      Sharing. Torrance can be positive with Chloe, as was evidenced when he gave
      her an appropriate toy during the family interview.
      2. Problems
      Intense rivalry. Torrance has placed feces in Chloe's crib, bites her, pushes her,
      and so forth. During the family interview, no negative behavior was noticed.
   h. Individual System
      1. Strengths
      Peer interaction. Torrance has been attending nursery school for 3 months and,
      according to his mother, is doing well although his speech is delayed.

Box 11-4 Family Assessment Summary: The Hixon Family—*cont'd*

2. Problems
Health. Torrance has a speech delay of 8 months. He is below the third
percentile in height.

VI. Hypothesis/Summary
Torrance Hixon, 3½, and his parents present with difficulty controlling his behavior.
The problem has existed for 2½ years. One hypothesis is that the parents, unaware
of normal child development, use age-inappropriate techniques. It is also hypothesized
that a precipitating factor was the unexpected death of Mrs. Hixon's brother, a close
confidant of both Mr. and Mrs. Hixon. Although the couple stated that they tried to
separate their own feelings and not to displace them onto the children, it is my
hypothesis that when Mrs. H. is feeling sad, she handles this by getting angry with
Torrance. Mr. H. "gets after" Torrance, particularly when he sees his wife upset. Chloe
seems to stimulate and receive positive feelings from the parents, whereas Torrance
encourages and receives negative feelings. The children seem triangulated into the
marriage.

VII. Goals and Plans
   a. The parents and Torrance agreed to meet for four sessions to learn how to
      manage Torrance's behavior.
   b. Joint meeting with parents, Dr. Carpenter, and myself set for January 19 to
      discuss Torrance's health, that is, short stature, delayed speech, and normal
      growth and development.

VIII. Signature: Anne Marie Levac, RN, BS

In the family assessment summary, the nurse must synthesize theory
and practice. All the isolated questions and answers discussed in the
interview are woven into a synthesized pattern. For example, the nurse
hypothesized that the Hixon couple had a helpful, symmetrical relationship when they were both able to share emotionally with Mrs. Hixon's
brother. Since his death, they have had difficulty with emotional communication. They are attempting now to have a complementary relationship
with each other, whereby Mrs. Hixon cries and expresses her feelings to
her husband. It is her expectation that he in turn should provide her with
support. He attempts to do this by joking around with her. However, this
does not help to alleviate her sadness. Thus, they are experiencing
tension in their relationship. The nurse identified this pattern and
discussed it as a problem under the marital system level in the family
assessment summary.

Madsen (2007) suggests collaboratively reviewing the assessment
with the family so that all perspectives are acknowleged rather than
the imposition of a homogeneous, single perspective. Of course this
process takes more time and may not fit in some contexts, but this kind
of documentation becomes intimately connected with the process of the
interview.

Intervention—How to Use CFIM

After the nurse has reviewed the CFAM, identified and listed the family's strengths and problems, and prepared an assessment, he or she should develop an intervention plan. We have found the following three steps helpful when we develop intervention plans in our clinical practice:

1. Identify specific problems.
2. Review the CFIM.
3. Choose interventions.

Each of these steps is discussed separately.

Identify Specific Problems

A nurse will find it helpful to embrace the facilitating belief that all families have problems and strengths. The intervention plan that the nurse and family collaboratively co-construct depends on the severity and complexity of the family's problems and the richness of their strengths (Madsen, 2007). A problem list that indicates mild problems may reflect a family coping with a normal developmental crisis or a transient situation. If the problem list, however, suggests severe issues, it is essential that the nurse recognize the gravity of the situation and not offer placebos or unrealistic interim solutions for conditions that require more expert assistance. In these situations, the nurse may wish to refer the family for more specialized assistance. Suggestions for how to refer families are given in Chapters 5 and 12.

If the nurse is going to continue to work with the family, however, the nurse and the family should identify specific target problems. Attempting to solve all family problems is overly grandiose at worst and simply unrealistic or impractical at best! The nurse needs to understand in conversation and collaboration with the family which health problems, concerns, or risks are causing the greatest distress, suffering, or threat to their everyday functioning. Some problems never go away, but the family can learn to navigate around them. For example, if the family has a child with severe developmental and physical challenges, these problems will not go away, but hopefully the family can learn to navigate around them so that adequate family time is provided with the inclusion of the child as well as time for the parents' respite and focus on their marital relationship. Therefore, priorities need to be set. It is generally unwise for the clinician to move too quickly to work on marital issues unless the couple has specifically asked for help in this area. A rule of thumb is to start with the presenting issue and try to influence the most change in the system; that is, the nurse should promote change where the maximum benefit and healing will be realized by all family members.

In the situation of the Hixon family, the nurse and parents chose to work on changing Torrance's behavior because that was an area that concerned both parents. Also, it enabled the nurse to bring the couple together to discuss their feelings and beliefs about childrearing. In this way, the nurse indirectly fostered emotional communication between the spouses. In addition, she planned to have sessions with the father, the mother, and Torrance to foster positive feedback. The nurse reasoned that if the family had to travel to and from the pediatric clinic by themselves (without Chloe), Torrance would be likely to receive more attention. Thus, by choosing to work on behavioral controls, the nurse was stimulating change at several levels: whole-family system, parent-child subsystem, and marital and parental subsystem. Also, because the nurse worked in a pediatric outpatient clinic, she was simultaneously involved in addressing Torrance's speech delay and health issues with the parents.

Review the Calgary Family Intervention Model

The nurse should review the CFIM to stimulate ideas about change and to match interventions to the particular area or domain of family functioning: cognitive, affective, or behavioral. As we know from our own clinical practice, certain interventions are a better fit with some families than with others. Therefore, the fit between the intervention and family functioning is always most important. Nurses should address the specificity question—that is, "What intervention will most effect change and invite healing with this particular problem with this particular family at this particular time?"

We encourage nurses to review the CFIM, specifically the intersection of domains of family functioning and intervention (Fig. 11-2) before deciding on a specific intervention or group of interventions. We have found in our own clinical work that we are sometimes biased toward one particular domain of family functioning and thus are likely as a result of our own biases to choose certain interventions regardless of whether they match the family's style of relating. Over years of clinical practice, we have also become more aware of how ethnicity, race, class, religion, sexual orientation, and other diversity issues influence the effectiveness of interventions. Thus, we review the following list before choosing a particular intervention for a particular family situation:

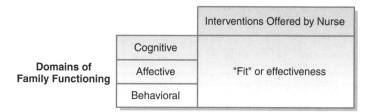

FIGURE 11-2: CFIM: Intersection of domains of family functioning and interventions.

- Questions as interventions
- Interventions directed at the cognitive domain of family functioning
- Interventions directed at the affective domain of family functioning
- Interventions directed at the behavioral domain of family functioning

When the nurse chooses interventions, he or she should focus on those interventions that best match the problem that the nurse and the family have agreed to change (Madsen, 2007). For example, the nurse and the Hixon family agreed to meet for three sessions to increase the family's skill in managing Torrance's behavior.

Another consideration in choosing an intervention is to pick one that flows from the nurse's hypothesis. Some interventions are more effective than others in bringing about change. One of the nurse's hypotheses regarding the Hixons was that Torrance was negatively triangulated into the marital subsystem. Thus she decided to choose interventions that would establish a more firm marital boundary while at the same time promoting effective parental controls of Torrance's behavior.

A further consideration in choosing interventions is to find those that match the family's strengths. How does change usually happen in the client's life? When? Where? With whom? We believe that families have tremendous resources to solve their own problems and that intervention by outsiders should be kept to a minimum. The nurse, in working with the Hixons, was aware of their belief about themselves as "special." They took pride in the fact that they were "survivors" and had overcome such adversity as unemployment after a serious motor vehicle accident. The nurse decided to build on such strengths in co-constructing the intervention plan with them.

A final consideration when choosing interventions is to pick those that match the nurse's competence level. We have discussed in Chapters 5 and 7 ideas for nurses to consider when evaluating their own competence level.

Choose Interventions
The following is a sample intervention plan for the Hixon family:
Problem: Parent-Child System: Difficulty with behavioral control. The nurse decided to have a meeting with Mr. and Mrs. Hixon to discuss normal 3-year-old child behavior, ways to set limits, and ways to positively reinforce good behavior. The nurse chose interventions aimed at the following domains:
Cognitive Domain: The nurse considered recommending parenting books on behavior management skills if the parents were interested in reading on this topic.
Behavioral Domain: The nurse thought about asking the couple to gather information about the available child-management courses sponsored by local community agencies (school board, parent-teacher groups, day-care centers, and so forth).

Affective and Behavioral Domain: The nurse decided to invite Mr. Hixon and Torrance to a session with the hope of increasing positive feedback and attachment between them. In agreement with the husband, Mrs. Hixon and the nurse planned to coach Mr. Hixon in improving his behavior management skills with Torrance. Chloe would be left at the grandparents' home during this session. In this way, the nurse hoped to draw forth more positive experiences of unique outcomes for father, son, and mother. At the same time, the nurse hoped that the grandparents, by babysitting Chloe, would be supportive of Mr. and Mrs. Hixon but not critical of their parenting abilities.

Use of Questions as Interventions: Every time the nurse met with the Hixons, she asked difference questions that invited the family to comment on the differences between their past, present, and future behavior management skills. She also used behavioral-effect questions to stimulate more solution-focused conversation about the positive effects of appropriate behavioral control of Torrance. That is, when Torrance responded to the parents' appropriate behavioral limits, the nurse hoped that the parents would recognize this.

We wish to emphasize that the nurse and the couple could have devised many other intervention plans to deal with the Hixons' difficulty with behavioral control of Torrance. For example, the nurse could have decided to focus more specifically on teaching the parents to control Torrance's eating patterns. Had the nurse chosen to do this, she might have invited Mrs. Hixon to meetings to discuss nutrition for a 3-year-old child. During such sessions, the nurse would provide support for the mother. There is the danger, however, that by having interviews only with the mother, the nurse might assume the role of "surrogate husband." The nurse would then exacerbate the difficulty between the husband and wife. Instead of choosing to work only with the mother, the nurse elected to work with both parents. In this way, she was choosing an intervention consistent with her hypothesis and goals of the family.

How to Record Progress Notes

After the nurse has developed an intervention plan and has continued to have contact with the family, he or she must maintain a record of the evolution of work with the family. In particular, it is important to record the specific work around the contracted presenting problem. A sample progress note is shown in Figure 11-3. The ideal progress note provides a structure for the nurse to identify his or her hypothesis, connect the assessment and intervention components, and maintain a sense of the evolving nature of the work with the family over time. Many hospital and agency progress notes are blank sheets of paper or check boxes. They are not easily conducive to stimulating the nurse to connect his or her hypothesis with the assessment and intervention plan, let alone providing an opportunity for the nurse to connect the family's responses

Family name: _____ Interview date: _____
Participants: _____ Interview place: _____
Nurse interviewer name and signature: _____

Hypothesis or plan pre-interview:

New information:

Content/process of interview (including interventions and family's responses):

New hypothesis:

Plan for next meeting:

FIGURE 11-3: Sample progress note.

to the intervention. We have found it helpful to address the areas listed in Box 11-5 when writing progress notes.

Some nurses find it useful to co-construct notes with family members. Some families and nurses each keep a record of the meeting. Other nurses have sent letters to families after a meeting outlining the content of the session. Nurses at one outpatient clinic send a summary of the clinical work to the family at the end of treatment, and occasionally they send a letter during the clinical work (Moules, 2002, 2003; Wright & Bell, in press). The letter provides general information about the dates and number of meetings. But most importantly, the letter recognizes the reciprocal relationship between families and nurses by routinely including two main areas: what

> **Box 11-5** Helpful Hints for Writing Progress Notes
>
> 1. Note the family members and the professionals who were present at the meeting, as well as the date and place of the meeting. This is particularly important if the interview takes place in a hospital setting because health professionals other than the nurse interviewer are commonly involved.
> 2. Record hypotheses or plan for the interview before the meeting with the family. We have found this invaluable in focusing ourselves for the meeting. It does not mean that we are slaves to, or become married to, the plan. For example, if the family comes in with a new crisis, we can alter the plan, but it does mean that we have an idea of how we will approach the meeting before the interview.
> 3. Record new information on what the family reports has happened since the last meeting. We are most interested in new information pertaining to changes in interaction around the presenting problem. These changes could be at the cognitive, affective, or behavioral domains of family functioning. For example, with the Hixon family, the nurse recorded the father's report that he and his wife had gone to a parenting class the previous week. After the class, they had stopped for a quick meal, which he said was "the first time we were out together in 6 months without the children."
> 4. Record the content and process of the meeting. We include the interventions and the family's responses to them. For example, the nurse used future-hypothetical questions to follow up on the information that Mr. Hixon reported about their going to the parenting class and out for a meal. The nurse asked the couple, "If you were to continue having time for yourselves to focus on parenting issues, what effect might this have on Torrance's behavior?" The parents' response that they thought Torrance would continue to be more compliant with them was recorded by the nurse.
> 5. Record a new hypothesis or a refinement of an old one. For example, as the Hixons progressed in achieving their goals, the nurse abandoned her hypothesis that the children were triangulated into the marriage. Rather, she developed a new hypothesis that focused on their strengths. She integrated the couple's previous history of positive coping (with the effects of a motor vehicle accident) and their need to deal with the effects of Torrance's health problems (delayed speech and short stature).
> 6. Address the plan for the next meeting. We jot down any ideas that we have for the next meeting and aim to review them just before or when we meet with the family.

the nurse offered the family (the interventions in the form of ideas, opinions, and recommendations) and what the nurse learned from the family. Many families have reported how much they have appreciated and gained from these therapeutic letters and stated that they frequently reread these letters to remind themselves of their accomplishments and to reinstill hope. A few families have even had the letters framed.

Moules (2002) has described a beautiful example of the impact of a couple receiving a letter after the wife met with a nurse. The husband had refused to come to the first meeting but found the nurse's recognition and understanding of their suffering significantly moving. He described his response to the letter:

> I think that when I read that letter, I found that they appreciated the fact of the illnesses we were fighting, the stresses that came along with having the illnesses like that. I can't say that it was ever put like the same way that this letter was…and in past…sessions it might have made mention of it but they didn't bring it to the forefront like this letter did like, you know, really appreciating that fact that we're putting up a big fight here, here every day, and that's what impressed me. Like, I wasn't going to go, I definitely was all set in not going but when I saw this letter, it changed my mind and I'll tell you I don't ever regret ever coming into, going to meetings and it was one of the best things I ever did…right there in that paragraph there, that's made up my mind just the way they addressed the fact that we had illnesses and how we were trying to combat them and, you know, find other ways to, you know, solutions to them, and that really impressed me, very much so, and that was, that sold me right away and then it just got better. (p. 106)

We do not have a particular preference for sharing or not sharing notes with families. What we believe is most essential is for the nurse and family to work collaboratively to solve problems, bring forth strengths, and promote health. If sharing records or writing therapeutic letters aids in this endeavor, it is useful to do so. There is no cookie-cutter approach to relational family nursing practice.

When learning how to work with families, it is important for nurses to conceptualize problems within a systems framework. Learning both the "thinking" and "doing" can be facilitated by an integrated approach to record keeping. The progress note presented in this chapter structures interview recording in a manner that facilitates systems thinking. It reflects the evolving connections between assessment and intervention. Hypothesizing, session planning, intervention, and family response are inextricably connected. The nurse reviews the previous hypotheses, questions, content and process themes, interventions, and family responses before each meeting with the family. By carefully recording the evolution of the therapeutic conversation, the nurse is more likely to remain focused on change in the presenting problem. This effectively leads toward closure with the family.

How to Record a Discharge Summary

Some nurses, particularly those in community health settings, have an opportunity to synthesize their work with families by doing a discharge summary. Other nurses, particularly those in hospital settings, have less of an opportunity to synthesize, in a written manner, their work with families. Nevertheless, we believe that where the opportunity exists, synthesizing information into a termination summary is a useful and meaningful event for both the family and the nurse. We highly recommend that nurses take advantage of this opportunity. A sample discharge summary is shown in Figure 11-4. There are many

Family name: _____ Date of first meeting: _____

Nurse's name: _____ Date of last meeting: _____

Nurse's signature: _____ Number of meetings: _____

Presenting problem and referral route:

Interventions and outcome:

Prognosis and recommendations:

FIGURE 11-4: Sample discharge summary.

ways in which one can record a discharge summary. (See Chapter 4, where we presented an excellent example of a therapeutic (closing) letter to a family, written by a student and her faculty supervisor.) In our own clinical work, we have found the areas listed in Box 11-6 useful to include in a discharge synopsis.

1. At the conclusion of the family sessions, is the presenting problem better, worse, or the same?

2. At the conclusion of the family sessions, to what extent (on a scale of 1 to 3, with 3 being a great deal) did the family's "thinking" about the problem change? Thinking may include ideas about the problem, understanding of the problem, or beliefs about the problem.

Box 11-6 Helpful Hints for Writing Discharge Summaries

1. Include the presenting problem or illness and referral route information in one or two sentences. We find that this focuses the report so that all the information written is relevant to the identified problem.

2. Focus on the interventions used and the outcome. By identifying the interventions used, we are able to learn more about what worked and what did not work to effect change in the presenting issue. For example, in working with the Hixon family, the nurse had recommended that the couple read books about effective behavioral management of children. She found that this intervention triggered a limited amount of change because neither the husband nor the wife was very interested in reading the material.

   Rather, they did benefit from the intervention in which the nurse asked them to "poll their friends, work colleagues, and relatives" about effective behavioral management strategies for young children. The couple enjoyed "survey research" and found time to discuss the results together. They reported that they enjoyed discarding some of the ideas. However, they retained and used the ones that were most consistent with their own childrearing beliefs. They also offered the nurse some information about websites that offer helpful parenting tips.

3. Address the area of recommendations. Given the limited resources in our health-care delivery systems, we find it useful to make recommendations that may be helpful if the family should come back for additional assistance. For example, the nurse who worked with the Hixon family recommended that, if they should ever need assistance in the future, it would be useful to inquire about what was most useful and least useful in this series of contacts with the pediatric clinic.

   In the future, the nurse most likely would not try to use bibliotherapy as an intervention without reassessing with the family whether this type of intervention might be useful. Rather, the nurse might recommend that the couple try experiments in soliciting others' ideas about how to handle the new issue. Once having done that, the couple could then come back and discuss with the nurse the advantages and disadvantages of adopting these solutions. By recommending such ideas, the nurse builds on the information gathered in working with the family this time. It does not prevent the new nurse interviewer from trying different ideas; it merely provides a tentative guide.

---

3. What specific changes in the family did you notice at the conclusion of the family sessions?

- Whole-family system: What changes did you notice in the family as a whole?

- Marital subsystem: What changes did you notice in the marriage?

- Sibling subsystem: What changes did you notice in the relationships between the children?

- Individual subsystems: What changes did you notice in the mother? Father? Child?

We suggest the following guidelines for a closing letter (Moules, 2002):

- Describe the presenting problem or issues dealt with. Do not highlight each session.

- Frame the changes experienced by the family as learnings. In other words, highlight what you learned from the family and working with the family.

- Describe the clinical interventions using the language of the family or language agreeable to the family. Highlight (in point form) what you offered or recommended to them (e.g., ideas, experiments).

- Provide closing thoughts (in point form). For example, "Finally, I would like to leave you with the following thoughts…"

- Keep the letter under two pages long.

See Chapter 12 for additional ideas about closing letters.

ISSUES IN RECORDING, STORING, AND ACCESSING RECORDS

Nurses are continually faced with issues about confidentiality. Who should have access to the family assessment summary or the discharge synopsis? Is it a family record or an individual record? Which family members can legally give consent for its release to another agency? Can the nurse talk to one family member about a meeting with another member when the first member is not present? These issues of confidentiality are becoming more numerous as a result of legislation and continuing advancements in communications technology. For example if the family meeting was recorded, family members sometimes request a copy so that they can play it at home. Family members and health-care providers are becoming more comfortable writing e-mails to one another or using text messaging; this also poses confidentiality concerns.

In the last decade, the subjects of human rights and confidentiality have increasingly come to the fore. In the areas of record content, release, consumer access, informed consent, records of minors, and compulsory reporting, nurses and other professionals have become increasingly more knowledgeable.

Guidelines regarding confidentiality exist in federal, state, and provincial regulations. Hospitals, clinics, and agencies also have guidelines for specialty areas. For example, in the area of mental health, there is a great variety of age designation and conditions under which minors may receive care.

In family nursing, confidentiality is a particularly complex issue. Data concerning more than one person are included in the file. Some of the family members are usually minors, and some are adults. When children and adults are in treatment as a unit, care must be taken to protect the privacy of each person. Nurses must be acquainted with the relevant legislation in their jurisdiction as well as the agency's or hospital's policies on confidentiality of family records.

Another practical issue concerning confidentiality is often raised. Family members sometimes try to obtain special attention by making telephone calls between sessions or by asking for private meetings with the nurse. The meaning of such behaviors should be carefully considered in the context of the nurse's understanding of the family system. For example, a nurse may be working with a family whose 25-year-old daughter, Puja, has a diagnosis of bipolar disorder. The father, mother, and daughter may agree during a family interview that the young woman should follow the physician's advice and take lithium. If, however, the father calls the nurse after the family session to discuss why he believes his daughter should not take lithium, the nurse should hypothesize about the meaning of the father's call. Could he fear disagreeing with his wife and daughter in front of them? Could he want the nurse to align with him against his wife and daughter? Generally, we recommend that nurses tell family members who request a private session that they should bring their concerns to the family interviews. In this way, the nurse avoids becoming triangulated between two or more family members. See Chapter 10 for additional ideas about how to avoid taking sides.

CONCLUSIONS

A particular format has now evolved in the process of family interviewing. The nurse ascertains whether a family assessment is indicated. If it is indicated, a family assessment is conducted. Box 11-7 provides some helpful hints for organizing and documenting family assessment data. After the nurse has assessed the family, we recommend that the nurse review the CFAM categories and delineate a list of strengths and problems. The nurse should then write a family assessment summary. A decision to intervene is made based on consideration of the family's level of functioning, the nurse's competence, and the work context. If intervention is indicated, the nurse

---

Box 11-7 Helpful Hints for Organizing and Documenting Family Assessment Data

- Identify and document a list of presenting problems and family strengths.
- Create a CFAM document that lists each category and subcategory. Enter reported and observed data in relevant categories and subcategories. Note information gaps to be filled at a future date.
- Include a genogram, an ecomap, brief family life cycle and family development data, and an attachment diagram for a significant family relationship.
- Formulate systemic hypotheses.
- Formulate an intervention plan.
- Continue to update the family assessment, using progress notes to document family changes and the impact of family nursing interventions.

Levac, A.M.C., Wright, L.M., & Leahey, M. (2002). Children and families: Models for assessment and intervention. In J.A. Fox (Ed.), *Primary health care of infants, children, and adolescents* (2nd ed.) (p. 17). St. Louis: Mosby. Copyright 2002. Reprinted with permission.

has to decide, in collaboration with the family, which issues are key and which ones are tangential. We recommend that the nurse review the CFIM. The nurse must also consider with the family which members will participate and what the frequency and length of treatment should be. An intervention plan should then be devised. The decision regarding which interventions will be used to facilitate change within this particular family is a critical one. The nurse then records on a progress note a record of his or her therapeutic conversations with the family and, at the time of discharge, synthesizes the work in a discharge summary.

We encourage nurses to adapt the documentation examples we have offered to fit their particular context and recording practices. However, if no family documentation is currently provided in their clinical setting, then we hope that nurses will persuade and champion the inclusion of family information so that the important care of families becomes more visible and valued.

References

College and Association of Registered Nurses of Alberta (2006). *Documentation guidelines for registered nurses.* Edmonton, AB: Author.

Goudreau, J., Duhamel, F., & Ricard, N. (2006). The impact of a family systems nursing educational program on the practice of psychiatric nurses: A Pilot Study. *Journal of Family Nursing, 12*(8), 292–306.

LeGrow, K., & Rossen, B.E. (2005). Development of professional practice based on a family systems nursing framework: Nurses' and families' experience. *Journal of Family Nursing, 11*(2), 38–58.

Madsen, W. (2007). Working within traditional structures to support a collaborative clinical practice. *The International Journal of Narrative Therapy and Community Work, 2,* 51–61.

Moules, N.J. (2002). Nursing on paper: Therapeutic letters in nursing practice. *Nursing Inquiry, 9*(2), 104–113.

Moules, N.J. (2003). Therapy on paper: Therapeutic letters and the tone of the relationship. *Journal of Systemic Therapies, 22*(1), 33–49.

Wright, L.M., & Bell, J.M. (in press). *Beliefs and illness: A model for healing.* Calgary, AB: 4th Floor Press.

Chapter **12**

How to Terminate With Families

Knowing how to conclude clinical work successfully with families is as important as knowing how to begin—perhaps even more so. When nurses part with families, they should do so in a manner that leaves the families with hope and confidence in their new and rediscovered strengths, resources, and abilities to manage their health and relationships. If the family has been suffering with illness, loss, or disability, then at the conclusion of the clinical work, a highly desired outcome would be softened or alleviated suffering and increased healing.

To end professional relationships with families in a therapeutic fashion is one of the most challenging aspects of the family interviewing process for nurses. Reed and Tarko (2004) make the interesting observation that, in nursing, "the issue of termination has been often discussed in psychiatric nursing texts, making it seem as if no other nursing situations have issues surrounding termination" (p. 266). Termination continues to be the least examined of the treatment phases in clinical work with families.

An important aspect of the termination stage is not only to end the nurse–family relationship therapeutically but to do so in a manner that will sustain the progress and foster hope for the future. Nurses commonly establish very intense and meaningful relationships with families and, therefore, may feel guilty or fearful about initiating termination. This is especially evident in nursing practice when the relationship has been a long-standing one, over months or even years, such as in nursing homes, extended-care facilities, and clients' homes. In this chapter, we review the process of termination by examining the decision to terminate when it is initiated by the family or the nurse or as a result of the context in which the family members find themselves. In many cases, the nurse's decision to terminate with a family does not necessarily mean that the family will cease contact with all professionals. Therefore, we also discuss the process of referring families to other health professionals. We provide specific suggestions for phasing out and concluding treatment as well as for evaluating the effects of the treatment process. We must emphasize that just as other aspects of family interviewing are conducted in a collaborative manner, so too should the termination phase. Termination should occur with full participation and input from the family whenever possible.

DECISION TO TERMINATE

Nurse-Initiated Termination

It is important to emphasize that termination may occur before the presenting problem or illness is completely "cured" or resolved. Rather, the family's ability to master or live alongside problems or illness, although hopefully with softened emotional, physical, and spiritual suffering, is the impetus for the initiation of termination. In most cases, it is unrealistic for nurses to attempt to completely eliminate the presenting concern or illness, and such a goal can frequently leave families feeling more discouraged and hopeless and nurses feeling inadequate or unhelpful. It is the softening of suffering with illness or increased healing and awareness that enables a family to live with their problems or illness in a more peaceful and manageable way. If the family's presenting concern is related to health promotion, then greater knowledge or increased expertise by the family might be an indicator for termination.

The termination stage evolves easily if the beginning and middle stages of engagement and treatment have progressed successfully. However, the most difficult decision for any nurse to make in regard to termination relates to time. When is the right time for termination? This question is directly related to the new views, beliefs, ideas, and solutions that have been generated by the family and nurse to resolve current problems. If new solution options have been discovered and consequently the family functions differently, particularly with the presenting concern, it is time to terminate because change has occurred. The skills necessary for nurse-initiated termination are given in a later section of this chapter ("Phasing Out and Concluding Treatment") and in Chapter 5.

In contexts where family meetings have occured over time, then the nurse and family may collaboratively decide that additional meetings are not necessary. In these situations, the termination phase of treatment has begun. First and most importantly during this phase, we prefer to help families expand their perspectives to focus on strengths, positive behaviors, and changes in beliefs or feelings that have occurred or re-emerged rather than focusing exclusively on troublesome or problematic behaviors. We encourage families not to associate these new behaviors with our work but instead with their own efforts. For example, we would ask a family what positive changes they have noticed over the last 3 months rather than asking what positive changes they have noticed since working with a nurse.

White and Epston (1990) offer another useful clinical idea for nurses terminating with families; they recommend that the interviewer "expand the audience" to describe and acknowledge the family's unique outcomes and progress. For example, we commonly ask families to tell us what advice they would have for other families confronting similar health problems. Sometimes we have families write letters to other families to offer suggestions regarding what has or has not worked in coping with a particular illness. For example, one woman, who was experiencing multiple sclerosis (MS) but was successfully living alongside her illness, wrote a letter to a younger woman who was not yet as successful in managing her illness. The younger woman, who gave her permission to receive a letter, found that it gave her hope and encouragement. The older woman expressed that writing the letter was a very "cathartic" experience for her. She went on to say, "MS is still here, but it does not dominate our lives and occupies only a small space over in the corner. I did experience a minor flareup after Christmas but it cleared quickly. I remain optimistic." The nurse should highlight and become enthusiastic about the family's ideas and advice as a way of both reinforcing positive ideas for change and the family's new beliefs about themselves and generating useful information for other families. Thus, the family's competencies, resources, and strengths are overtly acknowledged.

When termination is initiated by the nurse, the emphasis throughout the termination process is to identify, affirm, amplify, and solidify the changes that have taken place within family members. Consequently, it is essential that change be distinguished to become a reality (Wright & Bell, in press). One way to distinguish change is to obtain the perspective of other family members. The nurse can accomplish this by asking questions such as, "What changes do you notice in your wife since she has adopted this new idea that 'illness is a family affair?'" or "What else would your family or friends notice that is different in you since your depression about experiencing cancer has dissipated?"

Initiating rituals at the time of termination can also emphasize change and give families courage to live their lives without the involvement of health-care professionals. If the initial concern involves a child, we often have a party (balloons, cake, and all) to celebrate the child's mastery of the particular problem, whether it be enuresis, fighting fears, or putting chronic pain in its place. In addition, the child is given a certificate indicating that he or she has overcome the problem. This practice helps families to acknowledge change through celebration.

Other clinical nursing teams give families something to symbolize their progress. For example, one family was given a feather to indicate that their problems now only require "the touch of a feather" to be able to keep them in place. It is essential to mark family strengths and problem-solving capabilities as families continue their daily lives without the involvement of nurses.

In one outpatient clinic, a closing letter is routinely sent at the end of the clinical work to each family highlighting what the clinical nursing team has learned from the family and what ideas the team offered the family (Moules, 2002; Wright & Bell, in press). These therapeutic letters serve as closing rituals. They provide the opportunity to highlight the family's strengths and document in a personal way the family and individual interventions that were offered. The letters also acknowledge that family nursing is not a one-way street with nurses assisting families. Rather, by stating what the nurse and clinical team have learned from the family, the nurse honors the reciprocal and relational influence between the family and the clinical nursing team. More information about closing letters is provided in Chapter 11.

Family-Initiated Termination

When a family takes the initiative to terminate, it is very important for the nurse to acknowledge their desire and then to gain more explicit information regarding their reasons for wanting to terminate. This information helps the nurse to understand the family's responses to the interviewing process. Has the family discovered new solutions to their problems or challenged their beliefs to soften their suffering? For example, have they found a way to have respite from caring for their ill child without feeling excessive guilt? Has the family challenged some of their constraining beliefs about the illness experience (Wright & Bell, in press)? For example, have they now stopped blaming themselves for the husband suffering a coronary in part because of having to work two jobs? Are the family and nurse able to identify and agree on significant changes that have occurred in both individual and family functioning? Is the family also aware of how to sustain these changes? For example, if a son refuses to give his own insulin injections in the future, what will the family do differently?

If the family specifically states that they wish to terminate but the nurse believes this would be premature or even enhance their suffering, it is important for the nurse to take the initiative to review the family's decision. In so doing, the nurse reconceptualizes the progress the family has made and recognizes what problems remain and what goals and solutions might yet be achieved. One way to do this is to have family members discuss with one another their desires to continue or discontinue sessions and explore who most disfavors termination. Also, the specifics of the decision may be helpful, such as when the family decided to terminate and what prompted the decision. After establishing who is most eager to continue, the nurse can invite that family member to share with the other family members the anticipated benefit of further sessions. It is helpful for families to be specific and emphasize the benefits that could be achieved if family interviewing were to continue. However, there are times when termination is inevitable. At such a point, it is reasonable and ethical to accept the family's initiative to terminate and to do so without applying undue pressure, even though the nurse may disagree with their decision.

We strongly urge nurses not to engage in linear blame of either families or themselves when they believe that families have prematurely or abruptly left treatment. Rather, we encourage nurses to hypothesize about the factors that may have contributed to the termination. These factors may include such nurse-related behaviors as being too aligned with children, too slow to intervene, or too "married" to a particular hypothesis about the family's functioning, or not attending to the family's main concern (see Chapter 10 for elaboration of errors to avoid). Family-related behaviors such as concurrent involvement with other agencies should also be considered.

Nurses may also encounter cases in which a family states that they want to continue treatment but initiate termination indirectly. Indications include late arrivals for sessions, missed appointments, and the absence from sessions of certain family members who were asked to attend. Another indicator that families are perhaps considering termination is their expression of dissatisfaction with the course of treatment or complaints about the logistical difficulties of attending or the loss of time from work. In these situations, we suggest that the same steps be taken as when the family initiates termination directly.

The challenge of family-initiated terminations is to determine whether or not they are premature. In the nursing literature, there is a dearth of research to provide insights into reasons for premature termination. Therefore, nurses must rely on their own clinical judgment to ascertain if termination is premature. Hopefully, future research studies will address this area in nursing practice with families who are seen on an outpatient basis.

In our clinical experience, we have found that families who miss the first treatment session are at high risk for dropping out over the course of treatment. The implication of missed appointments refers back to the importance of the engagement stage and even to the initial contact with families on the telephone. We have also found that the referral source has a direct correlation with the family's continuing treatment. Families who are referred by institutions (such as a school or court) are more likely to discontinue treatment before achieving treatment goals than families who were individually referred (such as by physicians or mental health professionals). Families who are self-referred tend to complete the treatment process.

It is critically important to help families understand the nature of the treatment contract. Many families' understandings of what takes place in family interviewing are markedly different than the understandings held by nurses. Therefore, these families may relate to nurses as they do to physicians, imams, or clergy, whereby they use the services as they wish and discontinue when they desire. For this reason, we find it particularly useful when seeing families on an outpatient basis to contract for a certain number of sessions and then re-evaluate as progress occurs. This approach may help to prevent premature or abrupt termination.

Context-Initiated Termination

In some settings, such as hospitals (particularly those in managed health-care systems), it is not the nurse or the family who initiates termination but the health-care system or insurance company. In these situations, it is very important for the nurse to assess whether the family needs further treatment or can continue to resolve problems and discover solutions on their own. If the family needs to be referred, the nurse requires some specific skills in this area. The referral process will be discussed in a later section of this chapter.

PHASING OUT AND CONCLUDING TREATMENT

In Chapter 5, we highlighted some of the specific skills required for thera-peutic termination in the form of learning objectives. We will now expand on these particular skills.

Review Contracts

For families seen on an outpatient basis, we strongly encourage periodic review of the present status of the family's problems and changes. The use of a contract for a specific number of sessions provides a built-in way not only to set a time limit to the meetings but also to ensure periodic review. For example, at the Family Nursing Unit, University of Calgary, all families contracted for four sessions and then evaluated change. In some cases, four sessions were not necessary; families could put unused sessions "in the bank" to be used at a later time if desired. If the family required additional sessions at the conclusion of the four-session con-tract, then another contract was made between the family and the nurse and re-evaluation occurred again at the end of those sessions. Interest-ingly, families who contracted for more sessions rarely wanted another 5 or 10 sessions but usually requested just 1 or 2 more sessions.

Contracts help nurse interviewers to be mindful of the progress and direction of their work with families rather than seeing families endlessly and without purpose beyond the vague good intention of "helping." We prefer a designated number of sessions to open-ended sessions. However, nurses need to be flexible about the frequency and duration of sessions. Normally, the frequency decreases as problems improve, suffering has soft-ened, and confidence and hopefulness has increased. Periodic reviews allow family members the opportunity to express their pleasure or displeasure with the progress that is being made.

Decrease Frequency of Sessions

When adequate progress has been made, as evidenced by softened suffering, the time is ideal to begin to decrease the frequency of sessions. In our expe-rience, we have found that families are able to work toward termination more readily and with more confidence when they recognize the improve-ment in their own ability to solve problems. Many families, however, find it difficult to acknowledge changes. In these circumstances, we suggest the use of a question such as, "What would each of you have to do to bring the problem back?" to elicit a more explicit understanding or statement from family members regarding the changes that have been made.

Another significant time to decrease the frequency of sessions is when the nurse has inadvertently fostered undue dependency. We have had many family situations presented to us in which nursing students or professional nurses provide "paid friendship" with mothers. These nurses have become the mother's major support system because they have failed to mobilize other supports, such as husbands, friends, or relatives. In situations in which this dependency has occurred and is recognized, we strongly suggest that the nurse help foster other supports for the family and decrease the frequency of sessions. Regular consultation with colleagues or a supervisor will assist the nurse to ascertain if a dependent relationship has occurred between the nurse and the family.

If a nurse encounters hesitancy or reluctance to decrease the frequency of sessions or to terminate completely, the nurse should encourage a discussion of the fears related to termination and solicit support from other family members. It has been our experience that family members commonly fear that if sessions are decreased or discontinued, they will not be able to cope with their problems or their problems will become worse. Thus, asking a question such as, "What are you most concerned would happen if we discontinued our meetings now?" can get to the core of the matter very quickly. By clarifying family members' fears openly, other family members (who may be less fearful) have an opportunity to provide support.

Give Credit for Change

Nurses often choose the profession of nursing because they have a strong desire to help individuals and families obtain optimal health and soften their suffering. Their efforts are usually helpful, and they are commonly given all or much of the credit for the changes and improvements. However, it has been our experience in family work that it is vitally important that the family receive the credit for change. There are several reasons for this:

1. Families experience the tension, conflict, suffering, and anxiety of working through problems related to their health or illness and relationships; therefore, they deserve the credit for improvement.

2. If the identified patient is a child and the nurse accepts credit, the nurse can be seen to be in a competitive relationship with the parents.

3. Perhaps the most important reason for giving the family credit for change is that doing so increases the chance that the positive effects of treatment will last. Otherwise, you may inadvertently convey the message that the family cannot manage without you, and they will become indebted or too dependent. Termination provides an opportune

time to comment on the positive changes that have already happened during the course of treatment.

4. Praising the family for their accomplishments in having helped or corrected the original presenting problem provides them with confidence to handle future problems. Statements such as "You did the work" or "You people are being far too modest" can reinforce to family members the idea that their efforts were essential in making the change.

It is never possible to know for certain what precipitated, perturbed, or initiated the change that occurs within families. In many cases, nurses create a context for change by helping family members explore solution options to their difficulties or suffering. Wright and Bell (in press) suggest that creating a context for change constitutes the central and enduring foundation of the therapeutic process and further suggest that it is not just a necessary prerequisite to the process of therapeutic change; it is therapeutic change in and of itself. Sometimes the very effort of bringing a family together in a room to discuss important family issues and their suffering can be the most significant intervention (Robinson & Wright, 1995).

If families present themselves at termination with concerns about progress, nurses must express their appreciation for the family's positive efforts to solve problems constructively, even when no significant improvement has occurred. In such cases, we strongly recommend that nurses discuss with their clinical supervisors some hypotheses about why the interview sessions did not seem to be effective. Perhaps the goals of the family or the nurse were too high or demanding. If a family does not progress, it is usually the result of our inability to discover an intervention that "fits" the family. Too often, we excuse ourselves from making further efforts to intervene when we label families as noncompliant, unmotivated, or resistant (Wright & Levac, 1992). It is very important, however, that nurses believe that families have worked hard despite minimal progress, and it is important to praise them for having done so.

We do not mean to imply, however, that because we are encouraging nurses to give families the credit for change that the nurse cannot enjoy the change. Family work can be very rewarding, and certainly the nurse is part of the change process.

Evaluate Family Interviews

It is important to provide a formal closure to the end of the treatment process with a face-to-face discussion whenever possible. Madsen (2007) refers to this part of the termination process as a "consolidation interview." In a consolidation or termination interview, particular kinds of questions are asked that review the process not only of the work that the family and clinician have done together in the past but also of the work the family is seeking to accomplish on its own in the future. This kind of interview is a way to reduce feelings of anxiety, fear, or loss on the part of either the clinician, family, or both.

During this final session, it is very valuable to evaluate the effectiveness of the treatment process and the effect of changes on various family members. We recommend evaluating the impact not only on the whole-family system but also on various subsystems, such as the marital subsystem and individual family member functions. Questions such as "What have you learned about yourself and ALS?" or "What have you come to appreciate about your marriage?" or "What have you come to understand is the most effective way you can live with your grief?" invite reflections from the family about its changes.

We also believe in sharing the family's wisdom and will frequently ask: "When I meet with other families with chronic illness, from what you know now, what would you advise them or offer them?"

An even more dramatic evaluation can occur by having each family member and the nurse write about their reflections on the family meetings, emphasizing what they learned, what has changed, and what new ideas or beliefs they have about their problems or illness. One such family clinical nursing team wrote poignant descriptions about dealing with their grief (Levac, et al, 1998).

We also suggest asking family members the following questions: "What things did you find most and least helpful during our work together?" and "What things did you wish or were hoping would happen during our work together that did not?" or "Based on what you've accomplished and learned, what suggestions do you have for me or other nurses in trying to help other families suffering with similar issues?" This behavior demonstrates that the nurse is also open and receptive to feedback. It is important at this time that the nurse not become defensive to any of the feedback. Rather, the nurse can express appreciation to the family and inform them that this feedback will assist and educate him or her to be even more helpful in work with future families. Participatory evaluation research turns the traditional evaluation process on its head. Outsiders are no longer the "experts" but instead empower families to become leaders in evaluation and change throughout the interviewing process (Duhamel & Talbot, 2004).

Extend an Invitation for Follow-Up

Nurses often place themselves or are placed in situations of "follow-up." However, follow-up is frequently a negative experience for both the nurse and the family. For example, community health nurses (CHNs) have reported that they are often requested to "check" on family members to assess their functioning. However, those who request the visit (be they physicians or Departments of Child Welfare) often make no clear statement to the family about the purpose of the visit. Therefore, the nurse is in a very awkward position. We strongly discourage nurses from placing themselves in these kinds of situations unless there has been clear, direct communication with the family by the requesting party. Follow-up in this manner can give a very unfortunate and unpleasant message to the family that we anticipate further problems. It is better to make clear to the family that progress has been made and that the sessions are finished. However, if they would like input again in the future, indicate that you would be willing to see them. Families usually appreciate knowing that backup support by professionals is available to them in times of stress.

For nurses employed in hospitals, a follow-up session is usually not possible, but referral can be made to a CHN, emergency room outreach worker, or home-care nurse if deemed appropriate. Our experience has been that families do appreciate knowing whether they will have future contact with the nurse who has worked intimately with them.

Closing Letters

Another way to punctuate the end of treatment positively is to send the family a letter giving a summary of the family sessions. This letter provides the opportunity to highlight the family strengths, reinforce the changes made, offer the family a review of their efforts and what they have accomplished, and list the ideas (interventions) that were offered to them. At the Family Nursing Unit, University of Calgary, closing letters were routinely sent to each family on completion of treatment (Hougher Limacher & Wright, 2006; Moules, 2002, 2003; Wright, 2005; Wright & Bell, in press). Many families have commented about how much they appreciate the letters and how they frequently refer to them. Additional information about closing letters is provided in Chapter 11.

The following example illustrates a typical closing letter:

> Dear Family Barbosa:
> Greetings from the Family Nursing Unit. We had the opportunity to meet with various members of your family on eight occasions. I have also had several phone conversations with both Venicio and Fatima in recent months.
> **What Our Team Offered Your Family.** Throughout our work together, our clinical nursing team has been very impressed with your family. Although a great many challenges have been presented to all of you over the past years, your family was able to overcome many obstacles and search for ways of helping each other through these difficult times.
>
> 1. We offered you the idea that most families find it very difficult to talk openly about an impending loss or death of a family member but that talking can be very healing. You have shown us that this was the case in your family.
>
> 2. We offered you a few books to read about other families who have experienced a similar tragedy as yours.

3. We offered you the idea that resolving issues in a relationship that has been conflictual can bring great peace and comfort, particularly following the death of a loved one.

What Our Team Learned from Your Family. Our experience with your family has taught our clinical nursing team a great deal. The following is a synthesis:

1. Families dealing with a life-shortening illness in one of its members have the strength to deal with unresolved issues of blame, guilt, and shame. Even though there has been a great deal of pain and hurt in a family, they can heal their relationships and move on.

2. Although it can be a common response for family members to distance themselves from the possibility of death with a life-shortening illness and to be afraid of dying, it is possible for them to make peace with each other and find peace in themselves, giving them the courage to go on.

3. Although a mother and son may reside in different places and may not see each other often, they can still play a significant part in each other's lives. No matter how old a child and parent are, the knowledge that they love and accept each other for what they are can make a significant difference in their lives.

4. The uncertainty involved with a life-shortening illness can be the most difficult thing for families to handle. Family members can help each other with the uncertainty by discussing the situation openly among themselves.

5. Grandparents and grandsons have very special relationships that are different from those of parents and sons.

As you all continue to face the many challenges that are ahead, we trust that you will draw on your own special strengths as well as on more open communication to help you meet these challenges. It was truly a privilege to work with you. We wish you continued strength for the future.

Should you desire further consultation at any time, you can arrange this by contacting the Family Nursing Unit's secretary. A research assistant will be in contact with you in approximately 6 months to ask you to participate in our outcome study to ascertain your satisfaction with the Family Nursing Unit.

Sincerely,

Jane Nagy, R.N.   Lorraine M. Wright, R.N., Ph.D.

Masters Student   Director, Family Nursing Unit

Professor, Faculty of Nursing

Therapeutic letters, whether sent during clinical work with families or at the end of treatment, have proved a very useful and often potent intervention to invite families to reflect on ideas offered within the session as well as to reflect on changes they have made over the course of sessions (Hougher Limacher & Wright, 2006; Levac, et al, 1998; Moules, 2002, 2003; Watson & Lee, 1993; White & Epston, 1990; Wright, 2005; Wright & Nagy, 1993; Wright & Watson, 1988; Wright & Bell, in press).

REFERRAL TO OTHER PROFESSIONALS

Referral to other professionals may be advisable for various reasons. We will list some specific tasks that are required to make a smooth transition for the family from one professional to another. First, however, we will discuss some of the more common reasons for nurses to refer families to other professionals.

With the expanding specialty areas within nursing, including family systems nursing, it is becoming impossible and totally unrealistic to expect nurses to be experts in all areas. Therefore, when problems are quite complex, it may be appropriate for nurses to seek the input of additional professional resources. A nurse may refer families or specific family members for consultation or ongoing treatment. For example, if a senior within a family is experiencing temporal headaches, it is very important that any organic or biological origin of this problem be ruled out. Therefore, a nurse might refer the family for consultation with a neurologist and may suspend treatment until the consultation is complete. Similarly, the nurse may discover that a particular child has a learning disability that is out of the realm of the nurse's expertise. The nurse may suggest referring the child to an education center where personnel have greater expertise in dealing with children with learning difficulties. Nurses need to be open to referring individuals or entire families for consultation without perceiving this as an inadequacy in their repertoire of skills. To refer wisely, nurses need an extensive knowledge of professional resources within the community.

Although not as common, other situations nurses may encounter that require referral of families to other professionals include when the family moves, is transferred to another setting, or is discharged before treatment is over. It is very important that the nurse, especially in hospital settings, maximize opportunities to do family work. A beautiful illustration of this was given by one of our graduate nursing students. After some university seminars on the importance of family involvement, this student, who was working part time in a rural hospital, invited the parents of an asthmatic child to a family interview. The student obtained much valuable information regarding the interrelationship of the child's asthmatic problem with other family dynamics. Shortly thereafter, the child was discharged. The nursing student ascertained that the family was interested in changing the recurring problem of frequent admissions for this young child. The student made an appropriate referral to the mental health services within the community. This highlights the point that with only one family interview an assessment can be made and a significant intervention completed through referral for a recurring problem.

Some of the specific skills required in making appropriate referrals are described in the following paragraphs.

Prepare Families

Nurses must adequately prepare families so that they understand the nature of the referral to a new professional. This can be done by explaining directly to families the reason for the referral and why the nurse feels that the family would benefit from such a referral. Another method that can be useful for ensuring openness and clarity about the nature of the referral is for the nurse to write a summary and then to review this summary with the family. This summary can then be sent to the new professional and a copy made available to the family. In this way, the family is not left wondering what information will be shared with the new professional. Also, an important implicit message is given that this information is confidential and private about them and, therefore, they have a right to know what is shared.

Selecting a new professional can sometimes pose a challenge. If a nurse is known in the community, it is wise to solicit the help of colleagues for ideas and advice on which agencies or professionals are best for the type of treatment needed or to seek information from community information directories and booklets.

Meet the New Professional

It has been our experience that the transition to the new professional is much more effective and efficient if the nurse can be present with the family at the first meeting. In this way, a more personal referral is made. It often reduces the fears and anxieties that families may have about starting "fresh" with someone new. Before the referral, opportunities should be given to the family to express concerns or ask questions about the referral. At the first meeting, the family may wish to clarify with the new professional their expectations and understanding of the reason for the referral, and any misconceptions can be dealt with at that time. A conjoint meeting with the family, nurse, and new professional can also serve as a "marker" for the end of the nurse's relationship with the family.

Keep Appropriate Boundaries

Despite increased interdisciplinary collaboration in health care, it is still very important that when a family has been referred, boundaries of responsibility are clear. Otherwise, there is a potential for the nurse to inadvertently become triangulated between the family and the new professional. For example, a home-care nurse regularly visited an elderly patient who lived with her adult daughter. The purpose of the visits by the home-care nurse was to assist with colostomy care. The nurse observed and assessed a severe and long-standing conflict between the elderly parent and the adult daughter. This conflict was having a negative effect, deterring the elderly patient from assuming more responsibility for her physical care. Because of her family assessment skills, the nurse was able to make an important referral to a family therapy program where more in-depth work on the intergenerational conflict began. However, in future visits, the elderly patient expressed to the nurse complaints about the adult daughter that the patient was not discussing in the family meetings. Also, the family therapist called the nurse and asked the nurse to apply pressure on the elderly parent to be more cooperative in attending sessions. Thus, very quickly the nurse had become "caught in the middle" between the family and the therapist. The nurse dealt with the situation by requesting to join in a meeting with the family and the therapist to clarify expectations of all parties. In this one session, the nurse was able to "detriangulate" herself from any alliance by clarifying her present role with the family and the new professional. See Chapter 3 for more discussion about alliances and coalitions.

Transfers

In our more than 35 years of clinical experience, we have not found the practice of transferring families from one clinician to another to be very successful. We view the process of transfers as very different from referrals. A referral is usually made to another health-care professional with different expertise. A transfer, on the other hand, is usually made to another colleague of similar expertise and competence. We recommend, if possible, that nurses conclude treatment with the families they are working with rather than transfer them to another colleague. In our experience, families frequently disengage with the new nurse in various ways (by missing appointments, not showing up, or not stating any particular concern). It is understandable that families do not wish to "start over" with another nurse. We hypothesize that transfers are frequently made to assuage the nurse's feelings about leaving versus the family's desires about continuing treatment.

If, however, a transfer is necessary, we recommend that the "old" nurse use language indicating an ending of her relationship with the family. For example, she can say, "Now that my work with you is coming to an end, what would you like to work on with Sanjeshna (the 'new' nurse)?" In addition, we encourage the new nurse to directly ask the family about their relationship with previous nurses. Such questions as "What do you anticipate will be different in our work together versus your work with Li?" are useful. This type of conversation punctuates a change rather than a continuance of the same work. It fosters engagement and is important for the new nurse and the family in establishing a collaborative relationship.

Another way to increase engagement is for the current nurse to ask the family to take a break before the family initiates setting up an appointment with the new nurse. This again emphasizes the change in the working relationship and encourages the family to be self-directive in initiating the new contact rather than simply responding to the professionals.

Success of Treatment in Family Work

Although interventions may obtain positive and possibly dramatic results during treatment, the real success of family work is the positive changes that are maintained or continue to evolve weeks and months after nurses have terminated treatment with particular families. We strongly encourage professional nurses and nursing students to make it a pattern of practice to obtain data from the family regarding outcomes in order to determine best practices. When nurses focus on outcomes, they orient their work toward change, focus on problems that can be changed, and think about how families will cope without them in the future. We also suggest that nurses explain to families that follow-up is a normal pattern of practice (for example, by saying, "We normally contact families with whom we have worked within 6 months to gain information on how things are evolving"). It is also important to use this follow-up with specific goals in mind. A very useful reason for follow-up can be for research purposes. In our experience, beginning family nurse interviewers tend to be more focused on what is going on in the family, whereas more experienced nurses focus on more specific goals for treatment.

To facilitate evaluation, we suggest formalizing follow-up of families, particularly those seen on an outpatient basis, by live interview, questionnaire, telephone, or even e-mail. At present, we favor the use of a face-to-face discussion and questionnaire that is answered by all available family members.

At the Family Nursing Unit, University of Calgary, families were routinely interviewed 6 months after the last session by a research assistant who had no previous contact with the families (Wright & Bell, in press). This outcome study was designed to evaluate the services provided by the Family Nursing Unit. The variables examined by this study were the family's satisfaction with the services provided, satisfaction with the nurse interviewer, and change in the presenting problem and family relationships. A semistructured questionnaire designed for this study asked for each family member's perspective on each of the variables. Questions were asked in relation to two periods: at the conclusion of the family sessions and at the time of the survey. Results from the survey indicated that the most helpful aspects of family sessions were the opportunity to ventilate family concerns, thereby increasing communication among family members, and to obtain support from the Family Nursing Unit clinical nursing team. Families ranked the interview process and the suggestions from the Family Nursing Unit clinical nursing team as the second most helpful aspects.

Family members reported satisfaction with nurse interviewers, who were either master's or doctoral students or faculty members specializing in family systems nursing. They indicated that the friendly, professional, and nonthreatening manner of the graduate nursing students made them comfortable. More than 75% of the family members reported that the presenting problem was better at the time of the survey. Regardless of the presenting problem, positive changes in the marital relationship, such as increased communication, improved relationships, and decreased tension, were also reported, suggesting support for the systems-theory tenet that change in one part of the system affects change in other parts.

This type of outcome study suggests that change should be evaluated at the individual, parent–child, marital, and family system levels. We believe that a higher level of positive change has occurred when improvement is evidenced in systemic (total family) or relationship (dyadic) interactions than when it is evidenced in individuals alone. That is, individual change does not logically require system change, but stable system change does require individual change and relationship change, and relationship change requires individual changes.

Nurses can contribute significantly to family outcome research by focusing on follow-up with families in which particular family members experience a health problem. This area of family work is just beginning to be researched and lends itself beautifully to the active involvement of nurses in its evolution.

CONCLUSIONS

Concluding treatment in a therapeutic and constructive way is a challenge for any nurse working with families. Unfortunately, much more has been written in the literature about how to begin with and treat families than how to effectively and therapeutically terminate with them. However, we want to emphasize the extreme importance of terminating contact with families in a manner that will increase the likelihood that diminished suffering will be sustained and that changes and hopefulness in family relationships will be maintained, celebrated, and expanded.

References

Duhamel, F., & Talbot, L. (2004). A constructivist evaluation of family interventions in cardiovascular nursing practice. *Journal of Family Nursing, 10*(1), 12–32.

Hougher Limacher, L.H., & Wright, L.M. (2006). Exploring the therapeutic family intervention of commendations: Insights from research. *Journal of Family Nursing, 12*, 307–331.

Levac, A.M., et al. (1998). A "Reader's Theater" intervention to managing grief: Posttherapy reflections by a family and a clinical team. *Journal of Marital and Family Therapy, 24*(1), 81–93.

Madsen, W. (2007). Working within traditional structures to support a collaborative clinical practice. *The International Journal of Narrative Therapy and Community Work, 2*, 51–61.

Moules, N.J. (2002). Nursing on paper: Therapeutic letters in nursing practice. *Nursing Inquiry, 9*(2), 104–113.

Moules, N.J. (2003). Therapy on paper: Therapeutic letters and the tone of the relationship. *Journal of Systemic Therapies, 22*(1), 33–49.

Reed, K., & Tarko, M.A. (2004). Using the nursing process with families. In P.J. Bomar (Ed.), *Promoting health in families: Applying family research and theory to nursing practice* (3rd ed.). Philadelphia: Saunders.

Robinson, C.A., & Wright, L.M. (1995). Family nursing interventions: What families say makes a difference. *Journal of Family Nursing, 1*(2), 327–345.

Watson, W.L., & Lee, D. (1993). Is there life after suicide? The systemic belief approach for "survivors" of suicide. *Archives of Psychiatric Nursing, 7*(1), 37–43.

White, M., & Epston, D. (1990). *Narrative means to therapeutic ends.* New York: Norton.

Wright, L.M. (2005). *Spirituality, suffering, and illness: Ideas for healing.* Philadelphia: F.A. Davis.

Wright, L.M., & Bell, J.M. (in press). *Beliefs and illness: A model for healing.* Calgary, AB: 4th Floor Press.

Wright, L.M., & Levac, A.M. (1992). The non-existence of non-compliant families: The influence of Humberto Maturana. *Journal of Advanced Nursing, 17*(8), 913–917.

Wright, L.M., & Nagy, J. (1993). Death: The most troublesome family secret of all. In E. Imber-Black (Ed.), *Secrets in families and family therapy* (pp. 121–137). New York: W.W. Norton & Co.

Wright, L.M., & Watson, W.L. (1988). Systemic family therapy and family development. In C.J. Falicov (Ed.), *Family transitions: Continuity and change over the life cycle* (pp. 407–30). New York: Guilford Press.

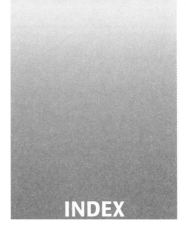

INDEX

Page numbers followed by "b" refer to boxed material; those followed by "t" refer to tables; and those followed by "f" refer to figures

THE "HOW TO" FAMILY NURSING SERIES

Available in DVD/.mov Files
Developed and Demonstrated by:
Lorraine M. Wright, RN, PhD, and Maureen Leahey, RN, PhD
Produced by FamilyNursingResources.com

This series presents live clinical scenarios that demonstrate how to do family nursing in practice. Interviews include a family with young children, middle-aged families, and later-life families. The health problems and health-care settings are varied, as are the ethnic and racial groups. Intended for practicing nurses, educators, undergraduate students, and graduate nursing students, these educational programs will increase nurses' skills to more effectively assist families experiencing illness.

These actual family nursing interviews are a perfect accompaniment to Wright and Leahey's highly acclaimed, award-winning text, **Nurses and Families: A Guide to Family Assessment and Intervention.** Further programs in this series are forthcoming.

#1: How to Do a 15 Minute (or Less) Family Interview (length 23:18)

Featuring real-life clinical scenarios, Wright and Leahey demonstrate key family nursing skills such as how to use manners to engage families in a short period; how to start therapeutic conversations with families; and how to routinely ask key therapeutic questions of families.

#2: Calgary Family Assessment Model: How to Apply in Clinical Practice (length 26:47)

Co-developers of the model, Wright and Leahey demonstrate the Calgary Family Assessment Model (CFAM) in clinical practice. Highlighting the structural, developmental, and functional categories of CFAM in clinical interviews, they present examples of specific questions the nurse can ask the family, illustrate the helpfulness of the genogram and ecomap, and demonstrate how to construct circular interactional diagrams in clinical settings.

#3: Family Nursing Interviewing Skills: How to Engage, Assess, Intervene, and Terminate with Families (length 22:32)

Observe the four stages of a family nursing interview from engagement through termination. Wright and Leahey define and demonstrate key perceptual, conceptual, and executive skills; show how to apply these skills in family nursing clinical practice; offer sample questions for nurses to explore family concerns/solutions; and show key interventions to help families change.

#4: How to Intervene with Families with Health Concerns (length 27:54)

Focus on intervention and change! Wright and Leahey demonstrate interventions in three new clinical interviews: encouraging the telling of illness narratives, validating affect, drawing forth family strengths/support, encouraging respite, offering commendations, and offering information/opinions. These interventions focus on strengthening, promoting and/or sustaining effective family functioning in cognitive, emotional, and behavioral domains.

#5: How to Use Questions in Family Interviewing (length 26:45)

Increase your interviewing skills by using questions that are effective and time-efficient! Wright and Leahey demonstrate how to use questions that engage all family members and focus the meeting, assess the impact of the illness/problem on the family, elicit family coping strategies/strengths, intervene and invite change, and request family feedback.

PURCHASE INFORMATION

Products are available in DVD format. For information about licensing agreements and .mov files, contact MDI at 1-800-661-1674 or mdi@mdicanada.net. These DVDs have been translated into Japanese and are available at www.igakueizou.co.jp

$259 DVD includes shipping & handling (per DVD)
Canadian residents pay in Canadian funds and add 5% GST ($12.95 per DVD)
U.S. and International residents pay in U.S. funds.

Payment can be made by: Visa, check, money order, or institutional purchase orders.
To order by Phone: 1-800-661-1674 No. America (8:30 am to
5:00 pm Mon-Fri Mountain Time)
To order by Fax: (403) 287-9053
To order by email: mdi@mdicanada.net
To order by Internet: www.FamilyNursingResources.com
To order by Mail: MDI-Canada Disc & Tape, Bay 7, 215 36th Ave. NE, Calgary, Alberta, CANADA T2E 2L4
Make check payable to: MDI-Canada Disc & Tape

Name:_____Dept./Title: _____

Organization:_____

Address: _____

City:_____ Province/State:_____ Code/Zip:_____Country _____

Telephone: (   )___Purchase Order#_____Signature: _____

Fax: (____)_____Email: _____

Name on Visa Card:_____

Visa Number:_____Expiry:_____Signature: _____

PROGRAM NAME	DVD	QUANTITY	UNIT PRICE	GST	TOTAL
15 Minute					
CFAM					
Nursing Skills					
Interventions					
Questions					
Total					

(Revised 2/18/09. Price subject to change without notice)